ANATOMICO-ROENTGENOGRAPHIC
STUDIES OF THE SPINE

ANATOMICO-ROENTGENOGRAPHIC STUDIES OF THE SPINE

Fourth Printing

By

LEE A. HADLEY, M.D.

Senior Attending Roentgenologist
Syracuse Memorial Hospital
Syracuse, New York

Lecturer in Radiology
Upstate Medical Center
New York State University
Syracuse, New York

Former Clinical Associate Professor of Public Health
Syracuse University College of Medicine
Syracuse, New York

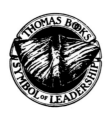

CHARLES C THOMAS · PUBLISHER
Springfield · Illinois · U.S.A.

Published and Distributed Throughout the World by
CHARLES C THOMAS ● PUBLISHER
Bannerstone House
301-327 East Lawrence Avenue, Springfield, Illinois, U.S.A.

© *1964, by* CHARLES C THOMAS ● PUBLISHER
ISBN 0-398-02818-4

Library of Congress Catalog Card Number: 64-11654

First Printing, 1964
Second Printing, 1973
Third Printing, 1976
Fourth Printing, 1979

Preface

THESE STUDIES were originally undertaken by the author as a means of coordinating the radiographic image with the anatomical structure of the spine.

So many anomalies appeared that it seemed desirable to review the embryological and post natal developmental processes of the structure.

The large number of cadavers from older individuals afforded an excellent opportunity of observing the degenerative changes in the spine incidental to the passage of time.

Of considerable practical interest were the serial studies of patients. These showed the anatomical effect incidental to trauma and the resultant changes thereto which were observable upon subsequent examination. Some of these were followed for periods varying from five to twenty-six years. Certain of the later observations were possible only through the gracious cooperation of radiologists in other distant cities.

Intervertebral foramen encroachment with consequent degenerative changes of the nerve roots, both in the cervical and lumbar regions, presented a worthwhile problem for study. Likewise, the crucial occipito-atlanto-axial region furnished many extremely important observations of interest to neurosurgeons and orthopedists as well as radiologists.

Different types of spondylolysis were observed, two patients being studied serially during the period while they were developing the condition.

Microscopic studies supplied additional information: sections of the intervertebral discs and the apophyseal joints as well as the vertebral bodies affected by various types of disease. Special staining methods were employed to visualize the nerves supplying the ligamentous structures.

These and various other studies of the spine accumulated over a period of some thirty odd years are presented here as a coordination of the roentgenographic image and the actual anatomical condition of that structure.

Acknowledgments

THE CONSUMMATION of this present work has been possible only through the generous cooperation of various individuals, institutions and publishers. For the specific illustrations indicated I extend my appreciation to the following doctors:

I:1 and I:3, Professor E. Carl Sensenig, Alabama University, Birmingham

I:18, Dr. E. M. Bick, New York City

II:29, Dr. Edwin Euphrat, Syracuse, New York

II:36, Doctors Newton Bigelow and Lucy Cobb, Marcy, New York

II:40, and II:41, Dr. Philip Rosenberg, Syracuse, New York

III:6, Dr. George Miyakawa, Charleston, West Virginia

III:7, Dr. D. L. McRae, Montreal, Canada

III:30, Dr. I. D. Harris, Wyandotte, Michigan

IV:13, Dr. F. J. O'Neil, Central Islip, New York

IV:17, Dr. J. J. Fahey, Chicago, Illinois

IV:20, Dr. James T. McMillan, DesMoines, Iowa

IV:21, Dr. J. M. Higgason, Chitanooga, Tennessee

IV:25, Dr. Nathan Kriss, Geneva, New York

V:10, Dr. Sam Gingold, Syracuse, New York

VII:27, Dr. John Hogan, Syracuse, New York

VIII:2, Dr. Ivan M. Woolley, Portland, Oregon
Mr. William Cornwell, Rochester, New York and the Lafayette Pharmacol Company

VIII:20, Dr. C. G. Otis, Townshend, Vermont

IX:15, Dr. Thomas J. Rankin, VA Hospital, Kansas City, Missouri

X:7, Dr. Dwight Needham, Syracuse, New York

XIII:9, Dr. Homer Pheasant, Los Angles, California

XIII:20, Dr. K. L. Mitton, Schnectady, New York

XV:8, Dr. Lotte Strauss, New York City

XV:10, Dr. Paul Riemenschneider, Syracuse, New York

XV:12, Dr. L. Luzzetti, East Bay, California

XV:12, XV:15, XV:16, XV:18, Dr. E. B. D. Neuhauser, Boston, Massachusetts

XV:19, Dr. Mark Harwood, Syracuse, New York

XV:21, Dr. Erich Lang, Indianapolis, Indiana

XVI:11, Dr. W. A. Redline, Utica, New York

I am grateful to the following Syracuse radiologists and medical faculty members for their suggestions and painstaking correction of manuscript: Doctors Alfred S. Berne, Edward W. Carsky, Daniel L. Doherty, Edwin J. Euphrat, Joseph A. Head, E. Robert Heitzman Jr., Herbert Lourie, and David B. Murray.

For the opportunity of making the anatomical studies I am indebted to Professor Philip B. Armstrong of the Anatomy Department, Upstate Medical Center at Syracuse. Appreciation is also extended to members of his staff including Mr. Ludwig Rimmler Jr., whose meticulous laboratory work produced the beautiful anatomical sections. The skillful work of Miss Stella Zimmer and Mr. Louis Georgianna of the Photographic Department aided materially in preparation of the illustrations. Professor Howard Ferguson and Staff of the Pathology Department as well as various other members of the faculty, and the Library Staff of the medical college, rendered invaluable assistance.

Additional material was supplied by the Department of Embryology, Carnegie Institution of Washington, at Baltimore, by the Warren Anatomical Museum at Cambridge, and through the courtesy of Dr. Mildred Trotter of the Anatomy Department at Washington University, studies from the Terry Anatomical Collection were made available. Illustrative material was also supplied by the Armed Services Institute of Pathology, Washington, D. C.

Appreciation is likewise acknowledged for the assistance and cooperation from members of the radiographic staffs and other departments of the following hospitals:

Syracuse Memorial Hospital
University Hospital of the Good Shepherd
V.A. Hospital of Syracuse
St. Joseph's Hospital, Syracuse
The Rome State School Hospital and
The Children's Hospital Home of Utica.

I am also deeply obliged to the publishers of the following periodicals for their gracious permission to reuse certain illustrative materials—

The American Journal of Roentgenology, Radium Therapy and Nuclear Medicine
The Journal of Bone and Joint Surgery
The Journal of the American Medical Association
The Journal of Neurosurgery

—and to my publisher, Charles C Thomas, for helpful suggestions and patient cooperation.

This is only a partial list of my obligations in the preparation of this work. I am also grateful to those cooperative patients who obligingly returned for followup examinations. To my friends and associates, as well as an understanding wife I am indebted for their kindly and unfailing encouragement. To all of these and others I dedicate this expression of my deepest appreciation.

L.A.H.

Contents

ANATOMICO-ROENTGENOGRAPHIC
STUDIES OF THE SPINE

Chapter I

Development of the Spine

A BRIEF REVIEW of spinal development provides a suitable background for later consideration of the anomalies which may be encountered at various periods throughout the life of the individual.

Three overlapping stages are recognized. The blastemal or membranous stage appears in embryos and continues up to about the end of the third month. The chondrogenous stage begins soon after the first month and continues throughout fetal life, while the ossification stage begins in the third month and is incomplete at birth.

The vertebral elements develop about the notochord which is the earliest evidence of the axial skeleton. Sensenig has shown this structure to be an evagination of the roof of the gut, appearing about the twenty-third day (Figure I:1). For the purpose of this discussion, the time mentioned in each instance represents the approximate gestation age from fertilization. Two weeks must be added to give the menstrual age.

By the third week of the membranous stage the dorsal surface of the embryo has invaginated and become closed over to form the neural canal (Figure I:1). Along each side of this structure the mesoderm is becoming segmented into somites separated from each other by the intersegmental blood vessels (Figure I:2). The sclerotome is the ventromedial portion of the somite and is the source of the connective tissue structures of the body. The rapidly multiplying mesenchymal cells migrate in the cephalic, caudal and medial directions joining with cells from the adjacent segments. Those cells which migrate ventrally toward the midline meet with those from the opposite side and surround the notochord. The perichordal tissue mass is thus formed from cells of mesodermal origin. Early disturbance of this growth pattern results in various anomalies to be discussed in Chapters II and III.

At the end of the fourth week, alternating zones of loose and densely packed cells are appearing within the axial mass of mesodermal tissue (Figure I:4). These become the primitive segments. Within the less dense zone—later to form the centrum of the vertebral body—occur the paired intersegmental blood vessels arising from the aorta. Well nourished by these vessels the large cells of the less dense area multiply rapidly to form the centrum. As growth occurs the centrum enlarges at the expense of the denser intervening zones of mesodermal tissue. From these more dense areas there develop: the intervertebral discs, the cranial and caudal surfaces of the vertebral body, the major portion of the neural arches and the ribs. The upper cervical spine and the base of the skull are one continuous mass of mesodermal tissue early before complete segmentation occurs. In (Figure I:4) the segmentation of this area is just beginning.

Separation of the mesodermal tissue into vertebral segments occurs at the chondrification stage about the end of the fifth week after fertilization. Cartilage develops rapidly about the intersegmental artery in the less dense primary

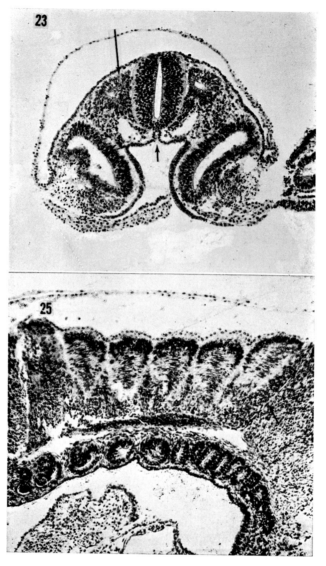

Fig. I:1. Human embryo about twenty-three days post-fertilization, magnification (X100). Transverse section of the upper thoracic region. No. 7611 from Department of Embryology, Carnegie Institution of Washington, comprising sixteen somites. The early notochord appears as a dorsal evagination of the gut roof and lies in contact with the ventral surface of the neural tube (short arrow). The mesoderm of the somite (long arrow) is to be seen with columns of cells migrating in a ventro medial direction toward the newly formed notochord. The long arrow crosses the amnionic sac. (Courtesy of Dr. E. Carl Sensenig, Professor of Anatomy, University of Alabama, Birmingham, and the Carnegie Institution of Washington, Baltimore, Maryland.)

Fig. I:2. Twenty-five day embryo (X95). Longitudinal section in plane shown by long arrow in figure I:1. The somites, composed of segmented mesodermal tissue, are seen at the top underlying the amnionic cavity. Arrow at the right indicates one of the intersegmental vessels arising from the aorta. The dark oval structures below are mesonephrons. (Courtesy of the Syracuse Memorial Hospital Laboratory.)

centrum of the definitive vertebra. The notochord which earlier traversed the centrum, becomes constricted by the rapid growth of the cartilaginous vertebra so that notochordal substance becomes crowded toward the intervertebral discs where it takes part in the formation of the nucleus pulposus (Figures I:6, I:7, and I:8).

Persistence of the notochordal structure may leave a defect through which herniation of disc substance may later occur forming the so-called Schmorl's nodes in the vertebral bodies. The apical ligament of the epitropheus is a functional remnant of the notochord (Figure I:6). Chordomata may subsequently develop from the notochordal rests which

occasionally persist in the base of the skull, the sacrum and rarely elsewhere (Figure XVI:11).

Early in the second month, multiple centers of chondrification develop within the less dense portion of each mesodermal segment. These quickly unite to form a complete cartilaginous provertebra comprising centrum, neural arches, transverse and articular processes all in one block (Figures I:5 and I:7B). The early failure of some chondrification centers to fuse may be partly responsible for the development of hemivertebra, cleft vertebra and certain other anomalies to be discussed in Chapters II and III (Figures II:25, II:26 and II:27).

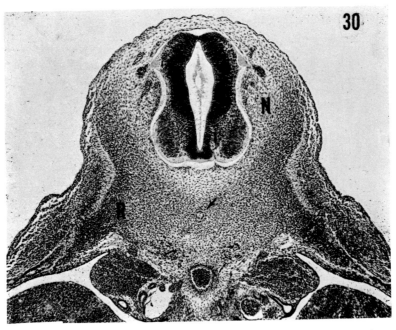

Fig. I:3. Thirty-day, 9 millimeter human embryo (X55). Transverse section of the thoracic region. The notochord (*arrow*) is now surrounded by the perichordal tissue mass made up of mesodermal cells which originated in the sclerotome or ventromedial portion of the somite and migrated to their present position. Condensation of cells which will form the neural arches are seen extending upward along each side of the neural tube. (N). The rib elements are visualized as condensations extending laterally from the mass (R). The artery is visualized in the midline near the bottom of the section. (Courtesy of Dr. E. Carl Sensenig, University of Alabama, Birmingham, and the Department of Embryology, Carnegie Institution of Washington.)

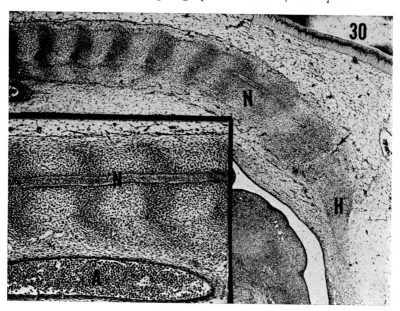

Fig. I:4. Thirty-day, 12 millimeter human embryo (X40). Sagittal section showing longitudinal segmentation of mesodermal tissue as alternating zones of greater and lesser density. This column of mesodermal tissue is seen to be continuous with and of similar character to the hypoglossal mass (H) which later forms the base of the skull. This is separated from the first cervical segment, by a cleft (arrow). The notochord (N), here seen at the second and third segments, appears in other sections to pass directly from the first cervical into the hypoglossal mass where it terminates. In a section cut more laterally there are visualized three nerves arising by multiple fibers from the brain stem and passing separately through this hypoglossal mass to its ventral surface. The inset is another section from the same specimen (X80) showing the notochord (N) passing through the adjacent somites. These mesodermal segments are alternating zones of lesser and greater density. Below is a section of the aorta (A) containing red blood cells, which are nucleated at this period. (Courtesy of Department of Anatomy, New York State College of Medicine.)

Fig. I:6. Sagittal section, cephalic end, from a 29-millimeter human embryo in the cartilage stage (eight weeks from fertilization) (X22). The rapid growth of the lighter zones has occurred at the expense of the more dense areas. Compared with the thirty-day embryo Figure I:4. The embryo has now at eight weeks developed the cartilaginous centra of the provertebra. Note base of skull (B), anterior arch of atlas (A), separate sections for odontoid (O) and body of the axis and centra for the third and fourth cervical bodies. The notochord is seen passing through the odontoid onto the dorsum of the base of the skull. The central nervous system appears dorsally (N).

Inset; same specimen, section taken somewhat more caudally (X13), showing the manner in which the notochord is being crowded into the disc spaces by the rapid growth of the centra. (From the Department of Anatomy, New York State College of Medicine.)

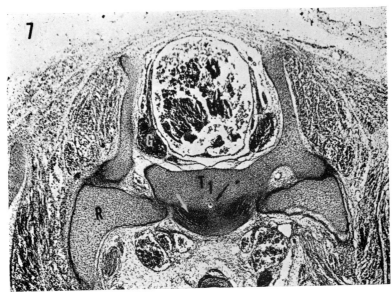

Fig. 1:5. Sixteen millimeter human embryo at about seven weeks gestation, in the cartilage stage (X21). The T_1 vertebral body, pedicle, transverse process and neural arch are one continuous cartilage. The arches are not closed over the dorsum of the spinal canal at this period. Dorsal nerve roots are seen entering the spinal ganglia (G). Ventrally are noted annulus fibrosis of the C_7 - T_1 disc (white arrow) while laterally appear the cartilaginous first ribs (R) articulating with the disc and the transverse processes of T_1. The notochord, seen in the mid-line (black arrow), was observed in the serial studies passing through all of the vertebral bodies, the odontoid and into the dorsal surface of the basal cartilage of the skull. The notochord is of greater diameter in the discs than in the mid-centra, where it later becomes entirely absent. There was some calcification in the clavicle but no other structures were visualized on a preliminary radiograph of this embryo. The soft tissues are somewhat disorganized but the cartilage structure is intact. Study of the other serial sections shows the cartilage of the occiput separate from that of C_1 at this time. There is no evidence of a separate rib element forming the anterior part of the upper six cervical transverse processes as held by certain authorities but there is a separate rib element forming the anterior part of the C_7 transverse processes (Figure I:14).

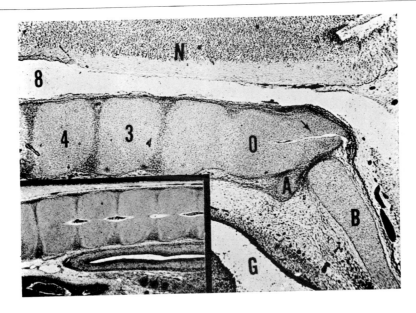

The spinal ligaments and the discs develop from the more dense, darker staining, closely packed cellular structure between the cartilaginous vertebra. (Figures I:4 and I:6).

For each segment there is a rapid enlargement of the cartilage cells and development of the ossification centers in the middle of the centrum and also within each neural arch. At first only calcium is deposited around the enlarged cartilage cells at those three points where the ossification centers will develop (Figure I:7A). There is some variation, but in general ossification will have appeared in each center by the end of the twelfth week. On each side there is a center in the neural arch for its pedicle with the transverse and articular processes and also in the midline a center for the vertebral body. This latter may at times be paired, a precursor of hemivertebra (Figure I:10B).

THE VERTEBRA AT BIRTH

Thus the vertebral body of a newborn comprises three bony elements: a spool-shaped centrum and the two sides of the neural arch. These latter consist principally of a pedicle and a spatula-shaped inferior articular process and lamina for each side. The superior articular process is very small. The pars interarticular is completely ossified. In the lumbar region this isthmus is not at all slender at birth as it is in the adult spine after assumption of the upright position. In the sixty-nine fetal and newborn spines examined by this author not a single example of dehiscence in the fifth neural arch was discovered (Figures I:15 and XIII:5).

The medial margins of the two spatula-shaped lamina approach rather closely at the midline posteriorly but do not joint until the first year. The notches seen on the anterior and posterior sur-

Fig. I:7. Ten weeks, 55-millimeter human embryo. The roentgenogram (A) X2 shows centers from C_7 to S_2 for the bodies and many of the vertebral arches. Microscopic study showed a deposit of calcium between and around the enlarged cartilage cells but there was no bone present, the calcium alone permitting radiographic visualization of the skeletal structures. The calcified areas in the neural arches were just dorsal to the transverse processes and all of the ribs were calcified.

B. Transverse section, same specimen (X14) shows the cartilaginous T_1 vertebral body, pedicle and transverse process (P) with calcific deposit (X) showing black on right side at the future location of the ossification center. The bifid C_7 cartilaginous neural arch is closed over but not continuous across the midline. Compare with the condition three weeks earlier, Figure I:5. At all levels the sides of the arch are united only by fibrous tissue in the midline. These sections are slightly oblique, being higher on the left side. In this section one sees on the left the head of the first rib (R) and the posterior articulation between the seventh cervical and first thoracic articular processes *(arrow)*.

C. Same specimen, lumbar area sectioned in the sagittal plane (X15.5). There were six lumbar segments. Other more lateral sections of the series showed the lowermost to be sacralized on one side only. Cartilage cells in the midportion of the centra are very large. The calcium deposit about the cells is visualized on the stained section as a dense black shadow but there are no bone cells present. By rapid growth of the centra the notochord has become crowded into the discs. In the fourth lumbar body it has partially persisted as a "notochord streak" *(arrow)*. These areas may constitute points of weakness

————————→

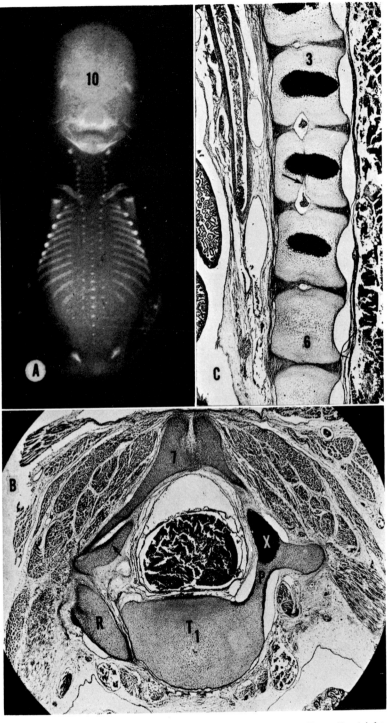

which allow subsequent herniation of the disc substance to occur. Dorsally (right side of illustration) the posterior longitudinal ligament is attached only at the discs while ventrally the anterior longitudinal ligament is more closely applied to the vertebral body and is continuous with the anterior disc margins.

faces of the vertebral body are spaces occupied by blood vessels (Figures I:10 and I:11). The pair of small openings seen near the midline on the frontal radiograph are venous channels on the posterior surface of the vertebral body.

Below C_2 the neural arch closes in the midline during or soon after the first year but the axis and atlas close at about the second and fourth years respectively. However at times the first arch may remain open. (Figure III:35). Closure of the neurocentral union between the pedicle and vertebral body does not occur until the fourth or fifth year. These latter junction lines may be mistaken for a fracture in a young child or they may even persist into adult life (Figures I:11 and I:14).

Ossification of the atlas, axis, sacrum and coccyx is somewhat specialized. The atlas develops from a pair of laterally placed ossification centers which give origin to the lateral masses and the posterior arch. A separate ossification center usually appears at the midpoint of the anterior arch cartilage during the first year. This arch and the lateral masses fuse about the fifth or sixth year (Figure I:14). If the anterior arch of the atlas does not develop the two sides of the structure may remain separate (Figure III:29).

The axis originates from a pair of lateral ossification centers for the arch, a midline body center, sometimes double, and a paired center for the epistropheus. These latter appear in the fifth month of fetal life and later coalesce. They unite with the remainder of the axis during the third or fourth year (Figures I:16 and III:3). The tip of the odontoid arises from a secondary center which appears by the fourth year and

fuses about the twelfth year (Figure I:22).

The sacrum is formed from five segments each corresponding to the separate elements of a single vertebra. These fuse into a single mass between the 12th and 25th year. In addition, two or three pairs of "costal" elements develop in front and later fuse to become the ala of the sacrum. There are also epiphyseal plate structures between the different segments as well as within the sacroiliac joints (Figures I:14, I:20, I:21 and II:21).

The coccyx is usually cartilagenous in the newborn, but an ossification center may be present in the proximal segment at birth.

By the seventh fetal month the osteoblastic center of the vertebra has acquired epiphyseal cartilage plates upon its cephalic and caudal surfaces. The growth area appears as a zone of columnar cartilage between the flat cartilage epiphyseal plate and the underlying invading bony trabeculae of the vertebra. Growth occurs at this zone by enchondral ossification, first calcifying and then ossifying (Figure I:12). These epiphyseal plates curve over the edges of the vertebra and dip into the notches which appear about the upper and lower margins of that structure within the first year (Figure I:17B). Radially placed vessels course along the surfaces of the epiphyseal plates within the cartilage. These latter are radially fluted for strength and fit accurately into grooves on the end surfaces of the vertebrae (Figures I:17F and I:19).

A wealth of blood vessels enter the centrum through the dorsal and ventral surfaces of the vertebral body (Figure I:9). Vessels passing from the vertebral

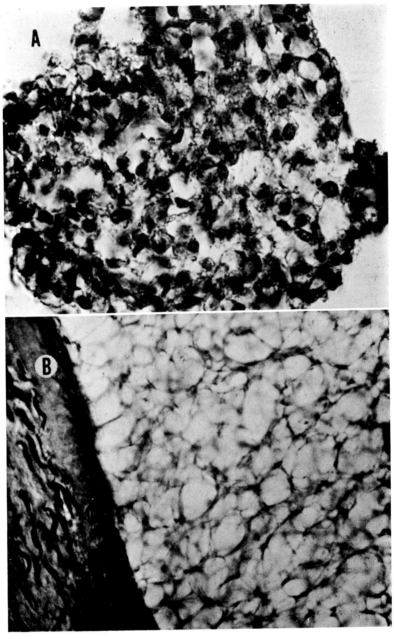

Fig. I:8. Photomicrograph (A) of notochord tissue from a ten weeks' embryo. X795. This is enlarged from the area just below the arrow head in Figure I:7C. There is some beginning development of the vacuolated physaliphorous cells and enlargement of the intercellular spaces. This is the tissue from which the nucleus pulposus develops. Section of a chordoma is seen in Figure XVI:11. Photomicrograph B, X795, shows the reticulated structure of the nucleus pulposus from a six months' fetus. This morphology provides ample space for the disc fluid of the nucleus. The darker area at the left is a portion of the annulus fibrosus.

body through the cartilage into the disc area in early life may subsequently constitute paths of weakness for herniation of disc substance. The notches at the upper and lower vertebral margins are occupied by cartilage into which are inserted the fibers of the longitudinal ligaments and the annulus fibrosus (Figure I:17). Later the epiphyseal ring forms at this point.

This ring may show calcification at ten years and ossification by adolescence (Figure I:18). As an epiphysis it allows the insertion of strong ligamentous structures without interfering with the underlying growth process at the time of life when the individual is very active. The ring may be absent posteriorly where the longitudinal ligament is weaker and less subject to strain because of the support of the neural arch structures. The ring fuses with the vertebral body at about eighteen years to form the elevated rim of the end plate of the vertebra (Figure I:19).

During the second decade the epiphyseal cartilages become gradually thinner until finally they form the upper and lower surfaces of the intervertebral disc. Immediately in contact with this cartilage is the end plate of the vertebral body which is perforated for transmitting nourishment from the vertebra into the disc. The latter is not normally supplied with blood vessels after growth is attained.

In Figure I:6 the tip of the odontoid is seen forming about the notochord (arrow) which then passes outward to continue through the apical ligament onto the base of the skull. At birth, Figure I:16 shows the two ossification centers of the odontoid together with the pointed cartilaginous tip of that structure. At first the tip of the odontoid appears bifid in the roentgenogram but soon after the third year a secondary ossification center appears in the apical ligament at the tip of the odontoid. This gradually enlarges in size and finally unites with the dens at about the time of puberty (Figure I:22). In case union does not occur the separate ossicle remains free, a possible hazard to the cord, as the so-called ossiculum terminale (Figures III:10 and III:11).

Secondary ossification centers develop during the second decade at points of ligamentous attachment. This allows growth to continue without interruption at the underlying epiphysis during this

Fig. I:9. Sagittal sections from a fourteen-weeks fetus (X28). The radiograph of this specimen closely resembled that of the ten-weeks embryo, Figure I:7A. Study of the sections showed ossification centers from C_3 to L_5 inclusive. Development of the sacrum lags somewhat. Its first three segments showed no ossification but there were distended cartilage cells surrounded by calcific material similar to the condition seen in the ten-weeks embryo.

The sagittal section (T_{11} upper left) through the eleventh thoracic vertebra shows very early ossification. Most of the center is occupied by distended cartilage cells surrounded by calcific material. The darker areas to the right in the ossification center are newly formed osteoid tissue. Ventrally (left margin of the section) are blood vessels between the aorta and vertebra. Venous channels are seen in both the dorsal and ventral portions of the vertebral body. Many of the sections show large venous sinuses within the ossification center. It is by way of these penetrating blood vessels that the osteoblasts reach the centers of the solid cartilage provertebrae.

———————————→

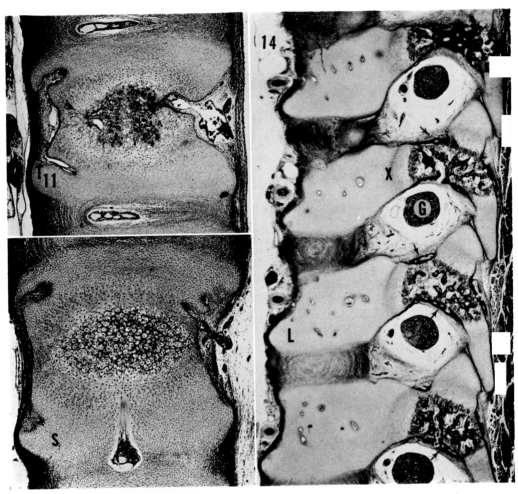

The parasagittal section (L on the right) of the lumbar vertebrae was made more laterally to show the pedicles and articular processes. The cartilage is continuous with that of the side of the vertebral body. Sections of the ganglia (G) are seen within the intervetebral foramina. The ossification centers in the neural arches, at the junction of the pedicle with the articular and transverse processes, are larger than they are in the corresponding vertebral bodies. In addition to the enchondral bone production seen at the ossification center, new dense surface bone is also being laid down by the nearby periosteum (black arrows). The neural arch is ossified by both enchondral and periosteal bone formation. The posterior articulations are composed entirely of cartilage at this stage. The annulus fibrosus (A) is well visualized within the intervertebral discs. The letter X indicates the site of the future neuro-central junction where bony union between the arch and the vertebral body will occur about the fourth or fifth year. This section was taken so far laterally that it does not show the ossification center for the vertebral body. The cartilage is well supplied with blood vessels at this stage. Sagittal section of the second sacral segment (S) shows enlarged cartilage cells in the pre-ossification stage. Bone has not yet formed but calcium was visualized by x-ray. Swollen cartilage cells surrounded by calcific material are normally seen at the site of the future ossification centers. Displaced notochord substance is collected at the centers of the intervertebral discs.

period of strenuous activity. For each vertebral body, in addition to the epiphyseal rings at the disc margins, there are seven additional secondary ossification centers, one for each of the processes attached to the neural arch (Figure I:23).

REFERENCES

Bick, E. M., *et al.*: 1950, *J. Bone & Joint Surg., 32A*:803–814, Anatomy.

Bick, E. M., *et al.*: 1951, *J. Bone & Joint Surg., 33A*:783–787, Anatomy.

Bardeen, C. R.: 1905, *Am. J. Anat., 4*:265–302, Development.

Brocher, J. E. W.: 1960, *Fortsch. a.d. G. d. Roentgens, 92*:363–380; Abst. *Am. J. Roent., 85*:208, Anatomy.

Cohen, J.; Neuhauser, E. B. D., *et al.*: 1956, *Am. J. Roent., 76*:469–475, Cleft vertebra.

Keibel, F., and Mall, E. P.: *Manual of Human Embryology*, Vol. I. J. B. Lippincott Co., Philadelphia, 1950.

Knutsson, F.: 1961, *Acta Radiol, 55*:401–408, Growth.

O'Rahilly, R., *et al.*: 1956, *Am. J. Roent., 76*:455–468, Anatomy.

Patten, B. M.: *Human Embryology*. Blackiston, Philadelphia, 1946.

Sensenig, E. C., *et al.*: 1957, *Proc. Zool. Soc. Calcutta*, 165–170, Embryology.

Sensenig, E. C.: 1949, *Carnegie Inst. Wash. Pub. 583*, Vol. *33*:21–41, Embryology.

Teissandier, J.: 1944, Thesis for Doctor of Medicine, Faculty of Medicine of Paris (French).

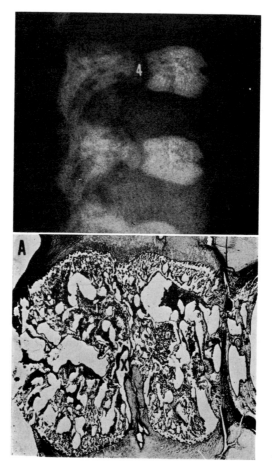

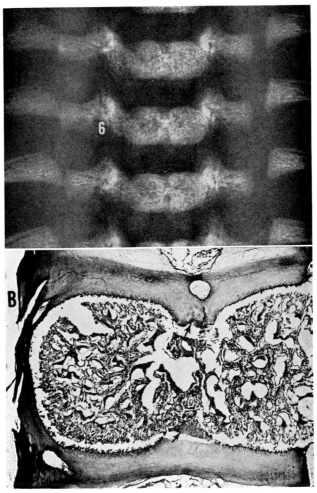

Fig. I:10. Radiographs and sections from the fourth lumbar vertebra (A) and the sixth thoracic vertebra (B) of a twenty-four weeks female fetus to show the occasional bifid character of the ossification centers. Rarely two separate ossification centers for a single vertebra may persist into adult life. However bifid centers are a more or less normal temporary condition, produced by prolongations of the disc substance into the ossification centers. Section A is a lateral projection and the ossification center is divided into an anterior and a posterior division by an upward projection of the epiphyseal cartilage enclosing remnants of the notochord (X). This is an example of the so-called "cleft vertebra" which has been described as occurring in early life. The condition, if present at birth, usually disappears after a few months. B is a frontal projection and shows the ossification center partially divided into lateral segments by inward projections of the adjacent cartilages (arrows). A much more complete and permanent division of the ossification centers into paired hemivertebrae is shown in Figures II:25 and II:26.

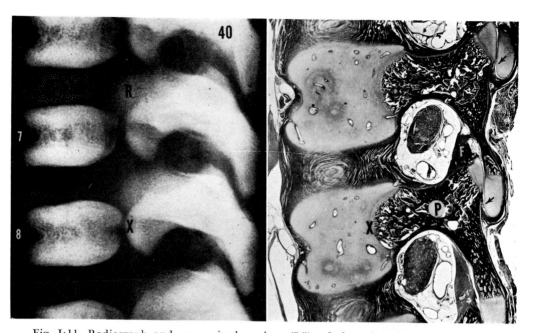

Fig. I:11. Radiograph and parasagittal section (5.5) of thoracic vertebrae of a fetus at term. The section was taken near the lateral margins of the lumbar vertebral bodies so that the ossification centers of the centra do not show. Note the excellent blood supply to the cartilage of the vertebral bodies during the growth period. The crisscrossing fibers of the annulus fibrosus of the discs are well shown. The oval intervertebral formina with sections of the nerve roots and blood vessels are bounded above and below by the darker, completely ossified pedicles (P). The motor portion of the nerve root is smaller than the sensory, darker in shade and appears on the ventral side of the nerve section. The neurocentral junction of the pedicle with the vertebral body appears on the left as a curved line (X). Final, complete bony union between the pedicle and the vertebral body does not occur until the forth or fifth year. On the extreme right are seen the superior and inferior articular processes with the apophyseal articulations between them. These latter are still largely cartilaginous but have already developed synovial structures (black arrows). The ligamentum flavum (F) forms the anterior capsule of the posterior joints. Compare this section taken at forty weeks with the same area shown at fourteen weeks in Figure I:9. The radiograph shows the seventh and eighth thoracic spool-shaped ossification centers more dense adjacent to the discs because of the large venous spaces at their mid-portions. The anterior and posterior notches transmit the vascular channels. Each side of the neural arch is a continuous bony structure comprising the pedicle, superior and inferior articular processes and the lamina, with the neurocentral junction at X. The head of the overlying rib shadow is seen at

R.

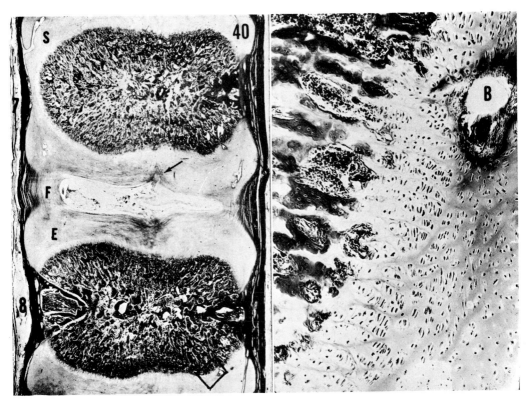

Fig. I:12. Sagittal section (S) of the seventh and eighth thoracic vertebrae (X10) segments from the same specimen at term shown in Figure I:11. The anterior longitudinal ligament is on the left side. The ossification centers contain many blood sinuses in their central areas and with notches on their anterior and posterior surfaces for these structures. As in the radiograph, one sees here that the bony tissue is more dense adjacent to the thick cartilaginous epiphyseal plates (E). These plates are relatively much thinner in adult life. Note the blood vessels penetrating the cartilage, some of them passing in from the surrounding ligamentous tissue while others originate in the ossification centers. Blood vessels do not persist within the disc structures after growth is complete. The disc space is bounded anteriorly and posteriorly by the annulus fibrosis (F). A notochordal streak defect is seen above and below, near the middle of the disc *(arrow)*. This constitutes a path for possible future disc herniation. The rectangle in the lower right corner indicates the epiphyseal field of higher magnification shown on the right.

B. Vertebral body epiphysis at term rotated about 60 degrees counter-clockwise (X125), showing enchondral bone formation. Above and to the left are the dark staining osteoid trabeculae with entrapped osteocytes and with marrow spaces between. Below and to the right of these are stacked columns of growing cartilage cells between streaks of collagenous material. The provisional calcification of this latter material forms a supporting matrix and is an intermediate stage of bone formation between cartilage and the final bony trabeculae. Below and to the right lies the epiphyseal cartilage with a blood vessel (B) in the upper right corner. For further discussion of bone formation see Chapter XV.

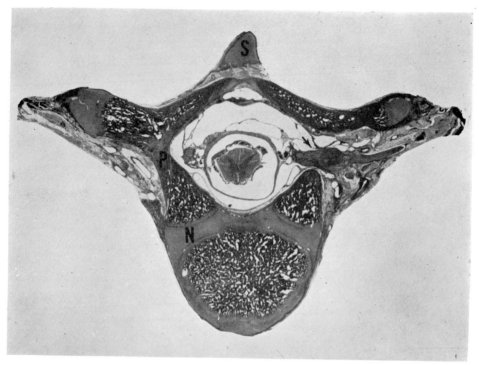

Fig. I:13. Transverse section of an upper lumbar vertebra at term X3. The spinal cord, surrounded by its arachnoid sac, has given off on the right side a nerve root which is seen with its ganglion passing through the intervertebral foramen (*arrow*). There is ample space within the spinal canal for the cord and its surrounding meninges. A cartilaginous center for the future spinous process appears at S. It will ossify by the age of two. Bony union of the two sides of the neural arch has not yet occurred at this stage. The pedicle (P) is separated from the ossification center for the vertebral body by the cartilaginous neurocentral junction (N). This will remain unfused until the fourth or fifth year.

Fig. I:14. Radiographs showing a group of vertebrae at term. The venous spaces may be seen as radiating dark linear shadows on C_4, T_6 and L_4. In the atlas there are three ossification centers: one for each transverse process and hemi-arch and a single one in the center of the anterior arch. This latter, however, usually appears later during the first year. C_2 shows the centers for the arches, the vertebral body and overlying paired centers for the odontoid. A photomicrograph in frontal section showing the bipartite odontoid is shown as Figure I:16. Note the foramina for the vertebral arteries in the lateral masses of C_4 and the centers for vertebral body, arches and ribs of T_6. The L_4 lumbar body is quite similar to T_6 but without centers for the ribs. Segments of the sacrum, comprising centers for the vertebral body and each side of the neural arches appear at the right. The first two sacral segments show rib elements in front which later become the ala of the sacrum (Figure I:20). The cartilaginous segments of the coccyx are faintly seen, attached to the fifth segment.

At the bottom, left, is a seventh cervical vertebra photographed from above with a short rib element on each side (*white arrow*). This condition is normal at birth. If the

————————————→

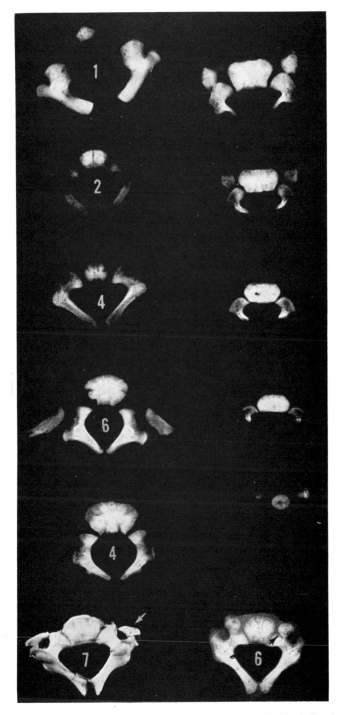

customary union with the pedicle of C_7 does not occur the individual develops a cervical rib.

At the bottom, right, is the radiograph of a sixth cervical segment at term showing separate rib elements (*black arrow*). I have been unable to find separate rib elements above this level.

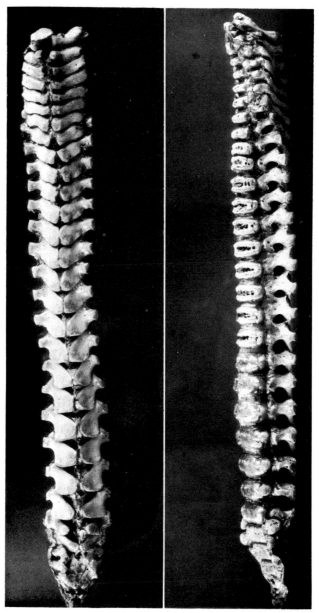

Fig. I:15. Posterior and lateral photographs of the spine at birth. None of the neural arches is closed. The lamina in the lumbar region are spatula-shaped with very small superior articular processes. An examination of sixty-nine fetal and newborn spines failed to show more than two ossification centers for any one neural arch. The intervertebral foramina are large and the sacral canal is open. In the lateral view one can identify the neurocentral union between the vertebral bodies and the neural arches. Note the many spaces on the anterior and lateral surfaces of the vertebral bodies for transmitting the generous blood supply to these structures. Large transverse processes develop in the thoracic region for articulation with the ribs and in the lumbar region for attachment of the muscles. Also see Figure III:5.

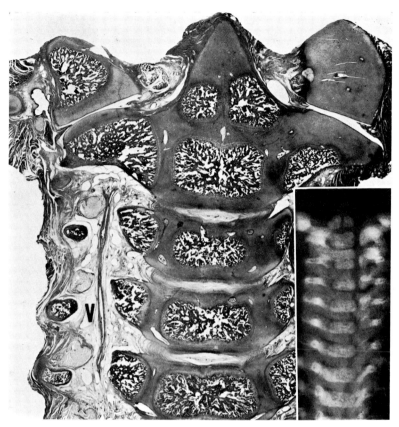

Fig. I:16. Coronal section of the cervical spine at term (X 3.5). There are at this time five ossification centers for the second cervical segment, two of them being paired centers for the odontoid. These latter show clearly in the radiograph (inset) which was made before decalcification of the specimen. The more caudad segments each have three separate centers of ossification, one for the centrum and one for each side of the neural arch. The vertebral artery (V) is seen on the left side of the section ascending through the foramina in the transverse processes. One side of the atlas has not yet developed its ossification center.

Fig. I:17. Studies from the thoracic vertebra of an eight-year-old male.

A. Lateral radiograph (X4). Note the characteristic notch formation at the anterior corners of the vertebral body (N). Calcification of the epiphyseal ring within this notch has not yet appeared.

B. The photograph of the fixed block of tissue (X) the anterior longitudinal ligament is at the left side and closely attached to the surface of the bone. Note how the white epiphyseal cartilage plate (C) dips into the marginal notches. The curved layers of fibers of the annulus fibrosus are seen joining the cartilage plates at the anterior portion of the intervertebral disc.

C. Sagittal section (X16), taken from the notch area showing the cartilage in the center with enchondral bone production along the epiphyseal line (X) between it and the bony trabeculae below and at the right. At the extreme left appears the anterior longitudinal ligament with Sharpey fibers from this structure penetrating the cortex of the vertebral body very near the bottom of the section at (S). Just above this point a small nutrient vessel penetrates the cortex. At the top of the section are alternating layers of annulus fibrosus with their fibers passing in different directions (F). Between the small blood vessel in the cartilage (V) and the anterior longitudinal ligament occurs a network of fibers originating from three sources: the annulus fibrosus above, from the anterior longitudinal ligament in front of the disc, and from that part of this same ligament attached to the vertebral body below. It is within this area that the epiphyseal bony ring develops during adolescence. (Figure I:18.)

D. Higher mangification of the network described under C (X55) rotated clockwise 90 degrees, showing for orientation the blood vessel (V) surrounded by the hyaline cartilage. Above is the network of fibers originating from three different directions and at the top of the section are layers of the annulus fibrosus.

E. Radiograph in the frontal plane (X5) showing in cross section the typical radiating grooves which normally develop at the epiphyseal line. This is the weakest point of a growing bone. The corrugated structure at this level contributes to increase the strength of the part, especially against shearing stresses.

F. Section in the frontal plane (X16) showing three of the bony corrugations surmounted by the epiphyseal line (X). The fibrous tissue of the annulus fibrosis (F) lies at the top of the section. Note sections of the vessel channels within the cartilage opposite each of the ridges (V). The epiphyseal bony ring is said to develop by calcification of multiple centers of hyaline cartilage, each corresponding to one of the radiating grooves. These centers later coalesce to form the ring epiphysis. Calcification within this structure may appear on the radiograph at about ten years and is somewhat earlier for girls than for boys. (Courtesy of the Pediatrics Department, Syracuse Memorial Hospital.)

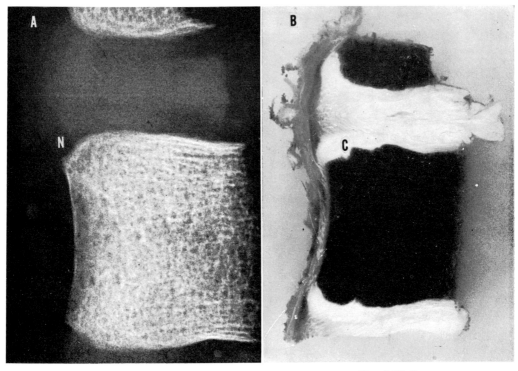

Fig. I:17 A   Fig. I:17 B

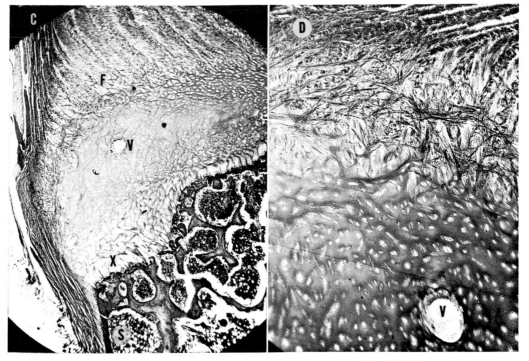

Fig. I:17 C   Fig. I:17 D

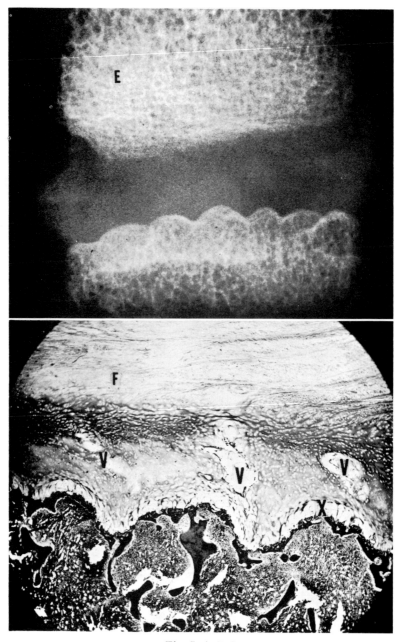

Fig. I:17 E-F

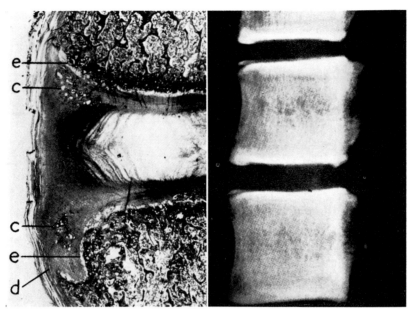

Fig. I:18. Section and radiograph of a thoracic disc from a thirteen-year-old female. The epiphyseal bony ring seen during the adolescent period is clearly visualized on the radiograph (*arrow*). This bony ring is seen in the section as a secondary ossification center at (c). The cartilage plate, covering the epiphyseal line (e) curves into the notches on the margins of the vertebral bodies. Fibers from the anterior longitudinal ligament (d) and from the annulus fibrosus are inserted into the epiphyseal ring. This structure later unites with the vertebral body to form the elevated margin of its plane surface. See figure I:19. Courtesy of Dr. E. M. Bick and the publisher of *The Journal of Bone and Joint Surgery*.)

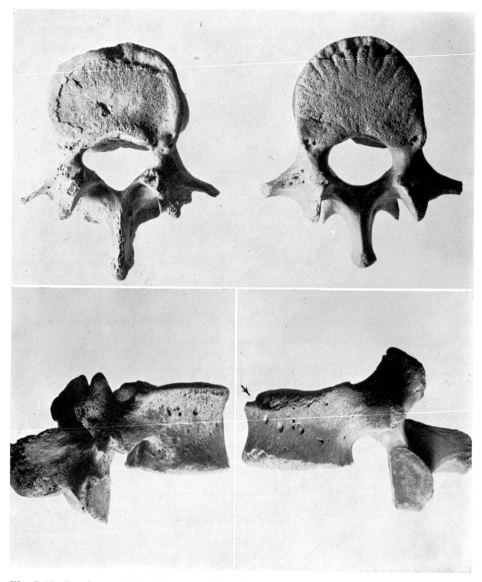

Fig. I:19. On the reader's right are axial and lateral photographs of a lumbar vertebra from an adolescent individual. Notches at the anterior margins of the vertebral plates (*arrow*) enclosed the epiphyseal ring. (Figure I:18). The vertebral plate is fluted in a radial manner as indicated in I:17 E and F.

On the reader's left are axial and lateral photographs of an adult lumbar vertebra. The flat surface shows many fine penetrations through the bony plate for the exchange of fluids between the vertebral body and the intervertebral disc. About the periphery of the vertebral plate, especially its anterior portion, is a smooth raised margin about 3/16ths of an inch wide (*arrow*). This corresponds to the former bony ring epiphysis which became united with the vertebral body after the cessation of growth. This raised margin limits the cartilage plate of the disc. Through this cartilage the fluids are exchanged between the disc and the vessels within the vertebral body.

Penetrating the lateral surfaces of both vertebral bodies are many openings for passage of the nutrient arteries.

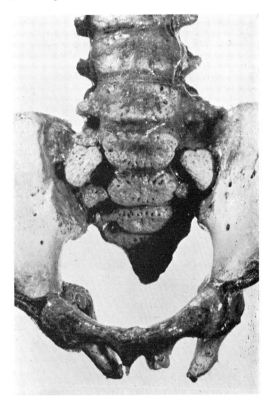

Fig. I:20 Photograph of the sacrum from a child of one year showing the four "rib" elements which form the ala of the sacrum. There are many openings in the various bony structures to accommodate the generous blood supply at this growing period.

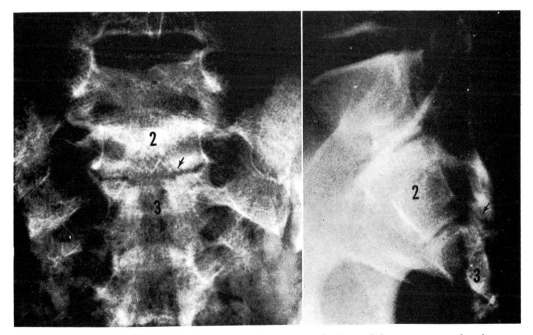

Fig. I:21. P. A. and lateral projections of the sacrum of a boy of fourteen years showing the partially fused segments which comprise the structure at that age. He had sustained a trauma nine days before which separated the second and third segments (*arrow*). Subsequent reexamination two months later showed evidence of healing.

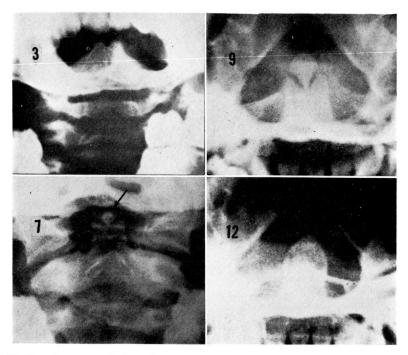

Fig. I:22. Development of the odontoid tip at three, seven, nine and twelve years. Compare with Figure I:16. Nine and twelve are from the same patient with the nine-year-old film retouched. A lateral projection of this same structure in this patient at nine years is seen in Figure III:3, as well as the ununited odontoid.

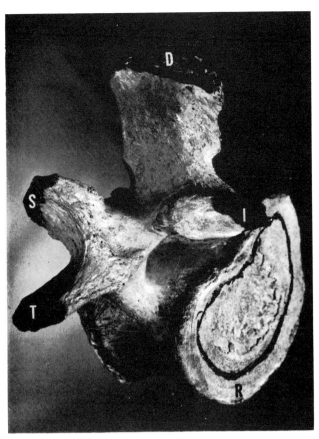

Fig. I:23. Photograph of the centrum and left neural arch of an adult vertebra. Certain areas have been darkened to indicate the locations of possible secondary ossification centers. These may develop about adolescence and fuse by the twenty-first year. They serve as points for attachment of ligamentous structures and permit underlying growth to continue in spite of strenuous activity. (R) Ring epiphysis, (T) Transverse, (S) Superior Articular, (D) Dorsal Spinous, and (I) Inferior Articular processes. Persistent secondary ossification centers are described in Chapter II.

Disturbance of Development

Congenital anomalies may appear at any level of the spine from the occiput to the tip of the coccyx. Many of these disturbances of development originate in the very early blastemal stage of the embryo and may be evaluated in light of the observations in Chapter I. Anomalies of the spine also result in connection with spinal cord maldevelopment.

Although incomplete and with some overlapping these interesting conditions will be discussed in the following order: 1. Agenesis or hypoplasia; 2. Lack of fusion and persistence of secondary centers; 3. Malsegmentation and non-segmentation; 4. Dysgenesis and 5. Miscellaneous anomalies.

AGENESIS OR HYPOPLASIA

Failure of development during the early blastemal stage may result in a partial or complete agenesis of any vertebral element. This may be due to a deficiency of the germ plasm, undernourishment or some other early influence. Early congenital deficiency may be in part compensated for as growth progresses. On the other hand deformity from a congenital anomaly may increase as the individual develops.

Postnatal bone growth is influenced by the various stresses to which the bone is subjected. Of these, to be mentioned, are tension or pulling stress as well as pressure and bending. This latter is an especially important factor at the lumbosacral level. Likewise, the spinal canal is in part moulded by the growth of the expanding central nervous system.

If some opposing part is absent the functional stimulus to later growth may be lacking. For instance, if an articular process is lacking the corresponding articular process, having nothing with which to articulate, will remain rudimentary.

By contrast to this observation it is interesting to note that when an agenesis is present the consequent weakness is compensated for by anomalous structures or by the development of increased strength in the adjacent vertebrae (Figure III:2). Multiple segments or parts of segments may be lacking. Agenesis or hypoplasia of varying degree is a common condition and may be encountered at any level of the spine from the absent odontoid to the lacking sacrum.

Anomalies are prone to occur at the transition levels such as the dorsolumbar or lumbosacral areas. Deficiencies in the articular processes at the lower spine level are not at all uncommon and present interesting compensatory features. These may be vicarious articulations between the neural arches or hyperplasia of the remaining structures. The ligamentum flavum and fibrous structures are found to be unusually tough in the presence of bony deficiencies (Figures II:1, II:2 and II:3)

Absence of all or part of the sacral

segments is frequently encountered, the sacrum and coccyx being the last part of the spine to develop (Figures II:4, II:5 and II:6).

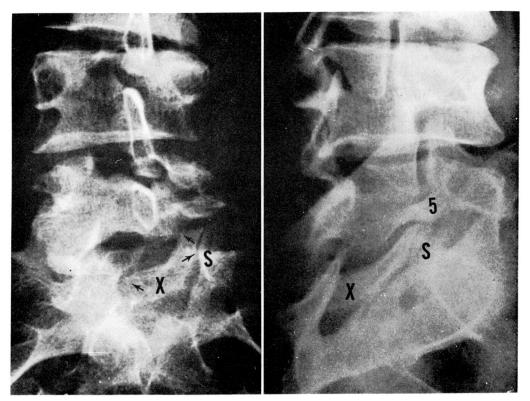

Fig. II:1. Female, thirty-four years old. For the past ten or twelve years she has complained of a steady dull ache in the lumbar region radiating down the right leg. This is aggravated by coughing, sneezing, rotation and certain other movements. The symptoms have gradually increased in severity. She has developed paresthesia in the right leg but the patellar and Achilles reflexes are normal. The fifth right inferior articular process is entirely absent. The right half of the first sacral arch (X) appears as an unfused separate ossicle with three articulations. It articulates with the fifth neural arch above, the first sacral articulation below and the left side of the first sacral neural arch medially *(arrows)*. This ossicle helps to stabilize the deficiency.

SECONDARY OSSIFICATION CENTERS

These ossicles appear as small epiphyses at the tips of the spinous, transverse and articular processes early in the second decade. They become united with the vertebral body between the sixteenth and twenty-first years. The bony rings at the upper and lower surfaces of the vertebral bodies likewise are secondary centers and furnish attachment for strong ligamentous structures during the period of underlying bone growth.

Any of the various secondary ossification centers of the spine may fail to unite or become avulsed. Ordinarily they offer only anatomical interest. However, following accident the question of fracture may arise. This is more likely if there has been an injury with the lapse of an

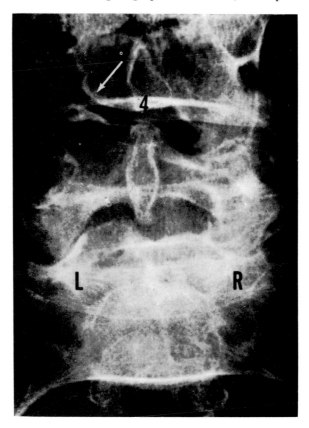

Fig. II:2. Male, fifty-six, complained of low back discomfort with pain and diminished sensation in the right thigh for the past five years. Radiographs reveal an absent left fourth posterior articular process with a vicarious articulation between the fourth and fifth laminae at this level *(white arrow)*. The unbalanced stress has resulted in hyperplasia of the posterior joints on the opposite side with arthrotic changes.

interval between it and the X-ray examination.

Non-union of the secondary ossification center at the tip of the first thoracic transverse process is said to occur frequently. It is ordinarily of no clinical interest but in the case here cited there was some question of possible trauma (Figure II:7). This problem is discussed by Schmorl and Junghanns.

Of common occurrence are those ununited secondary ossification centers occurring usually in males and at the tips of the inferior articular processes in the lumbar region. They have joint surfaces covered with cartilage and are normally asymptomatic unless they become wedged into the apophyseal joint space (Figures II:8, II:9 and II:10). Here likewise the question of fracture may arise following injury. Fractures of the inferior articular processes do occur following severe trauma of a rotary character, usually with the spine flexed. They produce severe pain and localized tenderness. A fracture, if present, appears as a detached fragment with the fracture line crossing the cortex of the articular process (Figure II:11).

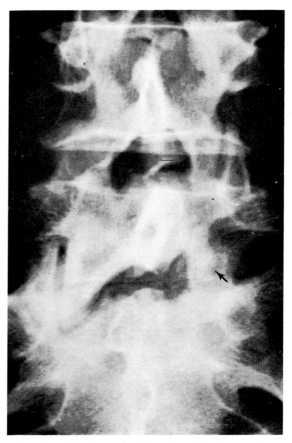

Fig. II:3. Female, thirty-nine. She has suffered attacks of backache referred to both legs intermittently for the past ten years, aggravated by lateral bending but not by coughing. The Achilles and patellar reflexes are normal. There is a congenital rudimentary fifth inferior articular process *(arrow)*. To compensate for this deficiency the patient has developed a marked hypertrophy of the fifth inferior articular process on the opposite side and a corresponding hypertrophy of the articular process of the sacrum.

INTRA-ARTICULAR OSSICLES

In the upper lumbar region certain of the ununited centers at the tip of the articular processes may be quite large. Some of the secondary ossification centers may become wedged in between the articular surfaces producing intra-articular ossicles. They cause the joint space to be widened. These joints are usually quite painful (Figures II:12 and II:13).

Small oval ossicles have been encountered in the upper lumbar region corresponding to unfused mamillary processes. They are only of academic anatomical interest (Figures II:14 and II:15).

The epiphyseal bony ring encountered during the growth period at the vertebral body margin, may remain ununited. This has been termed a limbus bone. In the lateral radiograph it appears as a triangular shadow replacing one of the anterior corners of the vertebral body. It should not be mistaken for a fracture or for one of the intercalary

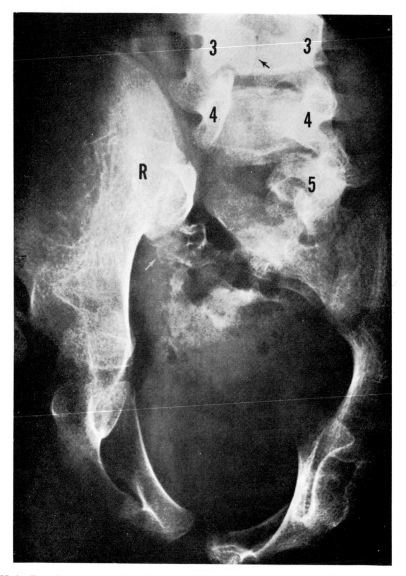

Fig. II:4. Female, age seven, bilateral club feet, also disturbed bladder and bowel control. The first three lumbar vertebral bodies appear normal. The third neural arch is unfused *(black arrow)* and the 4th arch is open. The right half of the fifth lumbar verte- bra and a part of the sacrum are absent. Opposite of this agenesis on the left side there is a hemivertebra for the 5th segment and the sacrum is intact. Fortunately, the lower part of the sacrum continued to develop on the right side *(white arrow)*. The patient has a dislocation of the right hip and the right ilium has remained rudimentary. Obviously, this condition arose in the blastemal stage of embryonic development.

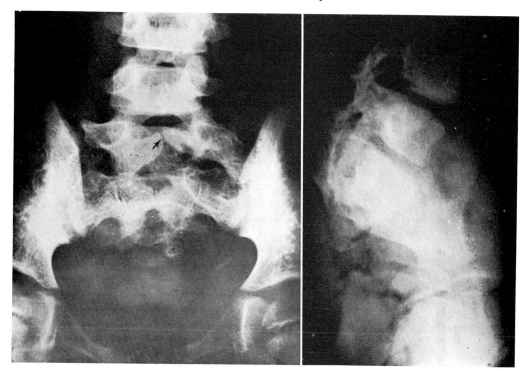

Fig. II:5. Female, twelve years old, with agenesis of the distal portion of the sacrum. There is sacralization of the left and probably of the right fifth transverse processes but the fifth neural arch is not yet completely fused (*arrow*). Anomalies of the sacrum are not uncommon. The sacrum forms last and not infrequently shows some deficiency of development.

bones that develop within the longitudinal ligament (Figures II:16 and II:17. Also XIII:23 and XII:20).

Non-union of the sides of a neural arch, either with or without a separate ossicle covering the mid-line deficiency, is a common finding, especially in the lumbar region. It has little or no clinical significance. The mid-line ossicles partially closing the gap of a spina bifida develop within the ligamentum flavum from a separate center like those on the tips of the spinous processes (Figure I:13). In the absence of such a center the unclosed spinal canal is well protected by the dense, tough ligamentum flavum. Occasionally such a defect is covered by a caudal projection of the spinous process from the vertebra above. This furnishes protection and ligamentous attachment.

The secondary centers at the tips of the spinous processes noted during the second decade may persist into adult life and be mistaken for fracture, especially after direct trauma (Figures II:18 and II:19). Fractures of the spinous processes are not uncommon but occur nearer the base of the structure. The spontaneous "shoveler's fracture" seen at the cervicodorsal level in workmen of inadequate physique is a fatigue fracture of the spinous process. In the cervical region these persistent centers are not to be confused with the ossicles which commonly develop in the nuchal ligament.

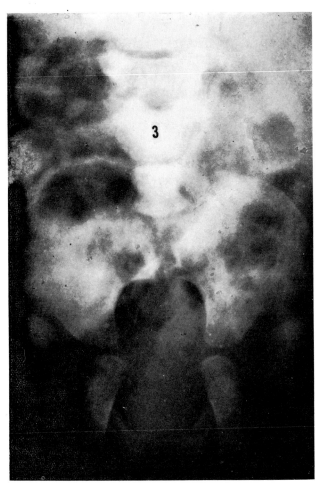

Fig. II:6. Agenesis of the sacrum in an infant. The first and second lumbar vertebrae are normal. The third is narrowed but possesses pedicles and a neural arch. The fourth lumbar segment is markedly narrowed and lacks a neural arch. The fifth lumbar vertebra and the sacrum are completely lacking. (Courtesy of Mr. Charles Turner).

The secondary ossification centers lying between the ilium and the ala of the sacrum have usually fused by the twentieth year. However, they may rarely be the site of a painful epiphysitis causing troublesome obscure low back pain during childhood (Figures II:21 and II:22). Discomfort and localized tenderness of lesser degree or even avulsion may be encountered in young men with ununited secondary centers who have undergone strenuous physical activity (Figures II:23 and II:24).

DISORDERED SEGMENTATION

Various types of bizarre spine development are predetermined in the early stages of the embryo.

At the end of three weeks' gestation one finds the mesodermal masses on each side of the neural tube separated ventral-

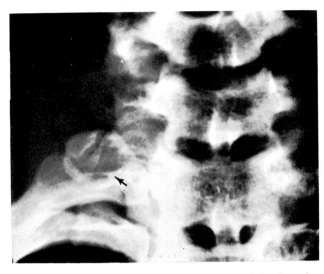

Fig. II:7. Ununited secondary ossification center at the tip of the first thoracic transverse process *(arrow)*. This is a common anomaly but caused some confusion in this case. The patient, a male of nineteen years, developed sudden pain in the right trapezius muscle while swinging a pick axe two days before. There was no evidence of a fractured spinous process.

ly by the gut and the beginning notochord. As we have seen, each lateral mass has its own arterial supply and is divided longitudinally into somites. The adjacent somites are separated by the intersegmental arteries (Figures I:1 and I:2).

During the next week the sclerotomes or ventromedial portions of the somites extend toward the midline to surround the notochord and join the corresponding sclerotomes from the other side. This occurs immediately ventral to the neural tube during the fourth week (Figure I:3).

Somewhat later in development if the two laterally placed primary centers of chondrification have failed to unite, paired centers of ossification may develop in a single vertebral body. In this manner a sagittal cleft vertebra results. After assuming the upright position pressure of the supraimposed weight may spread and distort the two halves, resulting in a bifid or so-called "butterfly vertebra."

The adjacent vertebrae or discs may develop a compensating triangular shape. Seen from the side these segments may be wedge-shaped with the narrow portion in front. As a consequence of their weakened attachment to the anterior longitudinal ligament the segments become displaced backward and a kyphosis is likely to result (Figures II:25, II:26, II:27 and II:28).

Through inadequate genetics the somite from one side may fail to develop at all. This leaves the remaining, unpaired somite to develop as a hemi-vertebra. It may take up a position in the midline posteriorly or parasagittaly on one side. Also, instead of joining with its corresponding fellow of the opposite side a somite may become united with the opposite one next caudad. This leaves an unbalanced hemivertebra on one side which may be balanced by a hemivertebra on the opposite side at a different level a few segments distant.

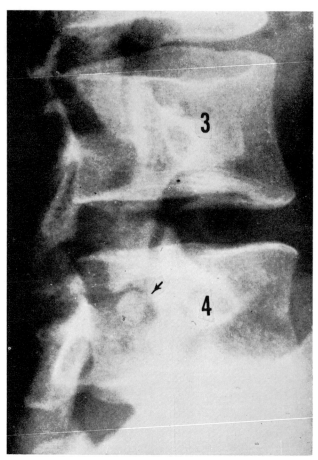

Fig. II:8. Female of nineteen years, low back pain of increasing severity aggravated by movement. Stands with the back inclined toward the left side. Tenderness to deep pressure in the right lower lumbar region. Right oblique roentgenogram reveals an ununited secondary ossification center at the tip of the right third inferior articular process (*arrow*). The condition was unilateral. This is the type of persistent secondary ossification center most commonly encountered in the lumbar region. These ossicles do not usually produce symptoms. Two years later this patient reported that the condition was no longer troublesome except upon fatigue.

Fig. II:10. Female, age forty-one. Partially intra-articular ossicle at the left third lumbar articulation resulting from the ununited fourth superior articular process tip (*arrow*). Occurrence at the superior tip is an unusual feature. The intra-articular ossicles are painful. (Courtesy of the *American Journal of Roentgenology.*)

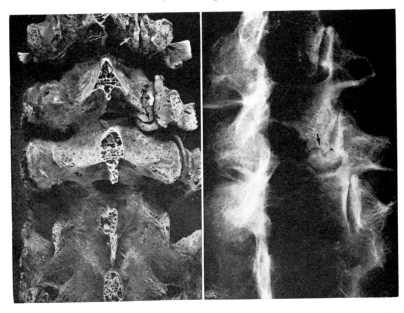

Fig. II:9. Specimen 2202, male, seventy-seven years old. Intra-articular ossicle in the right fourth posterior articulation *(black arrows)*. This has resulted from nonfusion of the secondary ossification center and it impinges against the fifth neural arch below. On the roentgenogram note the erosion and eburnation at point of contact. Rolled edges of the articular margins and extra-articular depressions for attachment of joint capsules are visible at certain joints *(white arrows)*. For a discussion of this feature see Chapter VI, Figures VI:7 and VI:12.

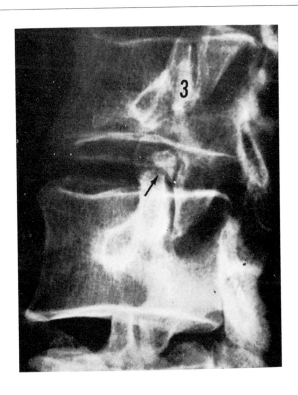

As a result scoliosis develops with the advent of weight bearing. These various maldysplasias occur during the fourth week of gestation (Figures II:29, II:30 and II:31).

In contrast to the anomalies resulting from the non-union of embryological elements, the failure of segmentation is a common cause of anomalies involving the somatic structure.

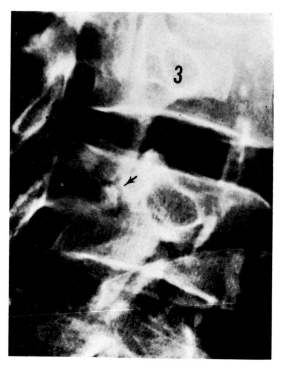

Fig. II:11. Male, age fifty. Accident two and one-half years before with fracture of all lumbar transverse processes on the left side. Separate fragment at the right L_3 inferior articular process (*arrow*). Note irregularity of the cleavage line. This is quite possibly a fracture and not a secondary ossification center. (Courtesy of the *American Journal of Roentgenology*.) See Mitchell J.B.J.S., *15*:608.

Fig. II:13. Male, age thirty-five (retouched). An intra-articular ossicle 5 x 9 mm is seen within a widened 4th lumbar posterior articulation (*white arrows*). There was some widening of the corresponding joint on the opposite side (*black arrows*). This intra-articular ossicle was painful. (Courtesy of the *American Journal of Roentgenology*.)

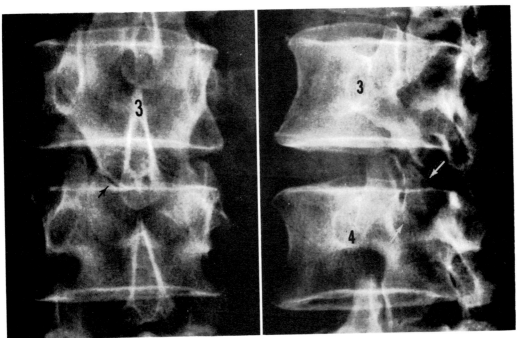

Fig. II:12. Female, age 49. Left lumbar pain, aching and "crackling" sensation aggravated by bending backward or to the left. Not painful upon bending forward or to the right. This patient has a cleavage *(black arrow)* between the 3rd left inferior articular process and the corresponding lamina. The ununited center has produced an unusually large wedgeshaped intra-articular ossicle which is seen on the oblique projection to be displaced downward. It acts as a painful bone block *(white arrows)*. This is one of a group of painful intra-articular ossicles. (Courtesy of the *American Journal of Roentgenology.*)

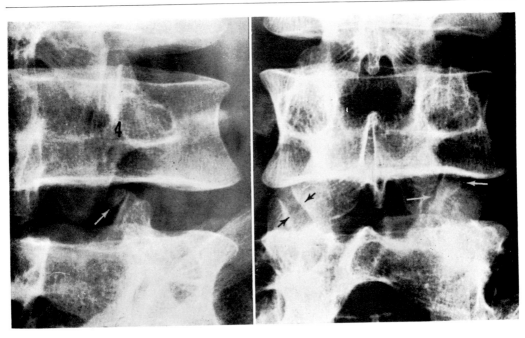

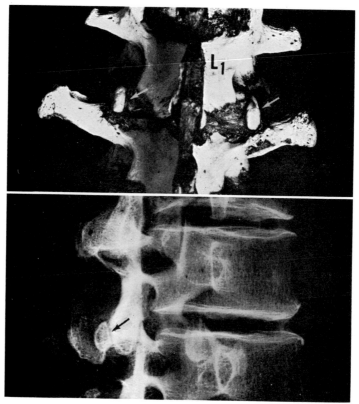

Fig. II:14. Specimen 53-13, male, age sixty-two. Bilateral ununited secondary ossification centers (*arrows*) 6 mm x 10 mm., for the mamillary processes of L_1. They were smooth and rounded, firmly incorporated in the capsular ligament and possessed a complete cortex. There was an articular surface covered with cartilage in contact with both the superior and inferior articular processes of the posterior articulation. (Courtesy of the *American Journal of Roentgenology*.)

NONSEGMENTATION

Possibly because some growth controlling influence in the embryo is lacking, the normal separation of parts of the organism into segments during the blastemal stage may not occur.

We have seen how the intervertebral discs develop within the alternating more dense zones of the sclerotomes (Figure I:4). During the rapid growth of the cartilaginous centra the dense zones between become relatively thinner and the notochord is forced into them from the adjacent provertebrae (Figures I:6 (in-set) and I:7). Later, during ossification, the disc begins to assume its final form with the nucleus pulposus in its center partly derived from the displaced notochordal cells (Figure I:12). If, for some reason, disc formation fails to occur, the cartilaginous masses of adjacent provertebrae are separated only by the epiphyseal plates. As a result, when ossification takes place the vertebrae are formed into a so-called "congenital block vertebra" consisting of two or more of the primary segments.

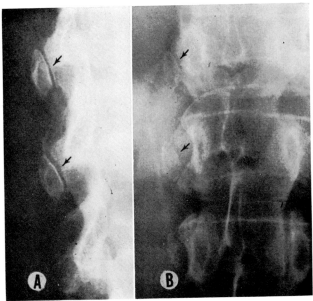

Fig. II:15. Female patient, forty-one. A and B show the ununited secondary ossification centers for the mamillary processes of the 1st and 2nd lumbar vertebrae (*arrows*). Compare with Figure II:14.

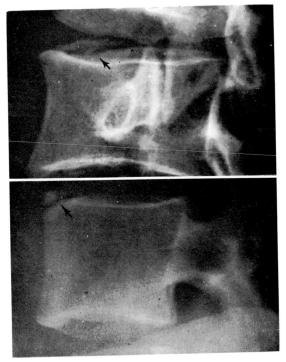

Fig. II:16. Female of twenty-three years with ununited vertebral epiphysis, the so-called "limbus bone" seen in the lateral and oblique projections (*arrows*). The condition is not to be confused with fracture or the intercalary ossicles that commonly form in the annulus fibrosis of the intervertebral disc (Figure XIII:23 and I:18).

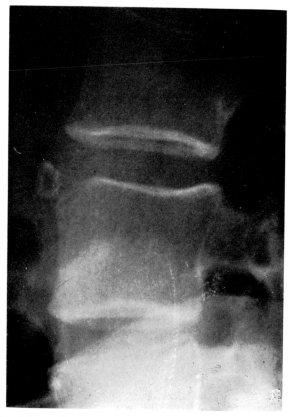

Fig. II:17. Female of forty-nine years with complete separation and displacement of the vertebral epiphysis. This is said to occur as a result of herniation of disc material into the area between the centrum and the epiphyseal ring (Figure VIII:21).

This growth deficiency and synostosis of the segments, at times called a fusion, cannot truly be termed a fusion because separation of the segments had never actually occurred. Non-segmentation is the preferable designation since the condition results from failure of segmentation of the mesodermal tissues.

Block vertebrae may be encountered at any level of the spine. If, because of hemivertebrae, the block comprises an unequal number of segments on the two sides or if one side is higher or if synostosis occurs on one side of the disc only while growth continues on the other side, a curvature of the block vertebra and consequently of the spine will result. Synostosis anteriorly produces a kyphosis but if it is at the side the patient will develop a scoliosis or torticollis (Figures II:32, II:33, II:34, II:35 and II:36, also figures III:17 and III:19).

Block vertebrae, in addition to being congenital, may be acquired. The acquired condition may result from trauma, disc degeneration, tuberculosis or other infective process, spondylitis deformans, or senile kyphosis. The latter is that type of fusion between the anterior margins of the mid-dorsal vertebrae caused from loss of disc substance (Figures IV:23, IV:25, IX:7E & F, IX:13, X:2, XI:5 and XI:11). A congenital block vertebra, as contrasted with a block vertebra secondary to trauma, disease or degenerative process, presents a flat smooth contour of the cortex on its anterior surface at the intersegmental level. Its A.P. diameter is likely to be less than normal for age and sex of the patient. The intervertebral foramen is small and round or oval in shape. A block vertebra on the other hand resulting from later fusion at the disc, shows a prominence at the disc level. The foramen is likely to be distorted and renal shaped, although it may be smooth and oval if the synostosis has been present for a long time.

Various disordered segmentations may occur in the same individual, apparently the stigmata of development. Their principal importance lies in the curvatures which they produce as well as any associated disturbances of the central nervous system.

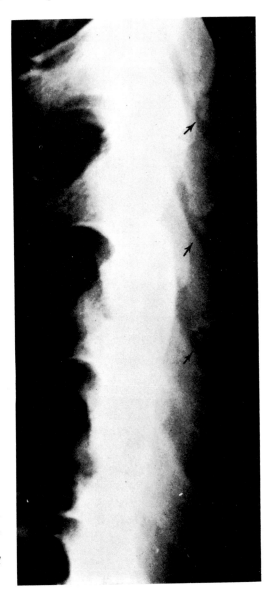

Fig. II:18. Male, age forty-six. Ununited centers at tips of the seventh, eighth and ninth dorsal spinous processes (*arrows*). The tenth and eleventh spinous processes are normal. The condition must be differentiated from fracture following trauma. A break usually occurs more proximally in the slender portion of the spinous process. (Courtesy of the *American Journal of Roentgenology*.)

SPINAL DYSRAPHISM

The median raphe of the neural tube is normally formed when complete dorsal closure of the cutaneous, mesodermal and neural tissues occurs early in the first month of development. Cutaneous dysraphic dysplasia results in a localized hypertrichosis, skin defect, pilonidal cyst, dermal sinus, nevus or some other superficial evidence of the underlying spina bifida. This latter develops from a non-closure of the mesodermal tissues dorsally in the midline (Figure III:18). Complete non-closure of the spinal canal is termed araphia. The canal remains widely open and the spinal cord develops as a flat plate, a condition incompatible with life (Figures II:37, II:38 and II:39).

The organism tends to adapt itself to

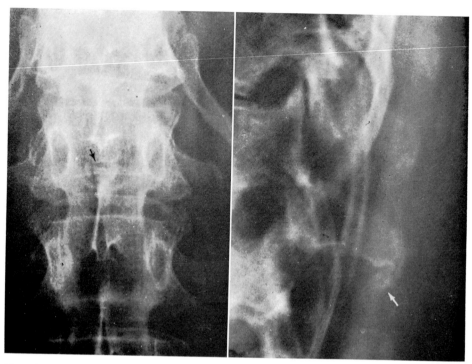

Fig. II:19. A small ossicle is seen at the tip of the T_{12} spinous process in a female of seventy-one years (*arrows*). The so-called shoveler's fracture which occurs at a somewhat higher level is an avulsion of the tips of the spinous processes in the upper thoracic region. It is caused by laborious use of the arms by individuals of inadequate musculature. The condition here shown is probably a persistent unfused secondary ossification center in an older individual.

Fig. II:21. Roentgenogram to show the normal sacroiliac epiphysis in a young man of seventeen years (*black arrow*). Epiphysitis of these structures may at times be the cause of obscure and confusing low back symptoms in early life. The iliac crest epiphysis is well shown at this time (*white arrow*).

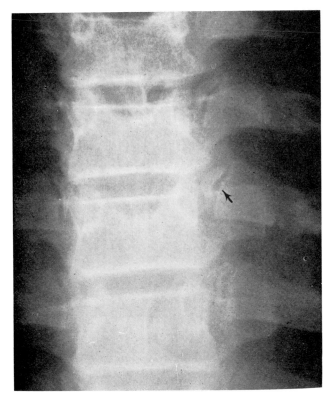

Fig. II:20. Roentgenogram to show the normal epiphyses of the heads of the ribs in a younger person. These will unite before the twenty-first year.

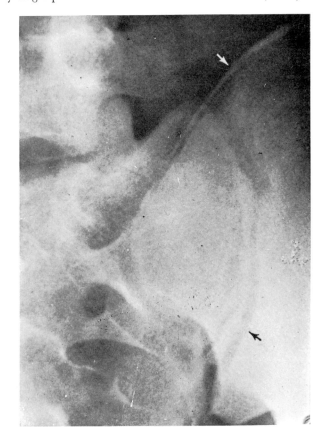

requirements. There is normally a dynamic relationship in growth between the brain and spinal cord on the one hand and the skull and spine on the other. If neural dysraphism occurs it is usually, though not always, accompanied by some type of spina bifida. In true spina bifida the spinal canal remains partially open. The dorsal portions of the neural arches curve laterally rather than medially. As a result of the open canal the exposed meninges and cord become attached to the superficial tissues with development of a meningocele. With longitudinal growth the usual as-

cent of the cord within the canal cannot occur without traction upon this structure. As a result of this traction during growth the Arnold-Chiari malformation and constriction of vascular and neural structures with increased intracranial pressure may develop at the foramen magnum. Various degrees of spina bifida, even with absence of vertebral body structures, may occur at any level of the spine. Complete separation of the two sides of the vertebra with presentation of the abdominal structures dorsally has been reported by Rosselet.

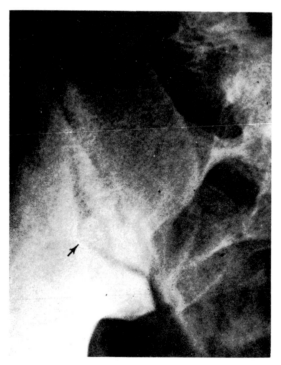

Fig. II:22. A persistent fragment of secondary ossification center in the right sacroiliac joint of a male twenty-two years old (*arrow*). Compare with Figure XII:24.

Fig. II:24. Avulsion of the ischial tuberosity in a boy of sixteen. This patient had sustained a severe fall at the age of twelve years resulting in a fractured skull. The avulsion was discovered during examination for a recent injury.

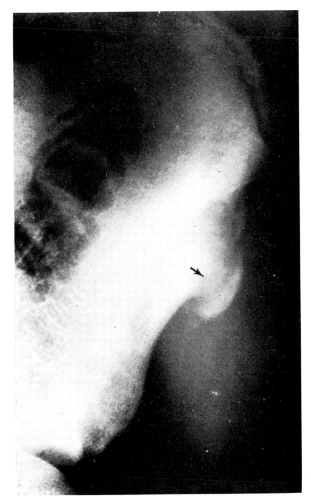

Fig. II:23. Avulsion of the epiphysis for the left anterior superior iliac spine (*arrow*). The patient, a boy of fifteen, stated that while running his left hip suddenly "gave out." He experienced only some discomfort upon walking.

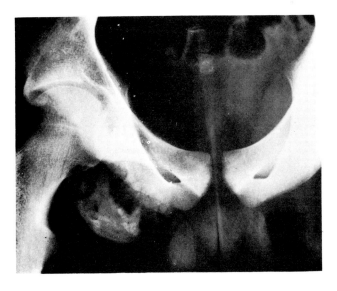

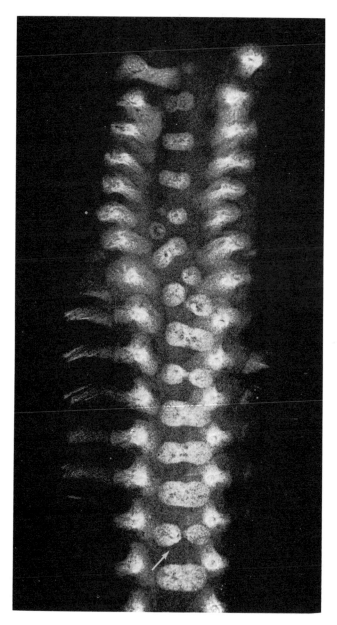

Fig. II:25. Specimen, female fetus at 6th month X4 bifid vertebra (white arrow) with asymmetrically paired centers for hemivertebrae in the cervico-dorsal region above. Had this individual survived she would probably have developed a butterfly vertebra like those in Figures II:27 and II:28 as well as a scoliosis at the cervico-dorsal level similar to that seen in Figure II:30.

In diastematomyelia the spinal cord is separated into two parts by a division through its central canal. Separation of the two lateral halves is maintained by the ingrowth of connective tissue elements between them, although they are both surrounded by a common dural sheath. From these mesodermal elements a spicule of bone may develop which tends to anchor the diastasis and prevents its upward migration as the child grows. The ultimate result of this traction may resemble that of a menigocele. In this extreme example of the dysraphic state there is widening of the canal but the roentgenogram fails to reveal destruction of pedicles or vertebral bodies to indicate intraspinal tumor.

Widening of the spinal canal without pedicle destruction is accomplished by increased transverse diameter of the vertebral body or by a laterally placed half vertebra. This latter may develop from the enlarged base of the pedicle directed medially so that the neurocentral junction occupies a para sagittal plane separating the two parts of the vertebral body (Figures II:40 and II:41).

The transverse diameter of the spine and the spinal canal may be widened by

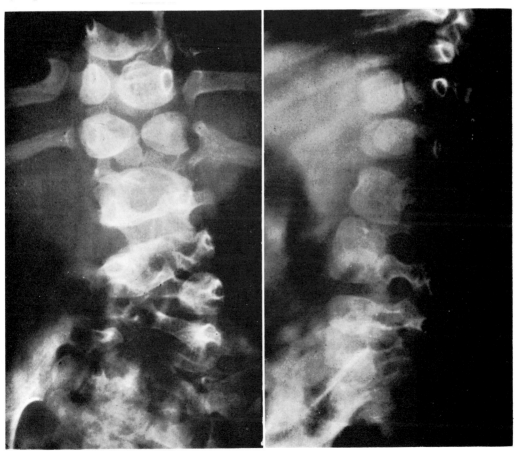

Fig. II:26. Male, age three years. Bifid vertebral bodies for the two lowermost thoracic segments. There are two upper lumbar vertebral bodies but the lower ones are represented only by hemivertebrae on the left side. This is an example of combined dysgenesis and agenesis not yet moulded by prolonged weight bearing.

an extra half vertebra. Even without a defect of the neural arch this indicates the possibility of meningocele or diastematomyelia. Diagnosis of the latter depends upon visualizing the septum between the two divisions of the cord. If a bony spicule, this may be seen on the film, but if it is cartilaginous or fibrous, myelography will be necessary for a differential diagnosis.

Various combinations of the anomalies already described or other developmental defects of greater or lesser extent may be encountered in any individual (Figures II:42 and II:43).

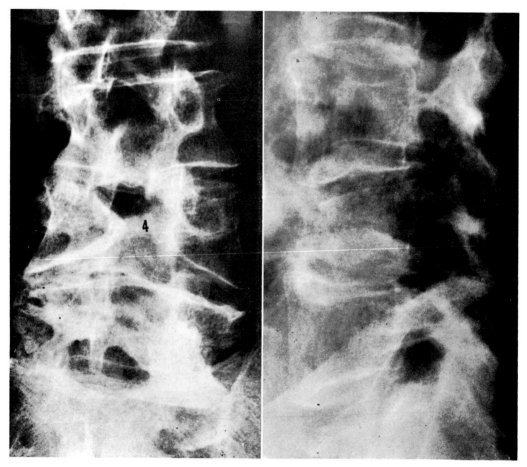

Fig. II:27. Female, sixty-nine years of age. Bifid or "butterfly" vertebra—"anterior spina bifida." In the postero-anterior view the fourth lumbar body is seen as two entirely separate, triangular-shaped hemivertebrae with a clear space between them. The upper and lower intervertebral discs are correspondingly distorted in shape and are joined by a zone of unossified tissue. The digit four has been applied to this area. The third and fifth vertebral bodies are also somewhat distorted. The neural arch is complete and connects the two sides of the centrum. In the lateral view the vertebra is seen to be wedge-shaped, higher in back, with its posterior surface on a plane behind the vertebrae above and below. The wedge-shape of the vertebral body has caused a straightening (relative kyphosis) of the lumbar curve. The condition is asymptomatic.

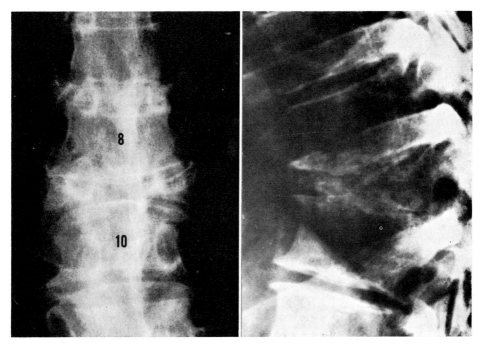

Fig. II:28. Male, forty years of age. Back pain aggravated by riding a tractor. Bifid T_9 with normal pedicles, neural arch and ribs. The side view shows the two lateral segments wedge-shaped and displaced backward because there is no attachment to the anterior longitudinal ligament. The same condition obtained in the patient in Figure II:27 and in both cases a kyphosis resulted.

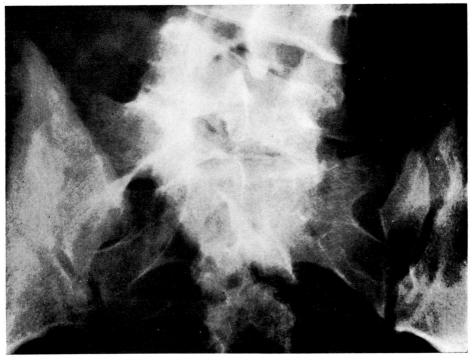

Fig. II:29. A hemivertebra constituting the right side of the first sacral segment in a young woman. This asymmetry, occurring at the basis of support, resulted in a moderate degree of scoliosis. (Courtesy of Dr. Edwin Euphrat, Syracuse, N. Y.)

REFERENCES

Secondary Ossification Centers

Bailey, W.: 1939, *Am. Jor. Roent., 42*:85–90.

Farmer, H. L.: 1936, *Am. Jor. Roent., 36*:763–767.

Hipps, H. E.: 1939, *J. Bone J. Surg., 21*:289–303.

Mitchell, C. L.: 1933, *J. Bone J. Surg., 15*:608–614.

Roche, M. B., *et al:* 1951, *Anat. Record., 109*:253–259.

Schmorl, G. and Junghanns, H.: *The Human Spine in Health and Disease,* Grune & Stratton, New York, 1959.

Sacral Anomalies

Blumel, J., *et al:* 1959, *J. Bone J. Surg., 41A*:497–518.

Calihan, R. J.: 1952, *Rad., 58*:104–108.

Dossel, P. M.: 1961, *Am. Jor. Roent., 85*:697–700.

Grand, M. J. H.: 1960, *Rad., 74*:611–618.

Katz, J. K.: 1953, *J. Bone J. Surg., 35A*:398–402.

Leigh, T. F., *et al:* 1954, *Am. Jor. Roent., 71*:808–812.

Zeligs, I. M.: 1940, *Arch. Surg., 41*:1220–1228.

Anatomy

Bingold, A. C.: 1953, *J. Bone J. Surg., 35B*:579–583.

Brailsford, J. K.: 1942, *Brit. Jor. Rad., 15*:213–223.

Cowie, T. N.: 1956, *Acta Rad., 46*:38–47.

Ehrenhaft, J. L.: 1943, *Surg. Gyn. Obst., 76*:282–292.

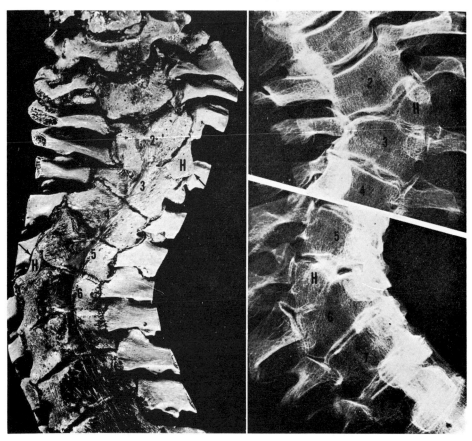

Fig. II:30. Photograph and radiographs of specimen with hemivertebrae (H) between T_2 and T_3 on the left and T_5 and T_6 on the right with resultant balanced scoliosis. The condition seen in this specimen indicates disturbed pairing of the mesodermal segments each side of the notochord during the blastemal stage.

McMaster, P. E.: 1945, *J. Bone J. Surg., 27*:683–686.

Neuhauser, E. B. D.: 1956, *Am. Jor. Roent., 76*: 469–475.

Stewart, T. D.: 1953, *J. Bone J. Surg., 35A*:937–950.

Neuhauser, E. B. D., *et al:* 1950, *Rad., 54*:659–664.

Sands, W. W.: 1954, *Am. Jor. Roent., 72*:64–67.

Seman, W. B., *et al:* 1958, *Rad., 70*:692–695.

Diastematomyelia

Bligh, A. S.: 1961, *Clin. Rad., 12*:158–163.

Campbell, J. B.: 1948, *Am. Jor. Surg., 75*:231–256.

Herren, R. Y., *et al:* 1940, *Arch. Path., 30*:1203–1214.

Holman, C. B.: 1955, *Ped., 15*:191–194.

Coronal Cleft Vertebrae and Butterfly Vertebrae

Cave, P.: *Brit. Jor. Rad., 31*:503–506.

Cohen, J., Neuhauser, E. B. D., *et al:* 1956, *Am. Jor. Roent., 76*:469–475.

Fawcitt, J.: 1959, *Proc. Roy. Soc. Med., 52*:331–333.

Fisher, F. J., *et al:* 1945, *J. Bone J. Surg., 27*: 695–698.

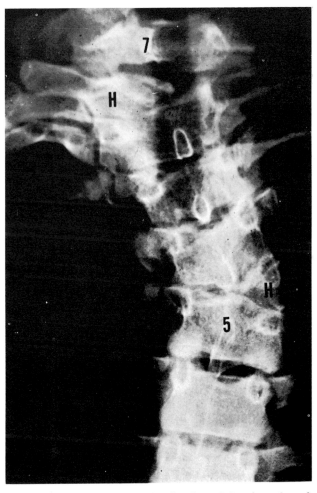

Fig. II:31. Female, age 13. There are a pair of balanced hemivertebrae between C_7 and T_5 (H and H). The first right rib is attached to the upper half segment and the fourth left rib is attached to the lower one. A balanced localized scoliosis results similar to that present in the previous specimen.

Dysraphia

Lichtenstein, B. W.: 1940, *Arch. Neuro. Psych.*,
  44:792–810.
Rosselet, P. J.: 1955, *Am. Jor. Roent.*, *73*:235–
  240.

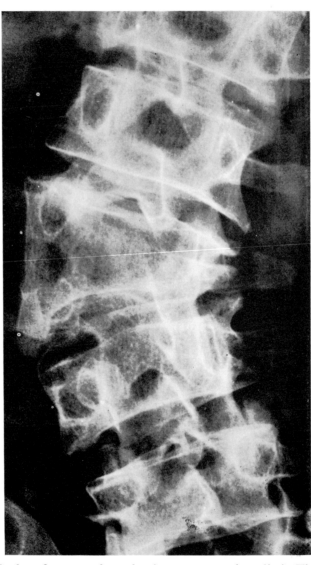

Fig. II:32. Male, forty-five years of age showing asymptomatic scoliosis. There is a wedge-shaped block vertebra consisting of two lumbar segments on the left side and one on the right with a resultant lumbar curvature. Note the absence of spinal rotation as seen in other types of scoliosis.

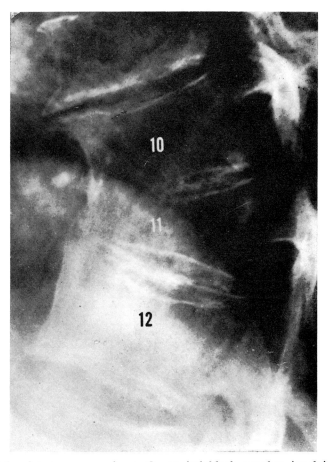

Fig. II:33. Male, sixty-two years of age. Congenital block vertebra involving the lower three thoracic segments with a complete anterior synostosis. Since early fusion had developed in front, a kyphosis occurred posteriorly as the vertebral segments continued to grow in back.

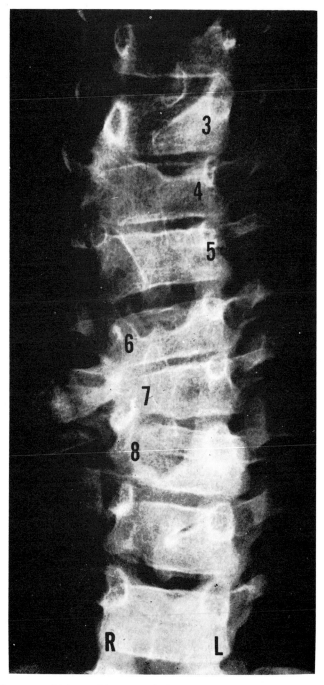

Fig. II:34. Nine year old boy with congenital non-segmentation of T_{3-4-5} into one block vertebra and T_{6-7-8} into another. There was also some asymmetry in the development of the neural arches. The ribs on the left side appeared normal while those on the right side are distorted and present a wide interval between the 4th and 5th ones posteriorly. The 8th rib is double. The two curves partially balanced each other so that only a minimal total curvature was present at the time. Since the lower block was fused on the right it continued to grow more rapidly on the left side. The reverse condition was true in the block above. A reexamination two and one-half years later showed that the angula-

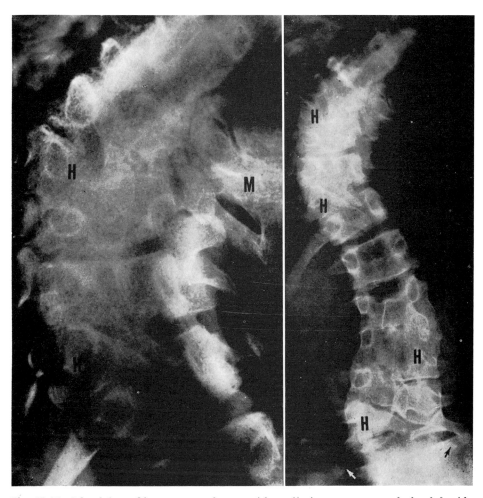

Fig. II:35. School boy, fifteen years of age, with scoliosis convex toward the left side caused by two hemivertebrae (H) in the thoracic region. The patient has twelve ribs on the left side and eleven on the right. Many of these latter have become fused into a single bony mass (M) which acts somewhat as a flying buttress to afford additional support on the side of the spinal concavity in the dorsal region. Unlike the condition in figure X:7, a secondary, compensatory curvature below is prevented by the fusion of the lumbar segments into a single block vertebra. In the lumbar region there are balancing half segments, one on each side (H & H). There is also sacralization of the lowermost lumbar segment on the left side *(white arrow)*. The lowermost neural arch on the right side is free, not joining the vertebral body by a pedicle but it does articulate with the ala of the sacrum *(black arrow)*. The fusion of ribs and of the lumbar segments has fortuitiously prevented further scoliosis in this case.

tion at each level had increased somewhat. However because of the balancing effect of the opposite curves the total curvatures had actually decreased during this interval. Compare this with a patient (Figure X:7) who had only a single thoracic block vertebra fused on one side and as a result developed a substantial curvature during her growth period.

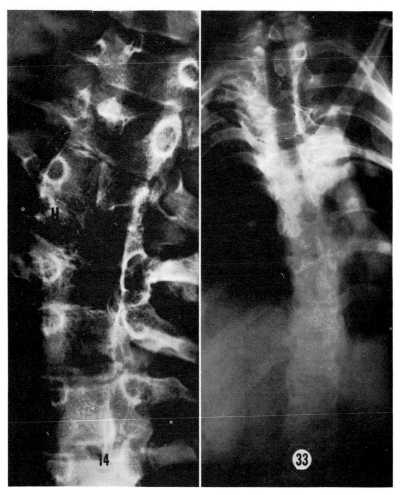

Fig. II:36. Adolescent school girl at fourteen years. The original film revealed a hemi-vertebra (H) on the right side between the 2nd and 3rd dorsal segments. This half section, together with the uppermost four complete thoracic vertebrae formed a single fused block vertebra. There was some resultant curvature, convex on the right side, caused by the extra half segment. The child had only eleven ribs on each side. Those on the left were somewhat distorted in shape and the eleventh one on the left was one vertebra below the corresponding one on the right. A reexamination (33) of the same patient made 19 years later reveals the curvature almost identically the same as it was during adolescence. The scoliosis was primarily the result of the hemivertebra but since the fusion was completely bilateral an increasing scoliosis did not result as it did in figure X:7. (The follow-up study was made by courtesy of Doctors Newton Bigelow and Lucy Cobb, Marcy, New York.)

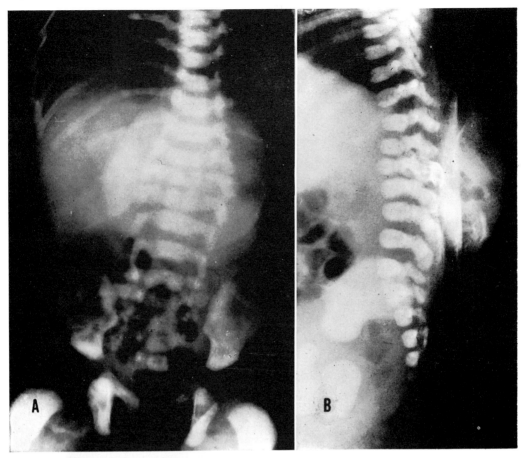

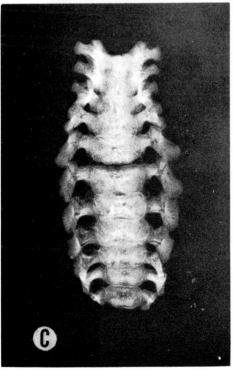

Fig. II:37. Roentgenograms of a female infant one month old with increased intracranial pressure, hydrocephalus and paralysis of both legs. The meningocele, extending from the 10th thoracic vertebra downward, became ulcerated and the child succumbed. The first three upper lumbar vertebrae and their discs are smaller than normal. The lateral (B) projection also visualizes six lumbar segments. The postmortem specimen (C) shows the everted neural arch elements which are typical of dysraphia. In this condition the sides of the arches spread apart and do not cover the spinal canal.

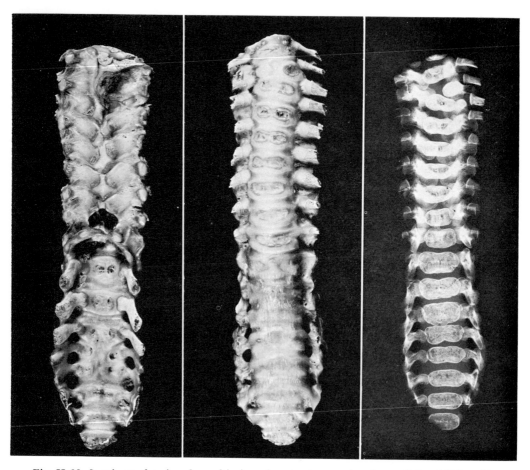

Fig. II:38. Specimen showing dysraphia in a female six months of age. Spina bifida with meningocele of lumbar and upper sacral region. As in Figure 37, the neural arches are directed outward. In spite of the hemivertebra in the mid-thoracic region, scoliosis had never developed as the child was unable to sit upright. Certain vertebrae show evidence of double ossification centers. (Courtesy of The Pediatrics Department, Syracuse Memorial Hospital.)

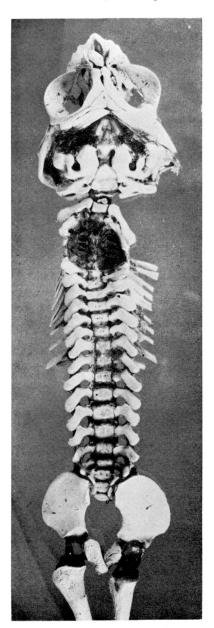

Fig. II:39 Araphia. Complete non-closure of the spinal canal in a six months' human, acephalic fetus. The sides of the neural streak did not close over to form the neural tube in the second week of development. The spinal cord developed as a thin, flat plate of neural tissue from which the spinal nerves passed laterally through the intervertebral foramina. All of the neural arches are everted. The darker portion in the cervical region represents a localized lordotic area.

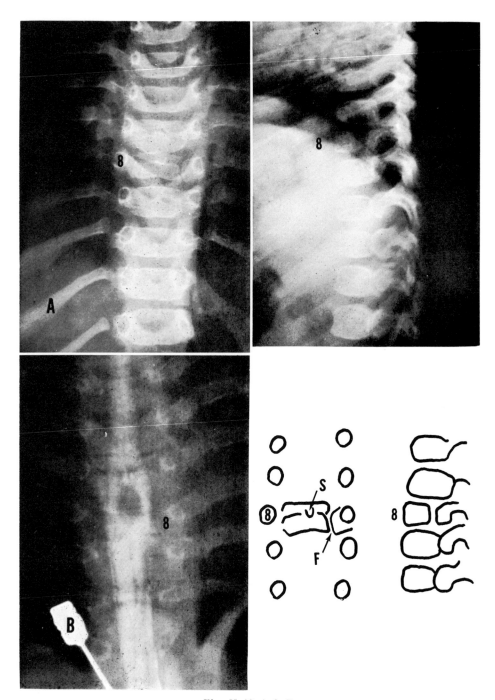

Fig. II:40 A & B

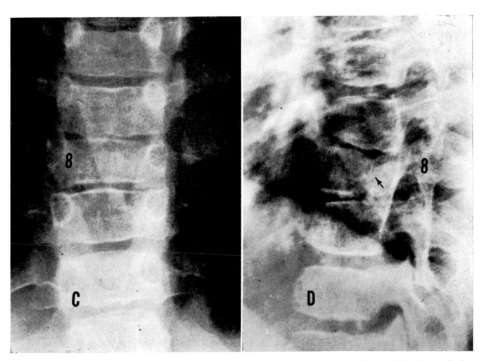

Fig. II:40. Female, one and one-half years of age. Diastematomyelia. Widening of the spinal canal at T_8 with a bony spicule in its mid-line attached to the vertebral body (S). In the lateral view the eighth thoracic vertebra is seen to comprise two segments, the larger one in front. These are separated by a cleft or column of soft tissue joining the seventh and eighth discs. In the A. P. projection one may note the enlarged base of the eighth pedicle on the left side joining the two segments of the vertebral body at a para-sagittal neurocentral fissure (F). A similar condition is present in this same patient at a lower level (Figure II:41A). The myelogram (B) shows the oil column and therefore the spinal cord divided by the bony spicule. At operation the cord had not yet become com-pletely anchored so that it was possible to free it. Through the courtesy of Doctor Philip Rosenberg this child was reexamined at the age of 8 3/4 years. A. P. and lateral studies (C and D) show evidence of fusion of T_7, T_8 and T_9, posteriorly with minimal kyphosis. The cleavage plane of the neurocentral junction is visualized (*arrow*). The spinal canal is open from T_6 to T_9 but the child is developing nicely. She appears healthy and attends school regularly.

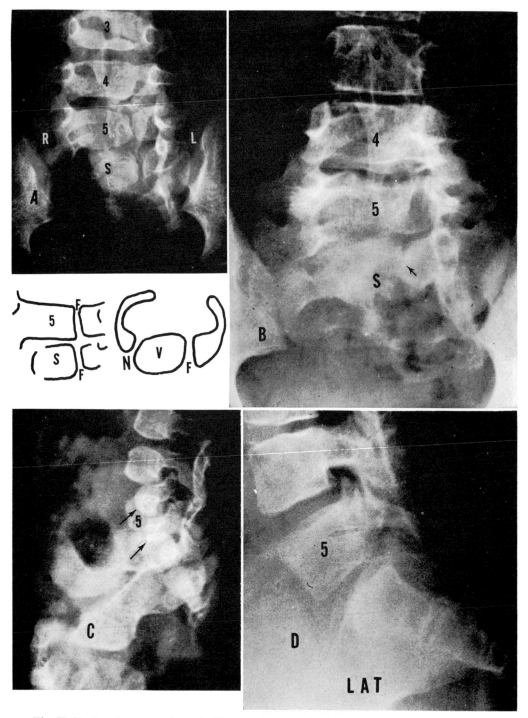

Fig. II:41. Female, one and one-half years old, same individual as Figure II:40. She has partial agenesis of the sacrum, only the first two segments are present and these are without neural arches on the right side. The sacral canal was wide open and myelography revealed a large meningocele posteriorly which was removed one year later. A number of other cases of incomplete development of the sacrum have been reported, complicated by socalled anterior meningocele, that is with the meninges herniating into the pelvic cavity.

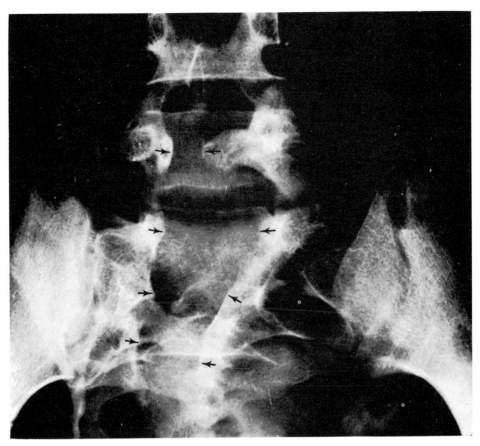

Fig. II:42. Spina bifida occulta in a female of seventeen years. The spinal canal and the 5th neural arch are open (arrows). This patient was the victim of left hydronephrosis, a left hydroureter 2 cm. in diameter and cystitis. (Courtesy of the University Hospital.)

Those patients have bladder symptoms, constipation, sensory and reflex changes. This patient had weakness of the left leg muscles with absent left Achilles and patellar reflexes. The roentgenogram shows some asymmetry of the lumbar neural arches. The fourth and fifth are rudimentary on the right side and the third right is united with the fourth left. An unusual congenital anomaly of some interest is seen at the L_5 and S_1 pedicles on the left side. Normally the neurocentral union is at the posterior lateral surface of the vertebral body. Rarely, as in the present instance, with a widening of the spinal canal the ventral end of the pedicle is considerably enlarged. This enlargement curves medially so that it forms a part of the widened vertebral body (see diagram). The neurocentral fissures (F) are seen in the P. A. view as lying in a parasagittal plane. The small diagram on the right below illustartes the condition as it would appear from the axial direction. In this diagram we see that the vertebral body (V) possesses a normal neurocentral union on one side (N) but on the other side the base of the pedicle is enlarged and forms a part of the widened vertebra, uniting with it at the fissure (F). This is similar to the condition seen above at T_8 in figure II:40, the site of the diastematomylia. The retouched lateral radiograph (C) shows the enlarged L_5 and S_1 pedicle bases (arrows).

The A.P. and lateral projections made at the age of 8 3/4 years show that the child has developed a functionally adequate sacrum. The site of the neurocentral union in the sacrum is still visualized on the A. P. view (arrow on B). The spinal canal remains open posteriorly at the sacrum but except for a slightly smaller left leg there is no evidence of a permanent neurological deficit. (Courtesy of the Syracuse Memorial Hospital.)

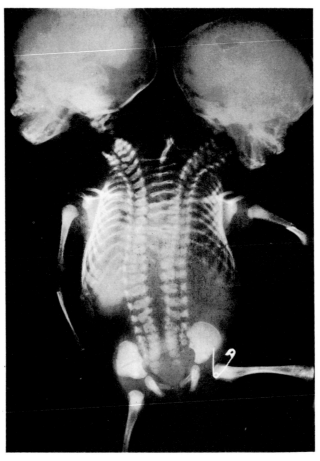

Fig. II:43. A dicephalic still born monster with two spines. There are hemivertebrae in the cervical region of each side. Some of the ribs are common. The lower vertebrae exhibit the parasagittal neurocentral fissures as diagramed in Figure II:41A.

Chapter III

Disturbances of Cervical Spine Development

Anomalies of the cervical spine, as elsewhere, may develop during the embryological period as a result of agenesis, non union or non segmentation. Dysgenesis may rarely occur also at a later period. Non development of certain elements may produce no particular disability or limitation of functions, Figure III:1. In other cases, since the condition originates so early, the organism may develop compensatory structures to offset the deficiency, Figure III:2. If a half vertebra is lacking others unite with the remaining hemivertebra to stabilize the structure (Figure III:4). For some unknown reason the growth stimulus of a structure may be delayed at first, later to appear, so that finally full development is attained (Figure III:3).

THE ODONTOID GROUP

Numerous examples of disturbed odontoid development are reported with increased amplitude of movement at the C_1-C_2 level. It has been shown that the odontoid arises from a bifid ossification center and that later a separate ossicle develops within its terminal ligament which normally becomes united to form the tip of the structure (Figure I:22). In case union does not take place the tip may remain as a separate bony structure, the so-called "ossiculum terminali." This may lie within and deform the foramen magnum.

Complete agenesis of the dens has been described as "absent odontoid." This condition must not be confused with congenital non-union of the odontoid with the body of the axis, the so-called os odontoideum. In these latter patients the upper surface of the body of the axis presents a cone shaped formation which serves as a pivot of rotation for the atlas (Figure III:5). The ununited odontoid is separate and may lie within the foramen magnum; it may be attached to the anterior arch of the atlas or it may come to lie in front of the axis (Figure III:6). This condition may easily be confused with previous fracture of the odontoid. There is, however, no history of injury, pain and muscle spasm are absent and there is no fracture line or break in the cortex. The separate ossicle with intact cortex shows a cleavage plane between it and the centrum of the axis. Dislocation of the atlas on the axis is the principal complication in either condition (Figures III:7, III:8, III:9, III:10, and III:11).

Persistence and non-union of the secondary ossification centers described in Chapter I may be the cause of some confusion, especially in the event of trauma (Figures III:12, II:18 and II:19).

NON-SEGMENTATION

In the cervical region the non-segmentation of two or more vertebral elements is not at all uncommon. The use of the term "fusion" is convenient although not exactly correct from the embryological standpoint. In areas of nonsegmentation the intervertebral foramina are round or oval and smaller than those at the levels of movable joints (Figure XIV:14).

With synostosis, the epiphyseal tissue remains imprisoned within the block. Growth continues so that both seg- mented and the non-segmented divisions contribute their proportionate share in the longitudinal development of the spine. The epiphyseal rest may persist within the block vertebra as a bony or cartilaginous plate throughout life (Figures III:13 and III:26). The condition

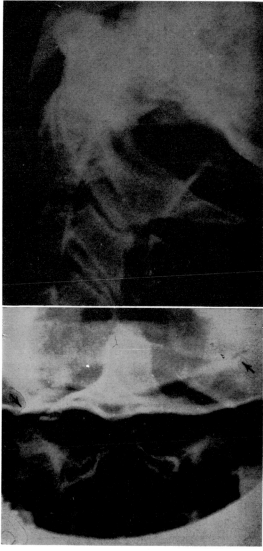

Fig. III:1. Male, thirty-one years of age. This patient has a partial agenesis of the first cervical neural arch, the structure being represented only by a cigar-shaped fragment of bone on the left side. The A.P. projection, however, shows both the lateral masses present and articulating with the occiput and the axis in the normal manner (*arrows*). The patient was at first thought to have sustained a fracture of the structure at a recent accident.

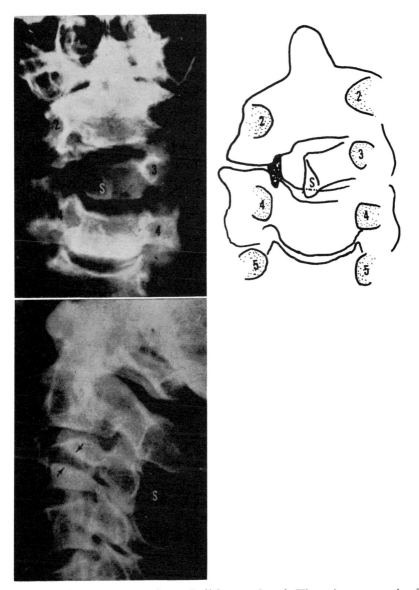

Fig. III:2. Male, forty-one years of age. Pedicles numbered. There is an agenesis of the third right cervical pedicle, neural arch and articular processes with compensatory, articulating bony columns from C_2 and C_4 which bridge this deficiency. The pedicle and left half of the third arch are present with the diminutive spinous process (S). On the lateral projection the joint surfaces between the compensatory bony columns are seen to separate when the cervical spine is held in dorsal extension (*arrows*) but upon forward flexion they make contact. This is an excellent example of a compensatory development secondary to a congenital deficiency. This condition originated during the first month of embryonic life when the mesodermal cells of the future third cervical segment failed to develop along the right side of the neural arch at that point. (Courtesy of the *American Journal of Roentgenology*.)

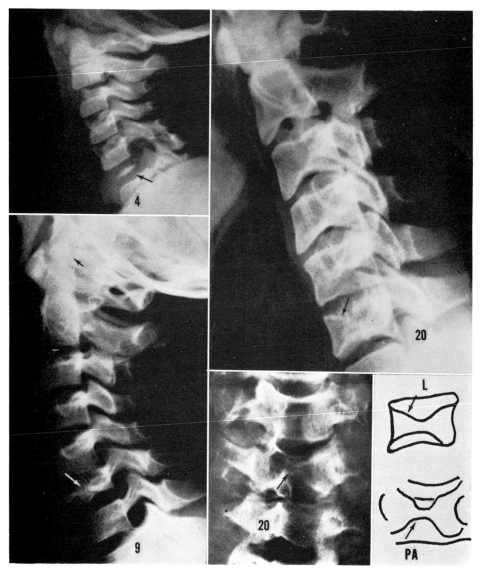

Fig. III:3. Male, showing development of platyspondylia in one individual studied from the age of four years to twenty. There was congenital hypoplasia of the sixth cervical vertebra. The centrum was represented radiographically only by a flat bony plate at four years (*arrow*). The pedicles were lacking but the posterior articulations and the laminae were present. The odontoid was still incompletely united with the body of the axis. Five years later at the age of nine (*lower left*) good development of the C_6 neural arch had now taken place. However, the centrum was incompletely developed (*white arrow*). The secondary ossification center at tip of the odontoid was ununited (*black arrow*). The A.P. view of this odontoid at nine and twelve years may be seen in I:22. At twenty years the lateral and posterior-anterior views showed the sixth cervical body to be of almost normal adult height peripherally but the vertebra was flat in the center. Following their initial delay the margins of the vertebral epiphyses at this level obviously functioned somewhat but since the periphery of the vertebral body develops from periosteal bone

may at times involve many vertebrae and even be confused with the late changes of juvenile arthritis or Still's disease. The latter condition however results from a destructive arthritic process causing an ankylosis of the posterior articulations (Figure III:14). Since no movement occurs between the segments of a block vertebra at the fused level, additional dynamic stress necessarily falls upon the structures of the adjacent joints. In older patients with block vertebrae these ad-

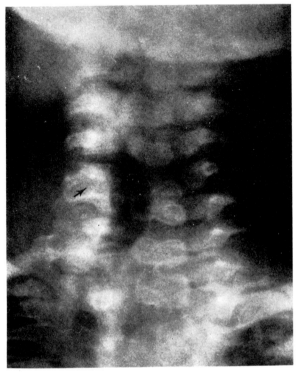

Fig. III:4. Roentgenogram showing dysgenesis of the cervical spine in an infant, X3. Unfused hemivertebrae are present in the upper cervical region. The fifth and sixth pedicles are fused on the right side (*arrow*) but separate on the left. A block vertebra at the C_{5-6} level is formed from two left and one right hemivertebrae. This condition dates from the first month of intrauterine life.

growth it would seem that the enchondral bone formation of the centrum may have been defective. Clearly visualized, are the concave upper and lower surfaces of the vertebral body (*arrows*). Obviously the 6th vertebra developed largely by periosteal growth. A tracing of the lateral (L) and (PA) views at twenty years shows the periphery of the sixth cervical vertebra to have reached nearly its normal height. Its central portion, however was only about 4 millimeters thick. At four years the posterior articulations for C_6 were present but the pedicles were lacking, apparently unossified. Five years later the sixth pedicles appeared essentially normal. The posterior articulations and the pedicle of each side normally develop from the same ossification center. See Figure I:9.

While the examination at four years presented somewhat the appearance of reticuloendotheliosis, there was no other evidence of Christian-Schüller's disease elsewhere. From the early deficiencies and subsequent course of the process it would seem that this child presented some localized congenital type of disturbed bone formation.

jacent articulations invariably show extensive arthrotic changes (Figures III:-15, IV:23 and IX:16).

Asymmetry in the shape of a block

vertebra is not at all unusual. In the presence of other cervical anomalies it is nearly always a factor in the deformity (Figures III:16, III:17, and III:27).

THE KLIPPEL-FEIL SYNDROME

This congenital non-segmentation of various cervical segments must arise within the first month of intra-uterine life. It is characterized by a short neck, low hair line, limited but painless movements of the neck and rounded back. The patient may have prominent trapezius muscles, the "webbed" neck or pterygium colli. The Scapulae are often raised (Sprengel's deformity) and the nipples are low. Various other findings

sometimes present are: depression of the skin surface in the mid-line posteriorly, torticollis, mirror writing, anterior or posterior spina bifida and scoliosis.

The non-segmented elements unite into a solid block often with a single large spinous process, neural arch and vertebral body. The intervertebral foramina persist but as in other cases of non-segmentation they are smaller than normal, smooth, and round or oval in

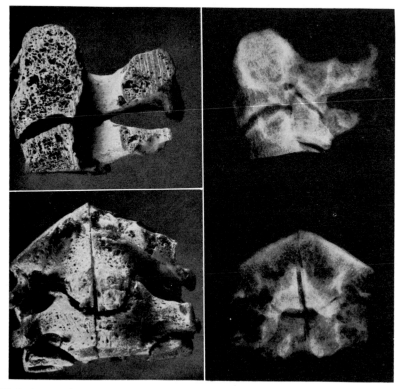

Fig. III:5. Anatomical specimen closely resembling Figure III:6 unfortunately not discovered until the atlas and skull had been discarded. Note the elevated mid-portion of the axis and its cone like shape which serves as a pivot for rotation of the atlas. The sagittal section does not show any definite cleavage plane between vertebral body and odontoid base. The cone shape suggests that this was probably a congenital anomaly, either an united or absent odontoid.

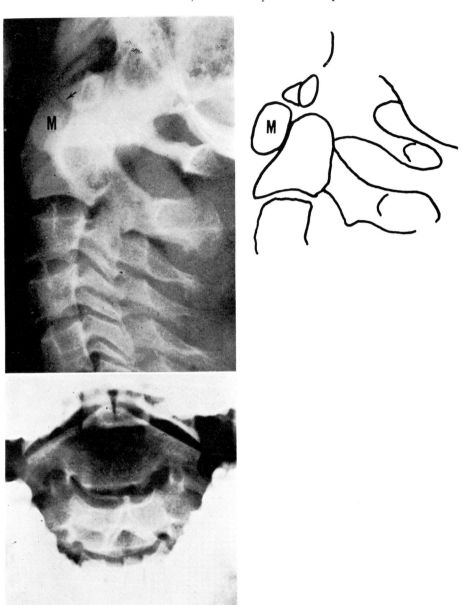

Fig. III:6. Male, thirty-two years of age. Congenital absence of the odontoid process. The A.P. view shows a complete absence of the odontoid with the mid-portion of the axis elevated to form a cone or pivot for rotation of the atlas. There is an oval-shaped mass of dense tissue, probably bone, lying immediately anterior to the upper surface of the axis. (M) There also seems to be a cleavage plane between this and a smaller triangular mass of tissue attached to the front of the anterior arch of the atlas *(arrow)*. Alexander reported from an autopsy upon a twenty-one-month-old infant a detached odontoid, entirely of cartilage and surrounded by a fibrous tissue. Such may be the origin of the oval mass here visualized. Temporary attacks of hyperesthesia, paresthesia and paralysis at various times followed injury. (Courtesy of Dr. George Miyakawa, Charleston, West Virginia, and the publisher of the *Journal of Bone and Joint Surgery, 34A:676.*)

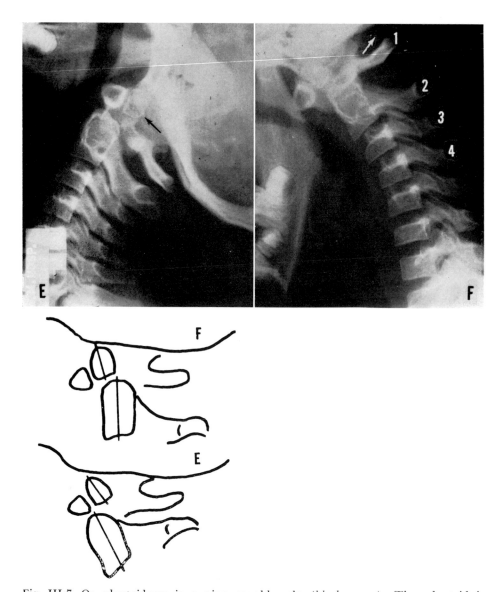

Fig. III:7. Os odontoideum in a nine-year-old male *(black arrow)*. The odontoid is entirely separate from the body of the axis but it is attached to the hyperplastic anterior atlantoid arch. Slight separation between the posterior arch of the atlas and the occiput is seen upon anterior flexion *(white arrow on flexion film)*. The tracings in flexion (F) and extension (E), with the axes of the odontoid and the second vertebra indicated, reveal a substantial degree of forward-backward gliding between these two upper cervical vertebrae.

There was a history of dizziness, occipital headache and wide base gait for three weeks. (Courtesy of Dr. D. L. McRae, Montreal, Canada, and the publisher of *Acta Radiologica 40:347.*)

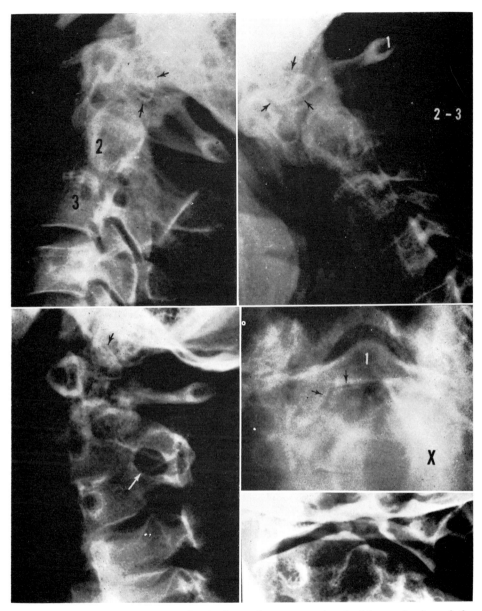

Fig. III:8. Male, age fifty, complained of muscle spasm and palpable crepitation of the neck the day following an auto accident. Radiographs show a triangular-shaped os odontoideum *(black arrows)*, attached to the anterior arch of the atlas but will separate from the axis. Instability, both lateral and ventro-dorsal, was minimal in amplitude. Open mouth projection shows the typical cone-shaped axis. Non-segmentation of C_2-C_3 has resulted in the round intervertebral foramen characteristic of congenital block vertebra. *(white arrow)*. In the base-vertex projection (X) note the os odontoideum *(arrows)* attached to the anterior arch of the atlas (1) slightly to one side of the midline.

outline. There is a foramen for each of the segments making up the block and each foramen is a complete bony ring unbroken by disc or posterior articulation. There may be one or more cervical ribs or an atlanto-occipital fusion, and asymmetry of some type is usually present (Figures III:18, III:19, III:20, and III:21).

ATLANTO-OCCIPITAL FUSION AND THE OCCIPITAL VERTEBRA

Disturbances of segmentation frequently develop in the upper cervical region. In a thirty-day embryo we have seen that the segments of the spine and the skull are continuous (Figure I:4). The sclerotomes which later form the cervical vertebrae are directly continuous with three or four postotic segments, together termed the hypoglossal or occipital mass. In the chondrogenous stage

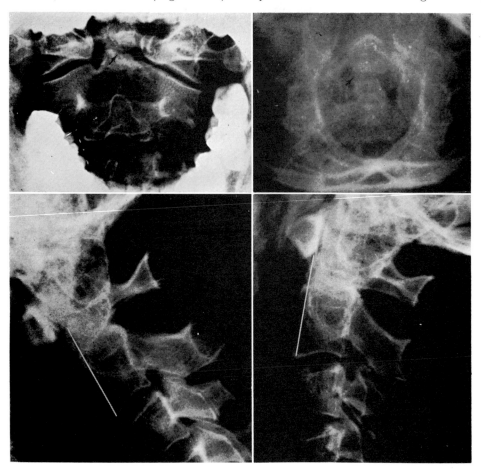

Fig. III:9. Male, thirty-one years of age. Pain in back of the neck with some stiffness and limitation of motion following accident one week before. Radiographs reveal the odontoid detached from the axis (arrow). This is obviously not a recent injury. The flexion study shows minimal forward gliding of C_1 on C_2. In the absence of a cone shaped axis as seen in Figures III:5, III:6 and III:8 this has more the appearance of an old fracture rather than that of an os odontoideum. Upon careful questioning the patient sepecifically denied any previous injury.

———————————→

Fig. III:10. Female, age sixty-five. Ossiculum terminale at tip of the odontoid (*arrow*). This center develops in the terminal ligament of the dens at about two years of age and normally unites at about twelve years to form the tip of the odontoid. In this individual, it has remained as a separate oval body 5 x 8 mm in size just above and behind the tip of the odontoid and probably does not encroach upon the medulla. There are two smaller ossicles in front of it, apparently within the atlanto-occipital membrane. The film through the open mouth, below, shows the cleavage line between the odontoid and the ossicle (*arrow*). See Figure I:22.

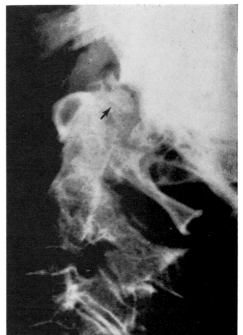

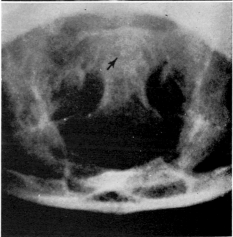

these segments form the occipital plates and later fuse to form the continuous occipito-sphenoid cartilage. Within this develop the three ossification centers of the occipital bone which partially surround the foramen magnum. Distinct bones can be developed in a continuous uninterrupted block of cartilage (Figure III:22).

If the posterior-most hypoglossal sclerotome is incompletely assimilated with the others forming the base of the skull the condition is described as "manifestation of an occipital vertebra." On the other hand, if segmentation is not completed between the occiput and the atlas, the so-called atlanto-occipital fusion is produced. Harrower believes these to be varying degrees of the same process. Assimilation of the atlas has been found in the human embryo and in newborn infants. Most of the cases are congenital but rarely a secondary acquired fusion of the atlanto-occipital joints may result from disease. Arthritis, osteomyelitis, echinococcosis, syphilis, tuberculosis and actinomyocosis have been mentioned in this connection.

CHARACTERISTICS OF THE OCCIPITAL VERTEBRA

An occipital vertebra is a morphological structure resembling a vertebral segment which surrounds the foramen magnum. There may be a hypochondral arch, partially or completely fused to the anterior margin of the opening. This may bear a third condyle for articulation with the odontoid. This condyle may be

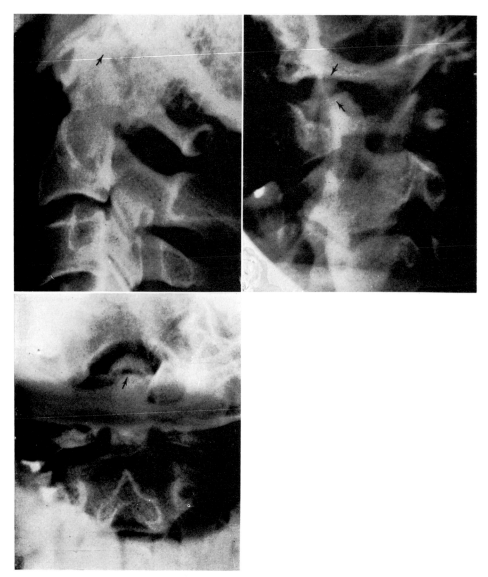

Fig. III: 11. Asymptomatic ossiculum terminale in a male of fifty-five years seen in the lateral, through mouth and Kasabach projections (*arrows*). See Figure IV:3C.

Fig. III:13. Female, typist, age twenty-three. Non-segmentation of the vertebral bodies and posterior articulations. Complains of pain in the neck and back of head. There is spasm of the trapezius muscles with limitation of all neck movements. Both the lateral and oblique projections show the first neural arch unfused posteriorly. (1). The most commonly observed type of non-segmentation, that of the cervical region, is seen at the 2-3 and the 5-6 levels. Congenital fusion of this kind invariably results in a narrowing of the block vertebra opposite the imprisoned discs and a smooth round or oval intervertebral foramen (*arrows*).

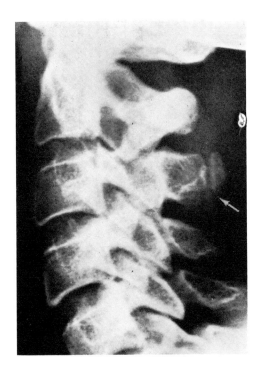

Fig. III:12. Female, age forty-six. Two ununited centers for the tips of the bifid third cervical spinous process *(arrow)*. These are not to be confused with the calcifications that frequently occur in the ligamentum nuchae. At a previous examination following an automobile accident these ossicles had been mistakenly diagnosed as ununited fractures. It is not unusual to encounter ununited centers at the tips of the spinous processes in the adult (Figures II:18 and II:19). (Courtesy of the *American Journal of Roentgenology.*)

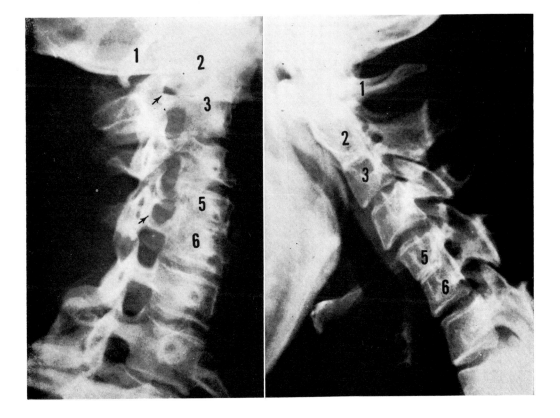

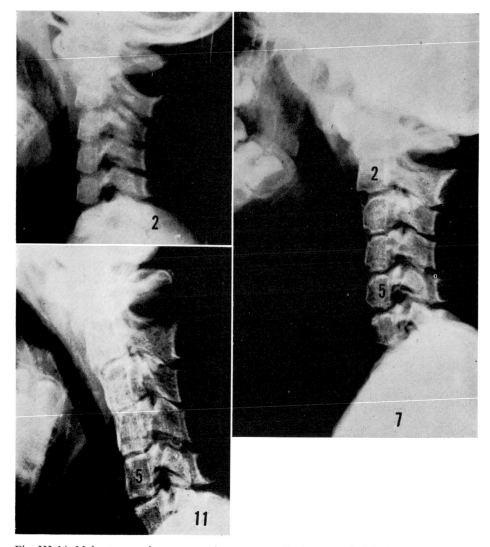

Fig. III:14. Male, two to eleven years. At two years. Early congenital fusion (non-segmentation) of C_2 to C_6 inclusive. No atlanto occipital fusion or foramen magnum constriction. First neural arch was not closed. At seven years the cervical bodies are growing. Epiphyseal notches are present anteriorly but no discs have developed. Other studies reveal non-segmentation of the fifth, sixth, seventh and eighth thoracic vertebrae as well as the tenth and eleventh. The first neural arch has now become closed. By eleven years (the film made in full anterior flexion) there was complete cervical fusion with fixation of movement below C_2. The notches are now occupied by the epiphyseal rings though not well seen on the reproduction. The posterior articulations have developed but have never functioned, there being apparently some growth-stimulation factor other than use. See figure III:31. In juvenile arthritis the posterior joints are destroyed and in congenital nonsegmentation the discs fail to develop. Since both conditions develope early they appear somewhat similar.

See Figures IX:15 and IX:16.

either an articular depression or a single tuberosity with an articular facet (Figure III:40). Bilateral bony masses or accessory eminences may seriously encroach upon the anterior part of the foramen magnum. These various bony tuberosities and masses develop in the ligamentous tissue about the opening. A partial or complete neural arch may be outlined about the dorsal surface of the foramen. Transverse processes may or may not be present, more or less fused with the bones of the skull. If present, they do not bear a foramen for the vertebral artery. The condyles resemble those of the normal subject and the atlas is present and normal in appearance and movement. The third condyle and basilar tubercles may be manifestation of the occipital vertebra (Figures III:40 and III:41).

An ossiculum terminale may be present in the anterior portion of the foramen magnum. This ununited secondary ossification center is developed as an ossicle within the terminal ligament of the odontoid and may produce some encroachment upon the foramen magnum (Figure III:23).

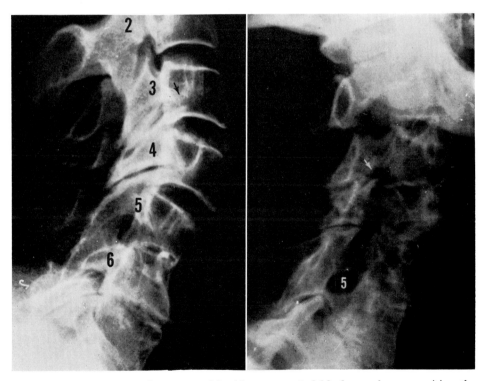

Fig. III:15. Male, seventy-four years old with a congenital block vertebra comprising the fifth and sixth cervical segments. Note the concave flattening of its anterior surface and the smooth oval outline of the intervertebral foramen (white 5). Compare with the shape of the foramina opposite the movable discs. The resultant fixation of movement at this most mobile part of the cervical spine has thrown additional stress upon the adjacent posterior articulation. The resultant posterior joint changes over the years have caused a substantial encroachment of the corresponding intervertebral foramina. Note especially the third articulation which has become enlarged forward so that it impinges beneath the pedicle and projects into the foramen *(arrows)*.

CHARACTERISTICS OF SO-CALLED ATLANTO-OCCIPITAL FUSION

As indicated by the name, in this condition there is an ankylosis between the atlas and the base of the skull. Some indication of the normal joints may persist. The condition may be unilateral with the two sides of the atlas separate and one of them remaining unankylosed (Figure III:30).

Flexion-extension studies will reveal absence of movement between the atlas and the occiput. The transverse processes bear foramina for the vertebral arteries and a space is present on each side between the dorsal arch of the atlas and the occiput for the passage of the suboccipital nerve and the vertebral artery. There is an articulation on the anterior arch for the odontoid. As with the occipital vertebra, the accessory eminences on one or both sides may encroach upon and distort the foramen magnum.

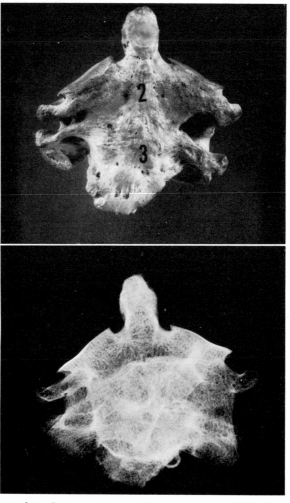

Fig. III:16. Photograph and roentgenogram of an asymmetrical block vertebra specimen. This one comprises the second and third cervical segments and is much lower on the right side. This type of asymmetry is not uncommon. There is ample space in the foramen, however, for the third right cervical nerve to leave the spinal canal. Compare with Figure III:19.

Asymmetry with tilting of the head is very common in congenital anomalies of the cervical spine. Ten of Dwight's fourteen cases were asymmetrical, some with distortion in the shape of the face, others with torticollis or rotation of the atlas on the axis. The atlas may be displaced laterally or forward on the axis. List reports a fatal case of forward dislocation of the atlas wherein the odontoid had

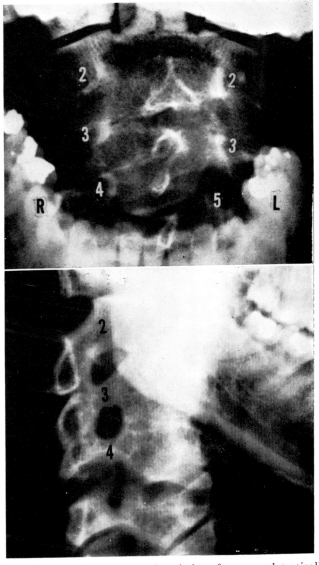

Fig. III:17. Female, age twenty-four, was the victim of structural torticollis. The right shoulder was higher than the left. There was some asymmetry in the shape of the skull and the head was carried well to the right of the midline. Rotation and flexion of the cervical spine toward the right side was about seventy-five per cent normal. The patient has a block vertebra comprising the 2nd and 3rd and 4th segments on the right side but only the second and third on the left. The 4th segment is a hemivertebra with pedicle and neural arch elements. There is an agenesis of the 4th left pedicle with its articular processes so that on that side the 5th process articulates with the 3rd. Note the shape of the 2nd and 3rd right foramina as characteristic of congenital non-segmentation.

compressed the spinal cord to a band 3 millimeters wide and 2 millimeters thick.

Non-segmentation is common at various levels below the fused atlas and produces torticollis when the block vertebra is higher on one side. Fusion may even be so extensive as to constitute the Klippel-Feil syndrome, a somewhat related condition. There are likely to be various other anomalies elsewhere such as club foot, hypoplasia of a lumbar articulation, syndactylism, etc. Both atlanto-occipital fusion and the occipital vertebra are of more than anatomical interest because of the constriction of the foramen magnum or because of basilar impression and resulting clinical symptoms.

Congenital anomalies of the atlanto-occipital region do not always cause neurological disorders. When they do

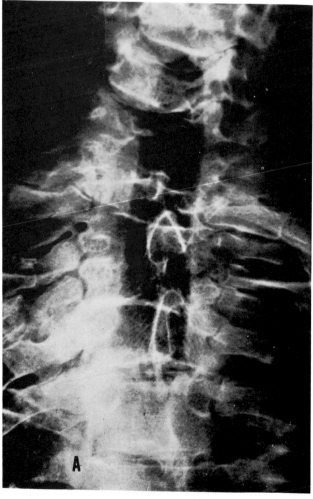

Fig. III:18. Male, age sixty-one. There is a massive consolidation of seven vertebral segments at the cervico-thoracic level with localized kypho-scoliosis and a defect in the neural arch. Note the proximity of the costovertebral articulations. The intervertebral foramina show the smooth round or oval configuration so characteristic of congenital non-segmentation. This case is somewhat suggestive of the Klippel-Feil deformity. There is a growth of hair at the upper thoracic level.

develop, however, the first symptoms are likely to appear as late as the second or third decade but may be progressive and even fatal. They are caused by: (1) constriction of the foramen with resultant pressure upon nervous structures; (2) adhesions; (3) ischemia from interference with blood supply; (4) interference with the dynamics of the cerebrospinal fluid between the ventricles and subarachnoid spaces causing hydrocephalus, and (5) increased pressure within the cerebellar fossa from basilar impression or invagination. Neurological symptoms, if present with foramen magnum encroachment, may be mistakenly diagnosed as indicating multiple sclerosis, spastic paralysis, amyotrophic lateral sclerosis, cerebellar or upper cervical canal tumor, Klippel-Feil syndrome, hydrocephalus or syringomelia. A lateral survey roentgenogram of the upper cervical spine made in full forward flexion to reveal possible fixation between the atlas arch and the occiput is indicated in all cases showing neurological symptoms of upper cord degeneration or compression. Such a lateral survey film should also be taken in all cases of torticollis or asymmetry of the head and neck. Some of those cases previously diagnosed syringomyelia or multiple sclerosis have been discovered upon reexamination to be cases of foramen magnum encroachment, and as such, are entitled to surgical consideration.

If a congenital anomaly of this type is discovered in a young child not yet showing symptoms, his parents should be acquainted with the possibilities, and remain alert for the first appearance of neurological signs. These may not appear until the second or third decade.

Early suboccipital decompression

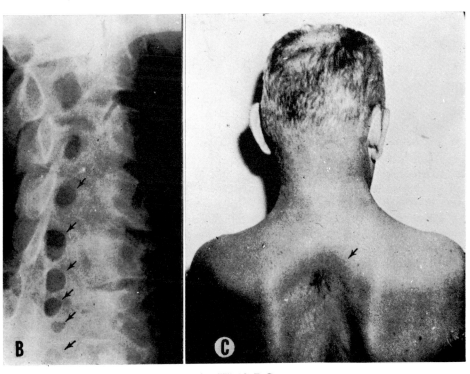

Fig. III:18 B-C

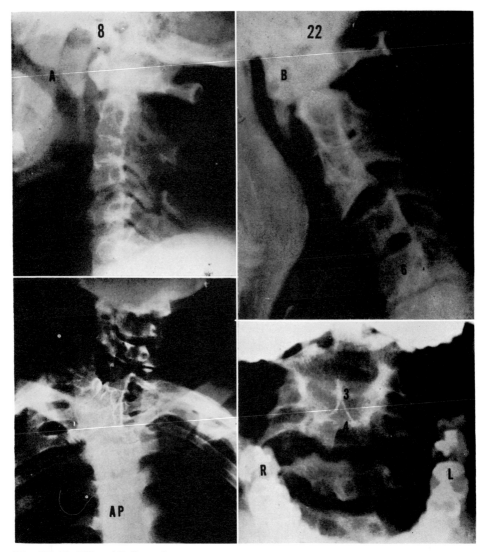

Fig. III:19. Klippel-Feil syndrome.

A. Female, eight years of age. Non-segmentation of the second, third and fourth cervical bodies and posterior articulations. There is a single neural arch with one large spinous process at this level and a spina bifida at the cervicothoracic level.

B. Same patient at twenty-two years of age in anterior flexion. More complete fusion has now developed during the fourteen-year interval. There is normal movement at the atlanto-occipital and atlanto-axial articulations and no evidence of basilar impression. The fifth and sixth vertebrae are separate and movable but the lowermost cervical and upper five thoracic segments constitute a single scoliotic massive block vertebra. This is convex toward the right side because some of the left segments are lacking. The A. P. *(retouched)* projection of the cervicodorsal level at twenty-two years shows the block vertebra causing scoliosis, convex to the right with synostosis of the upper three or four ribs and spina bifida outlined by a dotted line. The asymmetrical block vertebra seen through the mouth *(lower right)* comprising C_2, C_3 and C_4 is higher on the left side to partially compensate for the torticollis caused by the scoliotic block vertebra at the cervicothoracic level. The oblique views, "R"

———————→

operation with upper cervical laminectomy and opening of the dura has been
recommended in an attempt to arrest the
progressive compression and destruction
of nerve tissue. Of course, restoration of
normal bone relations or destroyed nervous tissue is impossible. Fusion should
be done if the atlas was dislocated. Respiratory embarrassment may be a troublesome complication (Figures III:24,
III:25, III:26, III:27, III:28, III:29,
III:30, III:31, III:32, and III:33).

BASILAR IMPRESSION-(INVAGINATION) VS. PLATYBASIA

Elevation of the floor of the posterior
cranial fossa may occur in cases of upper cervical anomaly. The first cervical
segment will be found above Chamberlain's line which extends from the hard
palate to the posterior margin of the
foramen magnum. In patients with basilar impression the elevated floor of the
posterior fossa and the foramen magnum
appear as a double sine curve on the anteroposterior view. That is, the lateral
portions of the posterior fossa curve
downward while the medial parts adjacent to the funnel-like foramen curve
upward on each side.

Easier to visualize is the curve seen

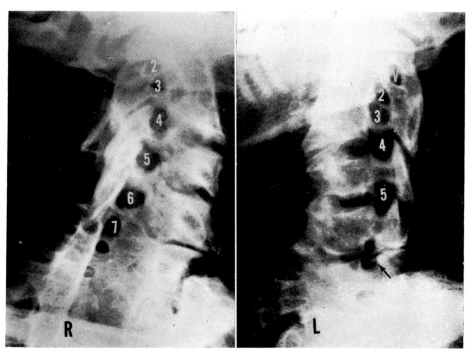

and "L", made at twenty-two years, show the small round or oval foramina at the fused
levels and larger normal-shaped foramina at the movable (4, 5, and 6) levels. Where movement occurs between vertebral bodies the foramen is larger because a cushion space about
the nerve is necessary to accommodate the physiological foramen constriction incidental to
these movements. Since this constriction of the foramen by movement does not occur
where the vertebrae are fused a much smaller foramen is sufficient at those levels. The sixth
left foramen of this patient, however, is encroached upon by a sharp bony arthrotic spur
projecting forward from the posterior articulation (*arrow*). The most cephalic foramen of
the block vertebra is for the vertebral artery (V).

from the lateral direction. Here, in place of the normal downward curve of the entire occiput, only the posterior part of the cerebellar fossa curves downward while that elevated portion about the foramen magnum curves upward (Figure III:34, 1 and 2).

Basilar impression can be differentiated into congenital and secondary types. The congenital type is frequently noted with atlanto-occipital fusion. Figure III:30. There are changes in the occipital bone, distortion in the shape of the foramen magnum and displacement of the odontoid process upward into this opening, decreasing its anteroposterior diameter.

The acquired type is secondary to a decreased hardness of the base of the skull as in Paget's disease, osteogenesis imperfecta, rickets, osteomalacia, or hyperparathyroidism. Here the softened skull is invaginated by the cervical spine thrusting the base upward into the posterior fossa. The basilar portion of the skull is thus convex upward showing as a

---

Fig. III:20. A.M.K. Female, fifteen years of age. Klippel-Feil, short neck, head sitting on the shoulders, torticollis, low hair line, kyphoscoliosis at the cervico-thoracic level. First thoracic and the cervical segments are fused into one solid mass. Visualized in this oblique projection are the small round intervertebral foramina characteristic of congenital block vertebra (F). The unusually large foramen magnum extends backward to the white arrow and is closely applied to the wide-open spinal canal. This funnel-shaped structure is enlarged both in the anteroposterior and lateral directions. Because the attachment of the tentorium is so low in the posterior fossa of this patient (*black arrow*) the cervical canal probably houses a part of the hindbrain. In the lateral roentgenogram there is no evidence of basilar impression or atlanto-occipital fusion. The first neural arch is seen entirely separate from the occiput and remains unclosed and widely open behind (N). Flexion-extension studies revealed 7 degrees of movement between the occiput and the fused cervical mass, most of it occurring at the atlanto-axial joint (X). The spinal canal measured 3.5 centimeters wide on the A.P. projection.

Fig. III:21. O.O.B. Female, sixty-four years of age. Os odontoideum and Klippel-Feil deformity. Somewhat similar to the previous case but in an older woman. The transverse diameter of the cervical canal is enlarged to 4 centimeters and is completely open in back. There are only three cervical arches, fused at the sides but open posteriorly. These are united below with the upper four thoracic segments into a single block vertebra. The stereoscopic studies show the atlas to be fused to the occiput. However, there are 32 degrees of flexion between the occiput and the fused cervical mass. This occurs at the C_1-C_2 joint which is clearly visualized (X) but is convex downward like the condyloid joints. This is apparently an example of adaptation to nodding movement. Just above this articulation is seen the upper surface of the axis where the base of the odontoid normally attaches. As in cases of absent odontoid this area is somewhat elevated and in profile has the same characteristic stubbed appearance (*black arrow*). In this patient, however, the odontoid is not fused with the upper surface of the axis. It seems to have developed as a separate ossicle, round in shape, the os odontoideum (O) articulating with the front of the axis and displacing forward the posterior pharyngeal wall (*white arrow*). Compare with Figure III:6.

The condition visualized in Figures III:20 and III:21 has been discribed by Edith L. Potter as an intermediate stage between iniencephaly and the Klippel-Feil syndrome. She describes iniencephaly as a defect in the occipital bone with an enlarged foramen magnum and absent laminae in the cervical region. The head is in extreme dorsal extension with the occiput in contact with the nape of the neck. The vertebral bodies are reduced in number, irregularly fused and abnormal in shape with the spinal canal widened.

reverse curve. The foramen magnum may be as high as the petrous pyramids and funnel-shaped. The occiput may develop a recess behind the foramen to accommodate the posterior arch of the atlas but the latter does not fuse with the occiput. Flexion-extension studies reveal movement between the base of the skull and the atlas.

In both types, the invagination of the occiput upward into the posterior fossa acts as a piston. The tentorium being fixed, pressure is exerted upon the cerebellum. Brain substance may be forced to herniate downward into the spinal canal somewhat as noted in the Arnold-Chiari syndrome. In secondary cases with widening of the skull base there may be traction upon the posterior five or six pairs of cranial nerves and deafness may be one of the symptoms.

PLATYBASIA-FLATTENED BASILAR ANGLE

The Martin's (or Welcker) basilar angle (root of nose—sella turcica—anterior margin of foramen magnum) as recorded by anthropologists is normally about 135 degrees. In one case of advanced acquired basilar impression secondary to Paget's disease the basilar angle measured only 110 degrees.

The anthropological term "platybasia" or flattening of the basilar angle

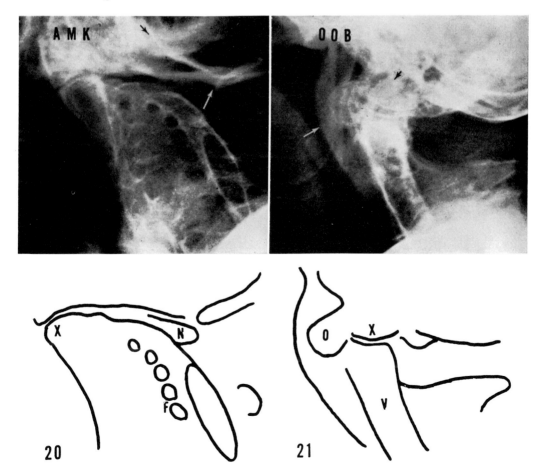

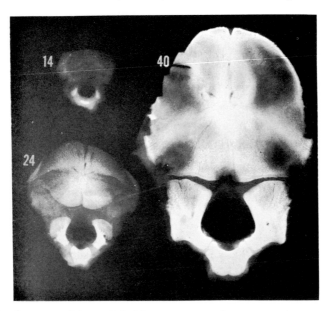

Fig. III:22. Development of the occipital bone as seen at fourteen weeks, twenty-four weeks and at term. The large supra-occipital ossicle develops in membrane but the two exoccipitals at the sides and the infra-occipital below develop in the hypoglossal cartilage. This originates from three segments, continuous with and similar to those forming the cervical vertebra (Figure I:4). There is a similarity between ossification of the vertebrae and this part of the occiput.

Fig. III:23. Female, eleven years of age. This is an example of occipital vertebra.

A. Radiograph at the full limit of anterior flexion showing the first cervical arch separated from the thinned posterior margin of the foramen and the cornua of the occipital vertebra (*white arrow*). A.P. studies showed the atlas apparently normal.

B. Kasabach 45-degree oblique view. The long arrow indicates the hypoplastic odontoid (O) which is shorter than normal. The three arrow-heads enclose a separate ossicle, the ossiculum terminale (T) which contributed to the foramen magnum encroachment. Atlanto-occipital and atlanto-axial articulations are indicated by the parallel lines on the tracing.

C. Constricted foramen magnum shaped like a bicycle seat. The anterior portion is distorted by bony masses projecting from each margin about one-third of the way across. The arrow points to the ossiculum terminale.

The child had complained of weakness for one-half year. On the left side there was hyperesthesia to tactile and pain stimuli with heat perception entirely lost and with cold producing a painful sensation interpreted as heat. The arm reflexes were exaggerated on the right side but absent on the left. Abdominal reflexes were present on the right side but absent on the left. The right patellar reflex was exaggerated, the left normal. Both Achilles reflexes were weak. There was a strong positive left Babinski with a questionable one on the right. The circumference of the right mid thigh was one inch smaller than the left. Movements were somewhat incoordinated. There was spasm of the right sternomastoid muscle and limitation of skull rotation toward the left side.

Operation revealed a thinned posterior margin to the foramen magnum and a small cornu each side of this constricted opening. These latter represented the rudiments of the posterior arch of the occipital vertebra. The opening was enlarged and a circular fibrous constriction of the dura similar to that described by List was uncovered and incised. The

does not properly apply to basilar impression since it designates only, as indicated above, that portion of the skull base anterior to the foramen magnum. "Basilar impression" more nearly describes invagination of the posterior cerebral fossa. On the other hand a true platybasia or flattening of the basilar angle to 150 degrees or more may occur without invagination of the posterior fossa (Figures II:34, 3 and 4).

OTHER MISCELLANEOUS ANOMALIES OF DEVELOPMENT

Various congenital anomalies of the atlas of possible medico-legal interest may be noted. The neural arch of this structure normally closes about the fourth or fifth year but it frequently remains open throughout life (Figures III:35, III:36, XIV:8B and III:13). Parts of one or both sides of the arch may be missing (Figures III:1 and III:37). The anterior arch of the atlas ossifies from a center which develops in the first year of life (Figure I:14). Failure of this center to appear may result in the two sides of the atlas remaining separate (Figure III:29).

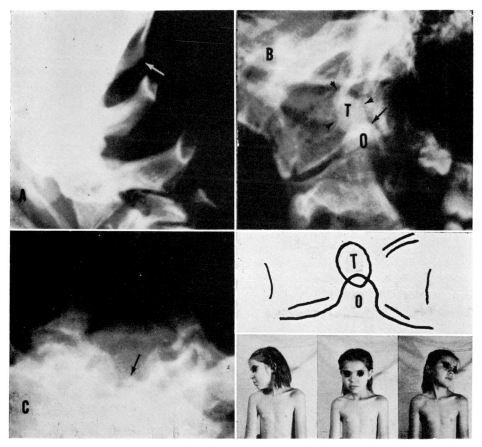

Babinski reflex disappeared but otherwise the neurological picture had remained entirely unchanged when the patient was examined five years later. (Courtesy of the *American Journal of Roentgenology.*) See Figure IV:3C.

Small bony masses, possibly remains of the hypoglossal arches, are frequently visualized lying alongside the foramen magnum. Separate ossicles lying between the occiput and the arch of the atlas or between the first and second arches are not at all rare. They are likewise of no clinical significance but may upon occasion present some legal importance (Figures III:1, III:38, III:39).

The third condyle appears as a tubercle and/or an articular facet on the anterior margin of the foramen magnum. It develops as an ossification within the terminal ligament or cruciate ligaments and may articulate with the odontoid or the anterior arch of the atlas. Specimens 13 and 14 millimeters in length have been reported (Figure III:40). Certain authors have erroneously called the ossiculum terminale and also the os odontoideum a third condyle.

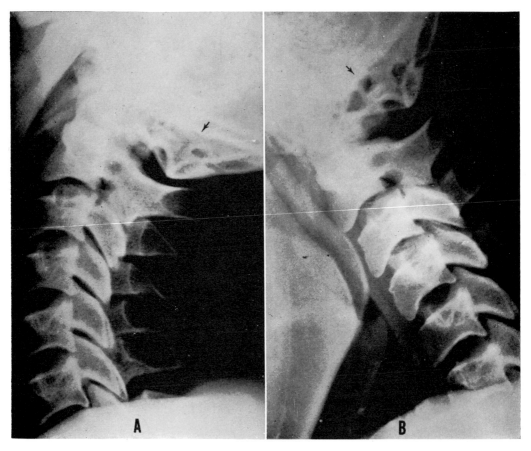

Fig. III:24. Male, thirty-two years old. There is a congenital non-segmentation between the first cervical segment and the base of the skull (arrows). Upon anterior flexion (B) the neural arch of the atlas cannot separate from the occiput. However, those spinous processes below C₁ separate in the normal manner. In the fused bony mass which incorporates the atlas note the foramina for the vertebral arteries. The oblique projection (C) is made with the head turned 45 degrees toward the right. The odontoid (O) lies between the left and right lateral masses of the atlas (L and R). Note in C that the transverse width of the C₂ lateral mass shadow (white line) is narrowest on that side toward which the head is

———————→

Other anomalies arise from abnormal ossification of ligamentous structures in this region (Figure II:41). The para- occipital process is a bony connection between the occiput and the first transverse process and lying close to the condyle (Figure III:33c). The paramastoid process is a bony column arising from the transverse process of the atlas and articulating with the base of the skull at the jugular process (Figure III:42). This is probably congenital (one case discovered by Dwight in a child, age nine months), and usually induces asymmetry in the posture of the head and neck. The pon-

ticulus lateralis is a bony arch extending from the superior articular surface of the atlas to its transverse process. The ponticulus posterius is a similar structure without clinical significance arising from ossification of the posterior portion of the atlanto-occipital ligament and commonly seen on lateral projections of the cervical spine. It is a bony bridge extending from the posterior margin of the superior articular surface of the atlas backward to the upper margin of the posterior arch of this bone. The ponticulus encloses the foramen arcuale (posterior atlantoid foramen) through which pass

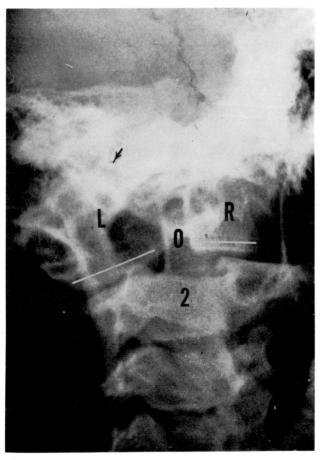

turned. This is because the condyles are oval in shape and are placed obliquely. See Figure IV:3C. The arrow indicates the point where the lateral mass is fused with the occipital bone. Radiographic study of the foramen magnum showed some encroachment upon the lumen of that opening.

the suboccipital nerve and the vertebral artery as they course over the upper surface of the first arch (Figure XIV-:6A & B).

Of greater clinical significance are the accessory eminences described by Le-Double and others as masses of bone lying along the anterolateral borders of the foramen magnum. They may be bilateral or unilateral and are believed to originate by ossification of the anterior portion of the atlanto-occipital ligament. They cause encroachment upon the foramen magnum as seen in Figures III:23, III:28, III:30, and III:32.

REFERENCES

Anatomy

Coventry, M. B.: 1959, *J. Bone J. Surg., 41A:* 815–822. Toricollis.

Dwight, T.: 1904, *J. Med. Research, 12:*17.
Harrower, G.: 1922, *J. Anat., 57:*178.
McRae, D. L., *et al:* 1953, *Am. Jor. Roent., 70:* 23–46.
McRae, D. L., *et al:* 1959, *Am. Jor. Roent., 84:* 1–25.

Odontoid

Fullenlove, T. M.: 1954, *Rad., 63:*72–73.
Gwinn, J. L.: 1962, *Am. Jor. Roent., 88:*431–442, Absent.
Schultz, E. H., *et al:* 1956, *Rad., 67:*102–105, Agenesis.

Agenesis

Berk, M. E., *et al:* 1961, *J. Bone J. Surg., 43B:* 77–86, Kyphosis.

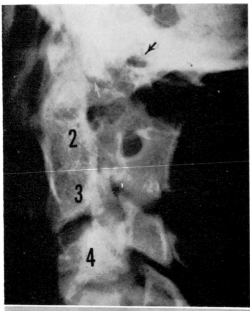

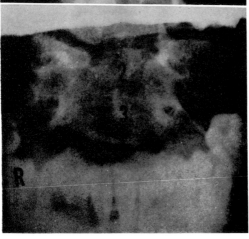

←————————

Fig. III:25. Male, age 15, hospitalized for neuromyelitis optica. There was bilateral nystagmus, inconstantly diminished left ankle and left biceps reflexes, also bilateral club foot and brachydactylism. The first cervical segment was fused to the base of the skull with foramina for the vertebral arteries (black arrow). With fusion of the atlas to the occiput, transverse processes for C_1 are present and are penetrated by the vertebral arteries. See Figure III:32. In this patient, segments 2 and 3 constitute an asymmetrical block vertebra surmounted by a short hypoplastic odontoid. Behind the tip of this structure is seen, in the lateral projection, the small unfused secondary ossification center for the tip of the odontoid (white arrow). Since the patient has reached the age of fifteen years this center will probably remain separate as an ossiculum terminale. (Courtesy of the *American Journal of Roentgenology.*)

Buetti, C.: 1953, *Radiol. Clin.*, 22:141–161; *Abst. Rad. 62:460*.

Steinbach, H. L., 1952, *Rad.*, 59:838–840.

Atlanto-Occipital Synostosis

Goettsch, H. B.: 1957, *Jor. Belg. d. Radiol.*, 40: 739–762.

List, C. F.: 1941, *Arch. Neurol. & Psych.*, 45: 577–616.

Lombardi, G.: 1961, *Am. Jor. Roent.*, 86:260–269.

McRae, D. L.: 1953, *Acta Rad.*, 40:335–354.

Basilar Impression

Bull, J. W. D.: 1955, *Brain*, 78:229–247.

Craig, W. M., *et al:* 1942, *Surg. Gyn. Obst.*, 74: 751–754.

Hinck, V. C., *et al:* 1961, *Rad.*, 76:572–585.

Peyton, W. T., *et al:* 1942, *Rad.*, 38:131–144.

Poppel, M. H., *et al:* 1953, *Rad.*, 61:639–644.

Platybasia

Furst, W., *et al:* 1942, *Am. Jor. Roent.*, 47:588–590.

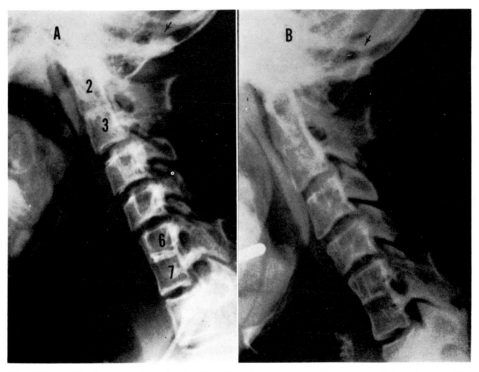

Fig. III:26. Twelve-year-old schoolgirl with atlanto-occipital fusion and fixed torticollis since birth. Radiographic studies showed a slender first cervical neural arch fused to the occiput each side of the foramen magnum *(arrow)*. This opening was distorted somewhat on the left side. There was non-segmentation at the 2-3 and the 6-7 cervical levels. The epiphyseal plates were visualized at this age, and even appear imprisoned within the block vertebrae. The torticollis was caused by an asymmetry of the uppermost block vertebra which was higher on the left side. She also had a partial agenesis of the sacrum. The patient was reexamined periodically during the following fifteen years during which the torticollis disappeared almost completely. Both films, A at age of twelve and film B at age of twenty-seven, were made at the limit of anterior flexion and show non-separation of the first neural arch from the occiput. In spite of non-segmentation the block vertebrae developed to normal height and configuration. The growth controlling factor may be associated with the development of the spinal cord. The patient accommodated for the torticollis and in spite of the distorted foramen magnum, she never developed any neurological symptoms. (Courtesy of the *American Journal of Roentgenology*.)

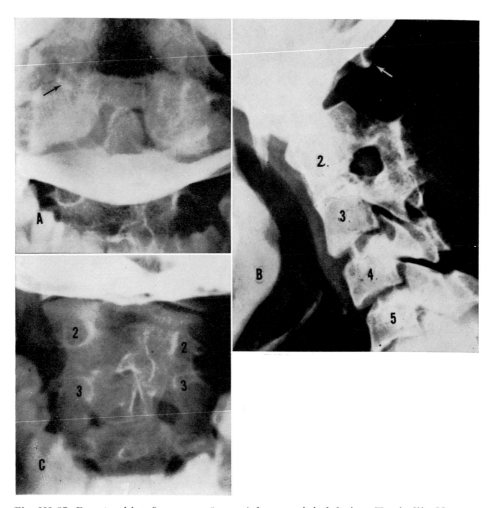

Fig. III:27. Female, thirty-five years of age. Atlanto-occipital fusion. Torticollis. No pertinent neurological symptoms.

A. Anterior-posterior view showing the odontoid and the atlanto-axial joints. The arrow indicates very slight vestige of right atlanto-occipital articulation. There is no indication of this joint on the left side.

B. Lateral projection in anterior flexion *(arches accentuated)*. The arch of the atlas remains attached to the occiput *(white arrow)*. There was fifteen degrees of flexion between the atlas and axis but movement was restricted elsewhere. The block vertebra comprised segments C_2 and C_3.

C. Anterior-posterior projection through the mouth showing the asymmetrical block vertebra much higher on the right side causing the patient's torticollis. Size of the intervertebral foramen (distance between the second and third pedicles) is greater on the right side than on the left. Compare with figures III:16 and III:19. This patient had a short neck and low hair line suggestive of the Klippel-Feil deformity. (Courtesy of the *American Journal of Roentgenology.*)

Gustafson, W. A., *et al:* 1940, *Arch. Neurol. &*
    *Psych., 44:*1184–1198.
Laube, P. J., *et al:* 1941, *Yale J. Biol. & Med.,*
    *13:*643–648.
Lichtenstein, B. W.: 1943, *Arch. Neurol. &*
    *Psych., 49:*881–894.
Ray, B. S.: 1942, *Ann. Surg., 116:*231–250.

Occipital Vertebra

Gladstone, J., *et al:* 1914, *J. Anat. & Physol., 49:*
    190.
Gladstone, R. J., *et al:* 1924, *J. Anat., 59:*195.
Hadley, L. A.: 1948, *Am. Jor. Roent., 59:*511–
    524.

Text

Potter, Edith L.: *Pathology of the Fetus and the
    New Born,* Year Book Publishers, Inc.,
    Chicago, 1952.

Klippel-Feil

Rechtman, A. M., *et al:* 1940, *Am. Jor. Roent.,
    43:*66–73.
Shore, M. J., *et al:* 1952, *Am. Jor. Roent., 68:*
    369–385.

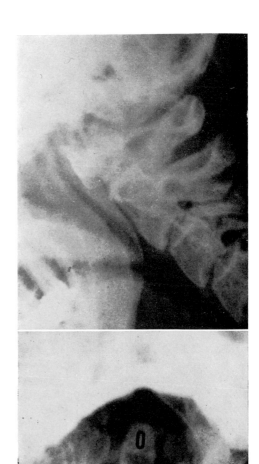

Fig. III:28. Female, age fifty-one. The atlas of this patient with atlanto-occipital non-segmentation remains in contact with the occiput upon anterior flexion. She has a bony mass encroaching upon the foramen magnum from the right side *(arrow)*. The odontoid (O) is actually in the midline although it appears to be displaced toward the right. In spite of this encroachment the patient presented no significant neurological symptoms. The foramen magnum was studied in eight patients showing characteristics of occipital vertebrae and/or atlanto-occipital fusion and of these, seven revealed some degree of foramen encroachment. In nearly all cases, there were present additional anomalies or stigmata of development. (Courtesy of the *American Journal of Roentgenology.*)

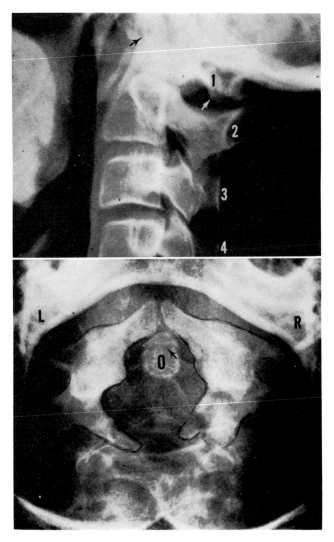

Fig. III:29. Male, thirty-two years of age with atlanto-occipital fusion. The lateral projection was made at the full limit of anterior flexion. The second, third and fourth spinous processes separate normally. There is little movement between C_1 and C_2 and the
atlas remains fixed to the occiput. In the vertex-submental projection below, one is able
to visualize non-union of the two sides of the atlas. A center of ossification in the anterior
arch probably did not appear. The radiograph, retouched laterally, shows the left side of
the neural arch somewhat more slender. The right side is shorter, thicker and encroaches
more upon the foramen magnum. In the lateral projection just below and behind the Fig-
ure:1, the right side of the atlas is seen to approach more closely the second neural arch
(*white arrow*). The odontoid (O) apparently articulates with a third condyle in front.
The fissure between these two structures is faintly seen (*black arrow*). (Courtesy of the
American Journal of Roentgenology.)

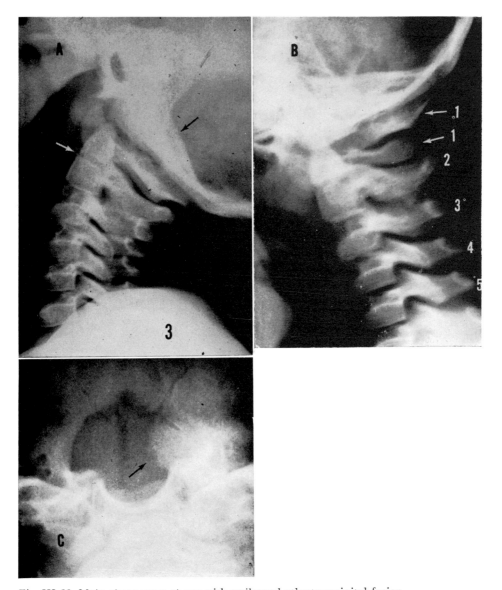

Fig. III:30. Male, three years of age with unilateral atlanto-occipital fusion.

A. Neck held in dorsal extension. The right and left sides of the first neural arch are in alignment. The black arrow indicates congenital basilar impression. The odontoid is still ununited with the centrum of the axis at this age (*white arrow*).

B. Neck in forward flexion. The lower cervical arches have become separated in the usual manner. The two sides of the atlas, however, are entirely separate. The right side only is fused to the occiput while the left side is free. In the forward flexion, therefore, the two sides of the arch no longer lie alongside of each other. The larger fused side is carried forward with the occiput while the free left side separates from that structure in the usual manner.

C. Foramen magnum. The arrow indicates a bony mass causing encroachment of the opening on the right side. This child had no symptoms at the time of examination.

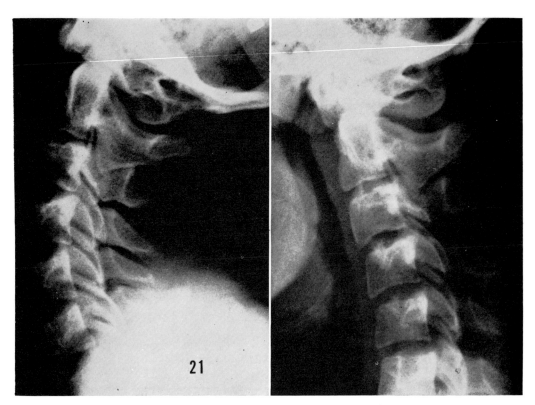

Fig. III:30 D Reexamination of this same patient at the age of twenty-one years was supplied by the courtesy of Doctor I. D. Harris, Wyandotte, Michigan. These flexion-extension studies show the one side of the atlas fused to the occiput with a foramen for the vertebral artery while the opposite unfused side separates as before upon anterior flexion. (Original studies courtesy of the *American Journal of Roentgenology.*)

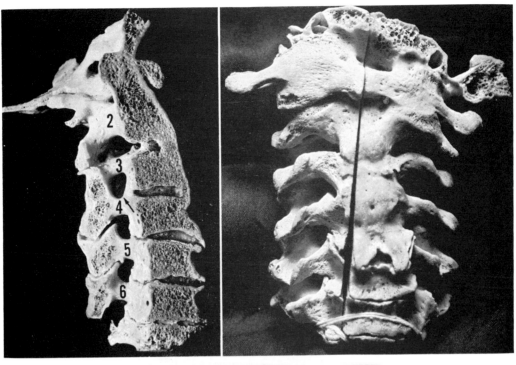

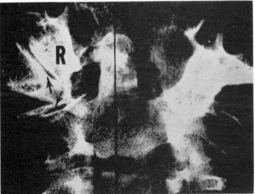

A

Fig. III:31. Anterior view and left side of a specimen showing congenital fusion between occiput and the first four cervical segments with acquired fusion between the sixth and seventh segments. As usual in congenital cases of this type there was some asymmetry, the right side of the atlas being higher than the left. Upon section one sees the fusion between the odontoid, skull base, first arch, the second and third discs anteriorly and their posterior articulations. The 3-4 foramen at the congenitally fused level is smooth and oval in shape (*arrow*). The foramina below this level, showing acquired fusion, are somewhat distorted in shape and the discs at levels of acquired fusion project beyond the anterior surfaces of the bodies. Upon the roentgenogram the outlines of joint surfaces are visualized even at levels where the joint margins are congenitally fused (*arrows*). Compare with Figures III:24 and III:27.

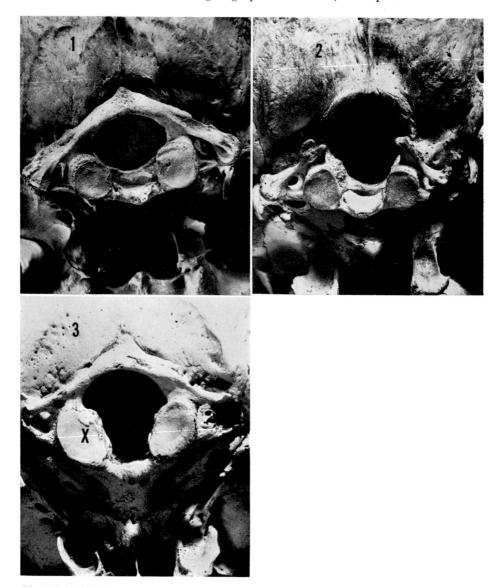

Fig. III:32. This is a group of cadaver skulls showing various examples of the atlas fused to the occiput. In each case the transverse processes were present, with foramina for the vertebral arteries. In number 3 the neural arch was fused to the occiput and the foramen magnum was distorted by the lateral masses.

Fig. III:33. Specimen showing fusion of the axis, atlas and occiput together with various other congenital anomalies.

A. Left anterior oblique view shows complete fusion of first cervical segment (1) to base of the skull, also congenital fusion of the fifth and sixth segments. Other discs show degenerative changes with thinning and spur formation of the disc margins.

B. Basilar view of the skull. The cervical spine has been removed below the second disc. Arrows indicate the point of congenital non-segmentation between the atlas and the occiput. The fusion between the lateral masses of the atlas and axis is clearly seen.

———————————→

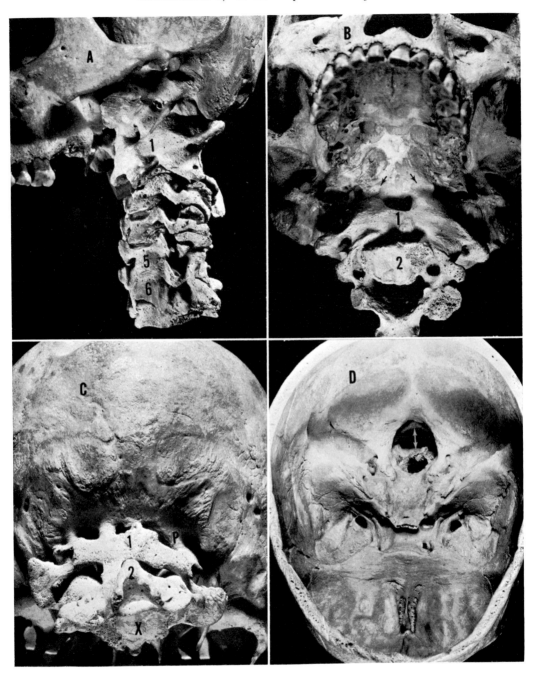

C. Posterior view with lower cervical segments detached at the second disc (X). Note the para-occipital processes (P) extending from the first arch to the skull base. Other areas of bony bridging developed within the ligamentous structures. Figures indicate the first and second neural arches.

D. Asymmetry of the cranial fossae. The right side is flatter and wider while the left side is more deep and narrow. The axis and the odontoid are seen encroaching upon the anterior half of the foramen magnum because of the forward displacement of the atlas and skull. The white arrows indicate the A. P. diameter of the narrowed passage remaining between the arch of the atlas in back and the odontoid in front.

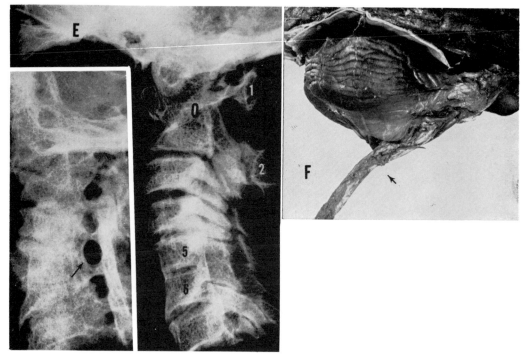

E. Lateral and oblique radiographs of this specimen. One may note the forward dis-location of the atlas, its neural arch being tipped upward and carried well in front of the second arch. The axis is distorted in shape with a short stubby odontoid (O). There is a congenital block vertebra comprising segments 5 and 6 with its concave anterior surface. The oblique view shows at this level the smooth oval foramen characteristic of congenital non-segmentation *(arrow),* with the distorted foramen of acquired fusion beneath it. Compare the anterior disc margins at levels of acquired and congenital fusion.

F. The hindbrain and cord from this specimen with flattening of the cord indicated by the arrow-head.

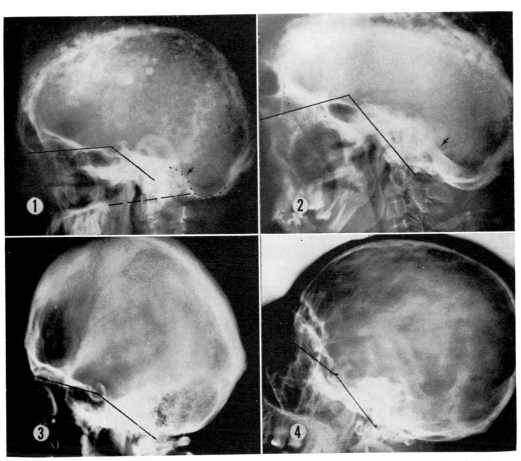

Fig. III:34. A group of patients contrasting basilar impression with platybasia. Number 1. Male, sixty-four years of age. Basilar impression (*dotted line*) secondary to Paget's disease (*arrow*). A normal basilar angle (root of nose, sella turcica, basion) of 140 degrees is shown by the solid line. Chamberlain's line is indicated by the dashes extending from the hard palate to the posterior margin of the foramen magnum. It will be seen that the odontoid and most of the atlas is above this line. The posterior arch of the atlas occupies a notch in the occiput just behind the foramen magnum. In the A.P. projection one was able to see the floor of the posterior fossa of the skull in its coronal plane with the central area elevated and with the funnel-shaped foramen magnum at its center. The cervical spine has become thrust upward into the skull. Number 2. Female, sixty-seven years of age. Advanced degree of skull flattening (tamoshanter skull) secondary to the softening of Paget's disease. There is basilar impression (*arrow*) but *a* subnormal basilar angle of only 110 degrees.

By contrast with the basilar impression of Numbers 1 and 2 the skulls of 3 and 4 are examples of true platybasia. The basilar angle is flattened to a value greater than 150 degrees. Number 3. A male of forty-nine years with turricephaly and a basilar angle of 158 degrees and Number 4 a male, fifty-two years of age showing true platybasia with increased Martin's basilar angle of 165 degrees. There is no basilar impression. In this patient with turricephaly the orbits are shallow with resultant exophthalmos and optic atrophy. The hands and feet showed both polydactylism and syndactylism.

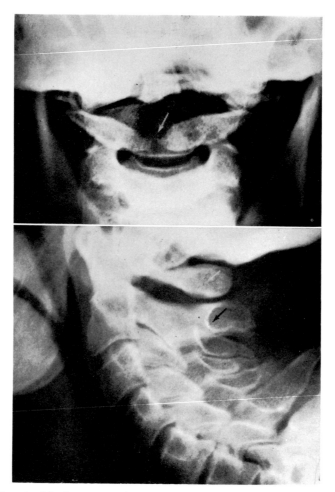

Fig. III:35. Female, fifty-four years of age. The PA view *(above)* shows the commonly observed non-closure of the first neural arch *(arrow)* which normally closes by the fourth year. This can also be easily recognized in the lateral projection. On the complete arch the cortex of the posterior wall of the spinal canal, here indicated below by a black arrow, normally appears as a white line. Note the absence of such a cortex in the lateral view of the first arch *(white arrow)*. The arches below C_1 have been retouched on this film. Observe the nesting of the neural arches in extreme lordotic position and the customary backward slipping of each vertebral body upon the one beneath it. This latter movement causes a normal physiological constriction of the intervertebral foramina and has a diagnostic value in the examination of a patient with possible cervical radiculitis. Compare with Figures III:13 and XIV:8.

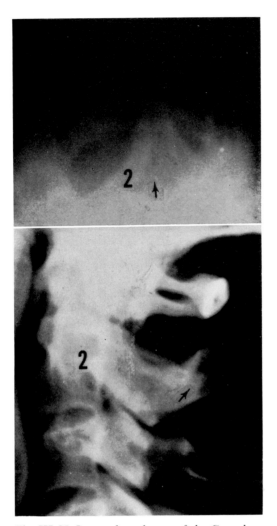

Fig. III:36. Incomplete closure of the C$_2$ arch as visualized through the foramen magnum (*black arrow*). On the lateral projection note the irregularity of the anterior cortex of the neural arch (*black arrow*).

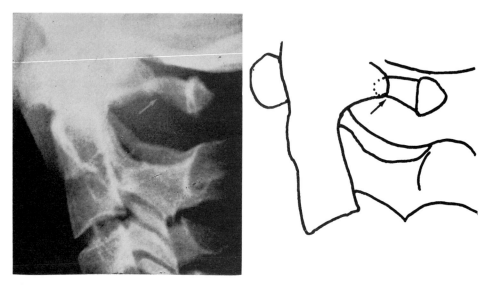

Fig. III:37. Female, thirty-one years of age. Deficiency in posterior arch of the atlas. On neither side is there bony continuity with the lateral masses. The arrow indicates the posterior portion of the arch which is completely detached from the anterior. There is some overlap just above the arrow as indicated by the tracing. This is a partial agenesis of the first cervical neural arch.

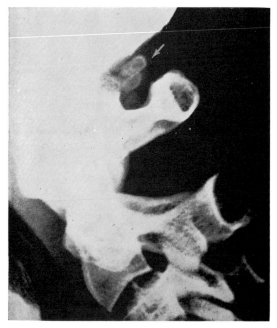

Fig. III:38. Female, twenty years of age. Ossicles each of the spinal canal, probably formed within the atlanto-occipital ligament (*arrow*). These ossicles are a common anomaly not to be confused with bony fragments following trauma.

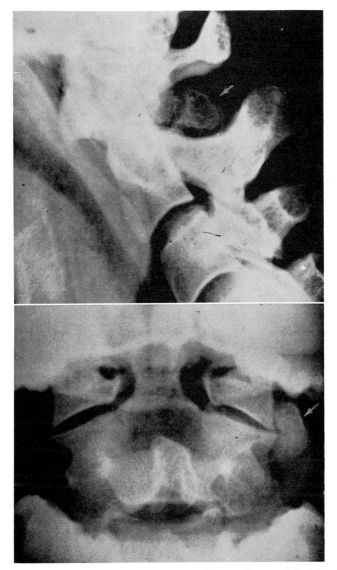

Fig. III:39. Female, forty-four years of age. Unusual anomalous ossicle lying between the first and second cervical arches on the side. This is closely applied to the atlanto-axial articulation. It projects somewhat into the spinal canal although not far enough to cause pressure upon the cord. The significance of these interesting congenital anomalies lies in the confusion which may arise following trauma and the medico-legal implications incidental thereto. There may be also the possibility of mistaking them as evidence of a neoplasm.

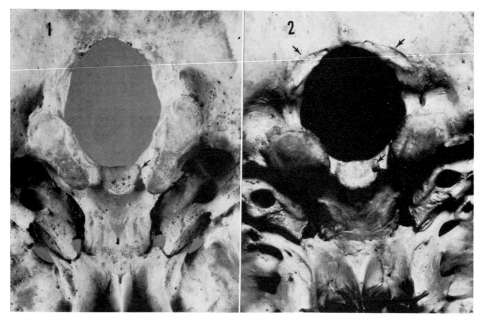

Fig. III:40. Specimens showing a third condyle for articulation with the odontoid appearing as a facet on the anterior margin of the foramen magnum between the anterior ends of the occipital condyles *(arrows)*. The presence of this anomaly indicates an encroachment upon the foramen magnum by the odontoid. In number two, rudiments of a neural arch *(arrows)* are said to represent "manifestations of an occipital vertebra."

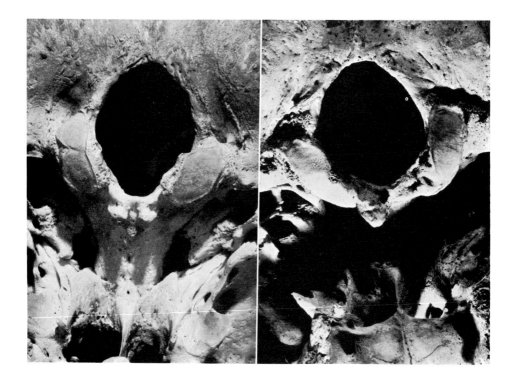

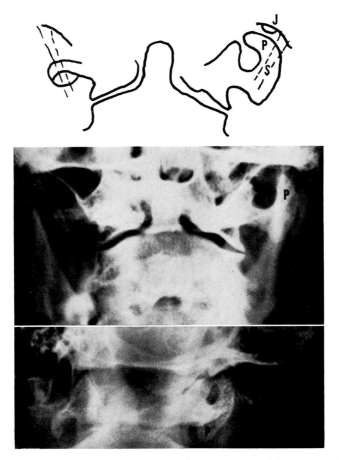

Fig. III:42. Male, fifty years of age. This patient has a paramastoid-process (P) on the left side originating on the transverse process of the atlas and passing upward to articulate with the jugular process (J) of the occipital bone on that side. The structure is also somewhat hook-shaped, thereby showing certain features of the ponticulis lateralis which arches over the foramen atantoidium through which passes the vertebral artery. On this roentgenogram the structure is crossed by the shadow of the styloid process (S) which lies anterior to it. The normal condition is present on the opposite side. The oblique projection at the bottom was retouched. See Figure IV:3C.

Fig. III:41. Basilar tubercles are said to represent a manifestation of occipital vertebra. There are various minor anomalies, ossicles, calcifications, etc. at this transitional area between the skull and cervical spine. Their importance lies in recognizing them as such, especially if the question of possible trauma arises.

Chapter IV

The Cervical Spine

T HE CERVICAL vertebrae are so formed as to allow the greatest possible degree of mobility. This is in contrast to the lumbar vertebral bodies which are designed to support the weight of the trunk and the upper limbs.

CERVICAL JOINTS

The posterior apophyseal articulations, with inclined coronal planes, permit flexion and extension upon a transverse axis as the articular surfaces glide upon each other (Figure IV:6). Some imbrication or telescoping of these surfaces also permits lateral flexion.

The biconvex occipital condyles situated upon elevations at the anterolateral margins of the foramen magnum are placed directly below the center of gravity of the skull (Figure IV:9).

Rarely there develops a mesially placed third condyle on the anterior margin of the foramen magnum for articulation with the tip of the odontoid (Figure III:40).

The concave upper articular surfaces of the atlas are usually bifid and are inclined with their mesial margins lower. However the inferior articular surfaces of this bone are somewhat higher mesially. As a result, the A. P. radiograph visualizes the lateral masses of the atlas as wedge shaped structures with the bases of the wedges directed laterally and the narrow edges toward the midline (Figure IV:1).

Maximum mobility plus stability and strength characterize the occipito-atlanto-axial articulations. Nodding and rotary movement occur at this level. These movements, together with a certain potential for lateral movement, qualify this as a universal joint. At the same time an adequate ligamentous strength maintains a firm attachment between the cervical spine and the skull.

Only nodding movement occurs between the atlas and the occiput. This together with the same nodding motion between atlas and axis totals twenty-five degrees or more of anterior-posterior movement at the upper cervical region. The atlas, carrying the skull, rotates to the right and left about the odontoid a total of approximately eighty degrees. The axis of this pivot lies between the condyles of the occiput. Since the lateral play between the atlas and the odontoid is about one-fifth the diameter of the latter, a certain degree of lateral movement is also possible between atlas and axis (Figure IV:3).

The amplitude of the rotary movement necessitates a relatively loose articular capsule between the atlas and axis. Posteriorly, the ligamentous attachment between spine and skull is much weaker than it is in front. However, from the sides of the odontoid the strong alar or check ligaments pass upward and laterally to the medial sides of the occipital condyles. These, the strongest of the attachment ligaments, are supplemented by the cruciate ligament, the weak apical ligament between dens and occiput, and the tectorial membrane. The latter is a continuation of the posterior longitudinal ligament upward separating the odontoid from the spinal canal and finally fusing with the dura and the periostium within the skull. The anterior longitudinal ligament of the spine is also prolonged upward past the anterior arch of the atlas to fuse with the periostium at the base of the skull externally (Figures IV:1, IV:2, IV:3 and IV:4).

The atlanto-axial articulation is a structure of considerable interest and importance both in traumatic and other conditions of the cervical spine. The very strong transverse ligament of the atlas crossing from one side of this bony ring to the other divides it into a smaller cylindrical socket in front for the odon-

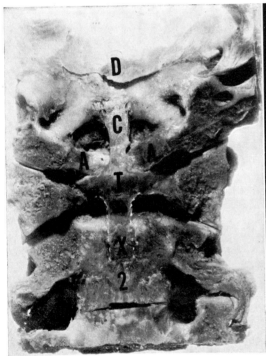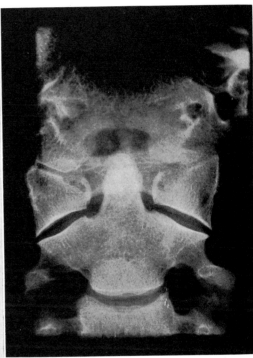

Fig. IV:1. Dissection and radiograph in the coronal plane depicting the cranio-cervical junction viewed from behind (partially diagramatic). The important transverse ligament (T) is seen bulging backward around the odontoid to be attached to the lateral masses of the axis. The superior (C) and inferior bands of the cruciate ligament, continuous with the transverse, connect the axis with the base of the skull. In this dissection the inferior crucial ligament had been detached at X. Its position is shown diagramatically between the dotted lines. The strongest attachments between the cranium and the cervical structures are the sturdy alar or check ligaments (A). These extend from the end of the odontoid laterally to become attached to the medial sides of the occipital condyles. They allow a rotary movement of about 40 degrees in each direction and prevent detachment of the skull from the cervical spine. Other lesser accessory ligaments (*not shown*) extend from the axis to the occiput. At D is seen the dural margin elevated from the base of the skull. The tectorial membrane has been removed. It is continuous below with the posterior longitudinal ligament and above with the dura. This structure serves to isolate the spinal canal at the cervico-occipital region from the articular compartment in front. Note the inclined planes of the occipito-atlanto-axial articulations.

toid and the much larger passage for the spinal cord posteriorly. For its size the transverse ligament is said to be one of the strongest in the body (Figure IV:3). As it bulges backward around the dens it is joined above and below in the midline by longitudinal bands. These structures together form the so-called cruciate ligament as seen in Figure IV:1. On the anterior surface of the transverse ligament there is a cartilaginous or bony facet for articulation with the odontoid. The surface of the odontoid normally exhibits a certain degree of irregularity for attachment of the alar ligaments. There is a notch posteriorly at the base for articulation with the transverse ligament (Figure IV:5). This must not be mistaken for a pathological erosion although erosions of the odontoid do occur in spondylitis deformans and Paget's disease (Figure IX:13).

The nuchal ligament, continuous with the interspinous and supraspinous ligaments, extends from the seventh spinous process to the external occipital protuberance. It serves as a check and gives origin to some of the muscles at the back of the neck. The ossifications which frequently form within its substance have no clinical significance.

MUSCLES

A high degree of coordinated muscle balance is necessary to support and move the head and neck. This is effected by the paired lateral groups of muscles

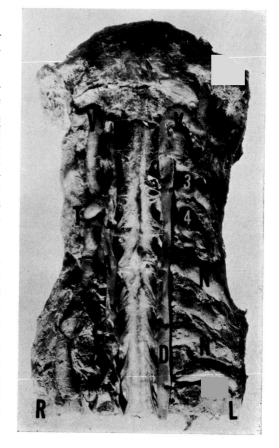

Fig. IV:2. Dissection showing the anterior surface of the spinal cord in the cervical region. The vertebral bodies up to and including a part of C_2 have been removed. Also the anterior portions of the lateral masses of the axis have been sacrificed to reveal the normal curvature of the vertebral arteries (V) as they loop through those structures. The dura (D) has been reflected to the left side while the more delicate arachnoid (A) has been displaced to the right. From the upper cervical cord the motor roots pass outward perpendicular to that structure while below they are directed obliquely and downwards. The lower cervical nerves (N) are much longer than those above. It was found, in turn, that the thoracic nerves were very much smaller than those supplying the extremities. This has a bearing on the question of foramen encroachment in the thoracic region. Tortuosities of the vertebral arteries were present in this specimen. The two cavities (3 and 4) on the left side were erosions of those pedicles by such tortuosities of the left vertebral artery. On the right side a complete 360 degree loop of the artery is shown at T.

which are attached to the spinous and transverse processes. Converging deep cervical muscles ascend in front of the spine to be attached in the midline to the vertebral bodies and the anterior spinous process of the atlas. These muscles, together with the sternomastoids and the anterior neck muscles help to resist any accidental sudden backward movement of the skull.

In the lateral radiograph one notes that the spinous process of the second

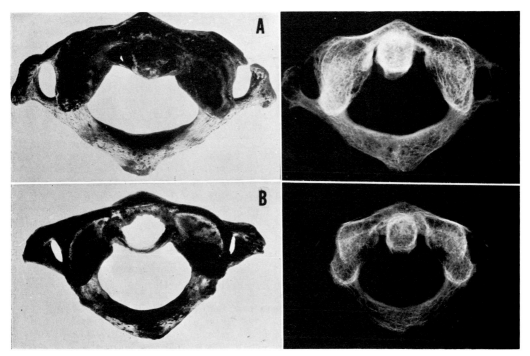

Fig. IV:3. Photo and radiograph (*reversed*) of the atlas seen from the axial direction (A). The odontoid was detached from C_2 and remans in situ. This cylindrical structure is seen articulating directly with the anterior arch of C_1. Since the odontoid forms the pivot of rotation directly above the spinal column it will be seen that the remainder of the atlas swings in an arc posterior to this point. In this manner one of its inferior articulations moves forward upon the axis below while the other rotates backward.

B is a second specimen in which the odontoid was removed after making the radiograph, leaving the strong curved transverse ligament in its normal position attached to the lateral mass on each side. This shows the relative portions of the bony ring of the atlas occupied by the odontoid and by the spinal canal. Note that the facets for articulations with the occipital condyles lie at each side of the odontoid and in line with the spinal column below. These structures are directly beneath the center of gravity of the skull. There is a space each side of the odontoid between it and the lateral masses of the atlas. The dotted lines on diagram C indicate that the lateral masses of the atlas are roughly oval in shape. They are situated anteriorly with their long axes oblique to the sagittal plane of the vertebra. In a direct AP roentgenogram their images are equal in width. On a projection with the vertebra rotated about the odontoid (O) as a center the image of the mass will be narrower on the side toward which the rotation occurs. The lines on C indicate the projection when the vertebra is rotated toward the left. This is clarified by turning the illustration forty-five degrees in a counter-clock wise direction (See Figures III:11, III:23, III:24, III:42 and IV:31.)

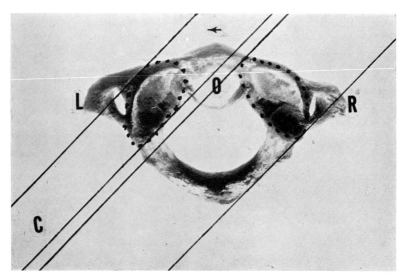

Fig. IV:3 C

cervical vertebra is much larger than those immediately beneath it. From this spinous process and its neural arch the various deep suboccipital muscles fan outward beneath the skull to be attached to the occiput. These serve to balance the skull on the upper end of the spine. More superficially, the semi-spinalis group, arising from the spine and attaching to the occiput constitutes the thick mass of muscle tissue at the back of the neck.

Fig. IV:4. This is a dissection in the sagittal plane of the cranio-cervical junction, a region characterized by a high degree of mobility adjacent to important structures and at the same time presenting strong ligamentous connections. The spinal cord was severed at the level of the foramen magnum (*arrow*) and the dura (D) was detached from the walls of the spinal canal both anteriorly and posteriorly to the cord. Above, it fuses with the periosteum of the skull. The odontoid (O) is held snugly in its rotation socket behind the anterior arch of the atlas (A). Note the dense bony articular facets between these structures. The strong transverse ligament (T) occupies its notch in the posterior surface of the odontoid. At times there is a bony articular plaque within this ligament at the point of contact. From the transverse ligament the superior and inferior elements of the cruciate ligament constitute a continuous union between C_2 and the base of the skull. The articular structures in front are separated from the spinal canal posteriorly by the tectorial membrane (M) a continuation of the posterior longitudinal ligament of the spine. This structure passes upward separated from the transverse ligament by a bursa. The tectorial membrane joins the superior band of the cruciate ligament and continues upward to blend with the dura and finally become continuous with the periostium lining the skull. There is a bursa (X) between these structures and the tip of the odontoid. Other structures visualized in this area are: S, the sphenoid sinus B, base of the skull; L, the apical ligament; and V, the left vertebral artery before joining its fellow to form the basilar artery. Below is seen the detached posterior wall of the pharynx (P). Above on the opposite side, at F is the posterior fossa of the skull. The numbers 1 to 4 indicate the spinous processes of the corresponding cervical vertebrae and posterior to these structures is the nuchal ligament (N).

———————————→

"WHIPLASH" TRAUMA

When not actually producing movement of the neck the tone of these various paired muscle groups, acting in balance somewhat like guy wires, tend to maintain a fixed position of the head and neck. However this becomes overbalanced by the sudden unguarded force of inertia in case of so-called "whiplash" accident. The term "whiplash" should preferably be applied to the type of accident rather than to the type of structural injury. The possible injuries include: muscle strain, ligamentous sprain, fracture, dislocation, vertebral body compression, and even brain concussion.

The skull, averaging about seven pounds in weight, is balanced on a slender, flexible column, the cervical vertebrae, which measure less than one inch in diameter. Structural damage may result either from sudden deceleration of momentum to the body in motion or from sudden acceleration applied to the body at rest. The inertia of this weight, balanced on so slender a support by muscle tone, offers a delayed response to the new force when it is suddenly applied. As a result, the head and neck flexes toward the force. A secondary reflex contraction of the overstretched

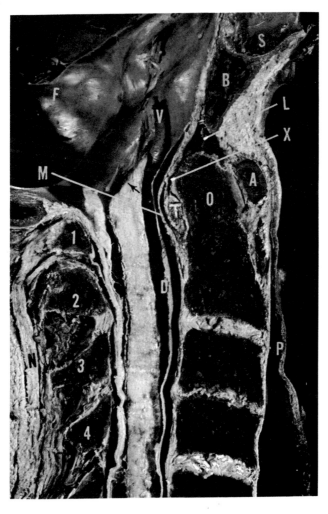

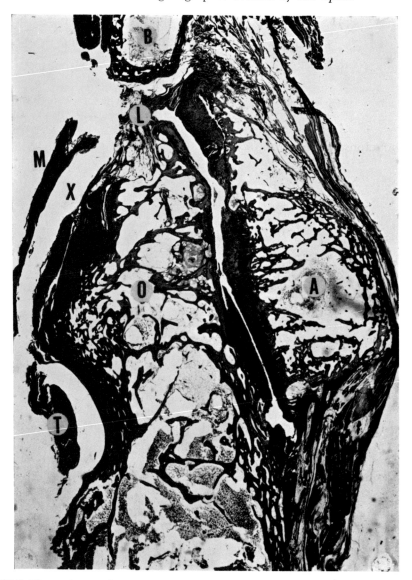

Fig. IV:5. Photomicrograph X5 of an atlanto-odontoid articulation showing the increased bony density at points of stress. The apical ligament (L) unites the tip of the odontoid with the skull base (B). There is a notch posteriorly for the transverse ligament (T) and the tectorial ligament (M) is separated from the tip of the odontoid by a bursa (X). The letter A designates the anterior arch of the atlas and O is the odontoid. This is not the same specimen as seen in Figure IV:4.

muscles produces a reverse movement, thus completing the whiplash cycle (Figures IV:9 and IV:10).

Almost invariably this results in a strain of neck muscles. This strain may be greater on one side if the head was turned sidewise at the time of the accident. Practically all patients complain of pain and soreness of the neck muscles at least by the day following the accident. This is usually a transient condition and subsides completely in two to four weeks.

Recovery is not so prompt if bony or ligamentous injury has occurred. Such injury may take the form of a forward angulation, dislocation or fracture.

RADIOGRAPHIC TECHNIQUE FOR EXAMINATION OF THE CERVICAL SPINE

All standard positions are utilized. Stereoscopic films are desirable and body section radiographs are helpful in certain cases.

The anterior-posterior projection of the atlanto-axial and atlanto-occipital joints can usually be obtained through the maxillary sinuses by aligning the tip of the mastoid and the zygoma with the central ray. The odontoid may be seen by superimposing it upon the foramen magnum and beneath the mandible or through the open mouth with the neck in an exaggerated backward extension. The oblique Kasabach method serves well to visualize the odontoid and the atlas. For this position the patient lies supine, with the saggital plane of the

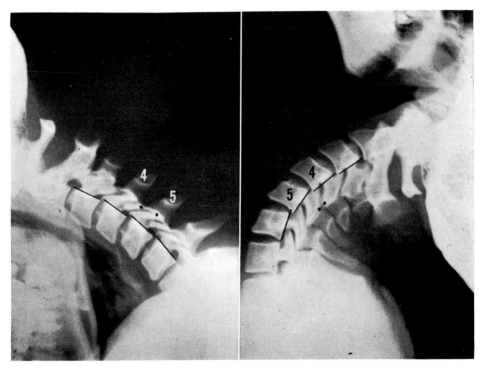

Fig. IV:6. Female, twenty-three years of age. Flexion-extension studies to show the normal forward-backward gliding movement of the mid-cervical vertebrae. For guidance, lines have been placed along the posterior surfaces of the vertebral bodies. One may note particularly that the greatest amplitude of movement in the adult occurs at the fourth and fifth discs. This mid-cervical region is the level where disc degeneration usually first appears and subsequently reaches its more advanced stage. Also note that all of the spinous processes separate widely upon anterior flexion while backward extension of the spine causes them to be closely approximated. There is also a gliding of the posterior articular surfaces upon each other. The dots indicate corresponding points upon the articular surfaces of the C_{4-5} articulation. The total angular movement of 86° between the plane of the skull and the axis of C_6 in this cervical spine is unusally high for an adult. See Figure IV:8.

skull turned forty-five degrees to the horizontal, the central ray is directed ten or fifteen degrees toward the feet and centered in the middle of the uppermost zygomatic arch. Stereoscopic films, preferably with a transverse shift, are especially valuable. The lateral mass of C₂ will appear narrower on the side toward which the head is turned, see Figure IV:3C.

An accurately positioned body section may be useful in visualizing the upper cervical region. Transverse movement of the tube and film will show best the outline of the odontoid. Tube-film movement in a cephalocaudad direction best visualizes the atlanto-occipital and the atlanto-axial joints. Without a thorough survey at different levels a detached, displaced odontoid may be reported as entirely absent.

Either the prone P. A. position centering from occiput to the tip of the mandible, or the supine A. P. chewing technique may be used to visualize the cervical spine below C₂.

The A. P. or P. A. roentgenogram will show the alignment of the spinous

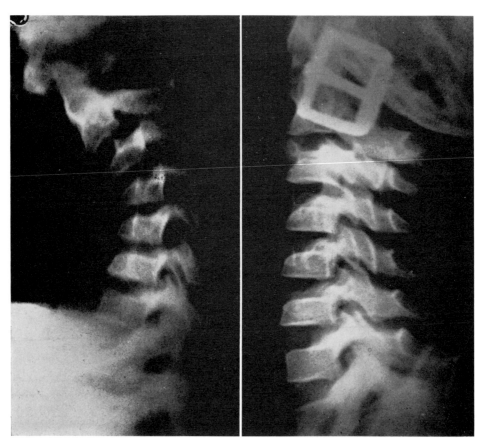

Fig. IV:7. In a young child the maximum amplitude of movement occurs in the upper cervical region. This five-year-old boy developed pain and stiffness of the neck while at play. There was no known trauma. The neck muscles were spastic and tender. After two weeks of support the alignment of the cervical spine was found to be normal. These studies, made on the same day, reveal a total of 86° of the angular movement measured by the method shown in Figure IV:8. (Courtesy of The Syracuse Memorial Hospital.)

processes, the thickness of the disc spaces, the covertebral joints, and finally the pedicles with the longitudinal interpedicular distance representing the size of the foramina. In some cases these foramina are constricted and the pedicles are closer together. The posterior articulations are seen laterally on each side. They sometimes show arthrotic changes or hyperplastic spur formations laterally. There may be an asymmetry in the direction of their planes. Normally the plane of the posterior articulation is transverse and slanting with its uppermost edge anterior and its lower edge posterior. However, it is not unusual for the articular plane on one side to be more horizontal or more vertical than its fellow. This condition necessarily results in some asymmetry of function. By contrast, the planes of the intervertebral discs are lower in front than they are posteriorly.

LATERAL STUDIES

A stereoscopic pair of lateral roentgenograms is made with the head in dorsal extension. A lead marker is attached on the cheek nearest the film for orientation. A single lateral is also made at the full limit of forward flexion. By rotating the head slightly toward or away from the tube, excellent stereo-

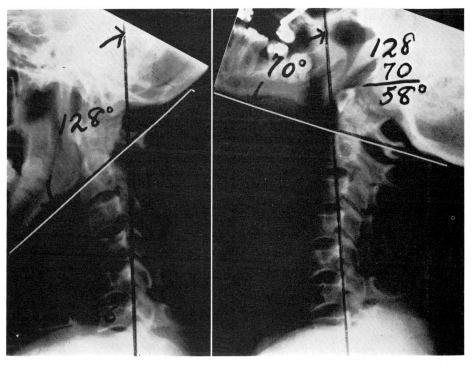

Fig. IV:8. Method used for recording the anterior-posterior movement of the cervical spine. This woman was forty-nine years old and showed an angular movement of fifty-eight degrees between the occiput and the axis of the sixth cervical vertebra. Measured in the same manner, she was found to have twenty-seven degrees of movement between the axis and the occiput, twelve degrees between axis and atlas and fifteen degrees between occiput and atlas. These values are about normal.

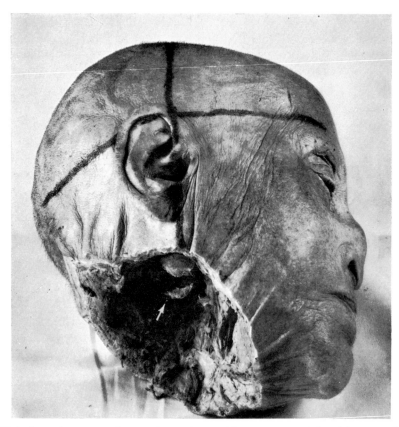

Fig. IV:9. One of a group of ten cadaver skulls with a average weight of 7.1 pounds. With the head in the upright position the center of gravity appeared to lie approximately above the occipital condyles (*white arrow*). The cross lines passing through the center of gravity were applied by a plumb line with the specimen resting upon a freely swinging platform suspended from above.

scopic studies are obtained of the posterior articulations upon that side toward which the rotation occurs. In cases of torticollis care must be used in centering the ray exactly perpendicular to that part of the structure to be studied.

A lateral roentgenogram of the normal cervical spine at rest reveals the bodies arranged in a symmetrical anterior curve. Their posterior surfaces form the anterior wall of the spinal canal while the posterior canal wall is marked by the profiles of the arches at their midpoints. These likewise are arranged in a symmetrical anterior curve. The diameter of the cervical canal increases from below upward toward the base of the skull to accommodate the medulla. In the absence of trauma the cervical spine maintains its anterior curve even in the presence of advanced disc degeneration. That is, as aging with disc thinning occurs, the vertebral bodies approach each other more closely and the posterior joints imbricate but the normal original anterior curve is still preserved. Upon anterior flexion of the normal neck, the curve is at first straightened and then reversed but it always remains symmetrical at all points.

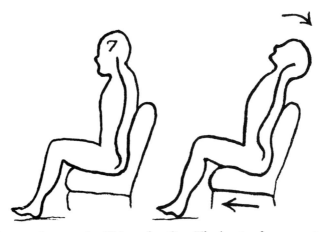

Fig. IV:10. Diagram of rear end collision, after Gay. The inerta of a compact skull weighing approximately seven pounds and supported upon a slender movable cervical column less than an inch in diameter is responsible for many injuries following so-called whiplash accidents. These may result from sudden unguarded deceleration of the moving body. Also, as shown in this diagram, they may occur by sudden acceleration of the patient's body when his car, not in motion, is unexpectedly struck from behind by another vehicle. They vary from minor strain of the neck muscles to severe injury of the skeletal structures. Also the possibility of brain injury, due to the impact of that organ against the unyielding inner table of the cranial bones must not be overlooked.

FLEXION-EXTENSION STUDIES

Lateral roentgenograms of the normal cervical spine made at extreme forward flexion will show the dorsal spinous processes widely separated. There is also a loss or a reversal of the normal anterior curve so that it becomes straightened or even convex backward. Upon dorsal extension the spinous processes become closely approximated and the curve is convex in front. This comparative examination reveals the normal movement between the various cervical segments (Figure IV:6). Arthritis or trauma may cause muscle spasm or fixation so that the flexion-extension studies will reveal a lack of movement between all the various segments. If the injury or pathology is local, two or three of the spinous processes will fail to separate upon anterior flexion. If the muscle spasm is general these dynamic studies will show fixation of movement between

all the various cervical segments. Upon subsequent examination it will be found in some cases that complete recovery of normal movement has taken place while in others the fixation seems to be permanent. By this method it is possible to record quantitative roentgen evidence of local or general ligamentous or soft tissue injury when the roentgenogram does not show other signs of bone or joint injury. By the same method any demonstrable recovery is evaluated.

The reference planes for measurement of this angular movement may be determined by: first, drawing a line tangential to the occiput and the tip of the mandible, and a second line, intersecting this, drawn tangential to the anterior or posterior surface of the 6th cervical vertebra. If the tip of the mandible is not visualized a point midway between the shadows of the lower margins of that structure will suffice. These two intersecting lines are drawn both upon the forward flexion and the backward extension roentgenograms made with the mouth closed each time. The same relative angles are measured upon the two films and represent the number of degrees of angular movement that occurs between the plane of the skull and the axis of the 6th cervical vertebra. Any other fixed reference points may be used. The 6th cervical vertebra is selected because that is the lowermost body that can usually be easily visualized (Figure IV:8).

An error of a few degrees in drafting may conceivably occur. However the method furnishes not only relatively accurate quantitative radiographic evidence of injury but upon later reexami-

nation produces a visual record of improvement or absence of recovery.

The normal range of movement varies with age and type of body structure. For the reference planes above described, between skull and 6th cervical vertebra, the angular movement between extremes of flexion and extension for a very young person may reach as much as ninety degrees. The usual figure for an adult of middle age however is in the neighborhood of about 55 to 60 degrees. The change, if any, upon later comparable reexamination is important. Care must be taken to insure that the full limit of both flexion and extension is recorded in each instance.

Other radiographic methods of recording such movement have been devised but this one has proven to be the most useful in the hands of this author.

GLIDING MOVEMENT

The flexion-extension studies reveal not only a forward bending of the cervical spine with separation of the spinous processes but also a gliding of each vertebral body backward and forward upon the disc cushion beneath it. The amplitude of this movement is, of course, much greater in early life. Such gliding movement of the weight-bearing disc in the lumbar region is taken to indicate instability of the disc. In the cervical region, however, with its greater mobility, this is a normal condition. Measure-

ments show that the point of greatest amplitude of this gliding in adults is about the mid-cervical area. In children it is somewhat higher. This is the level at which the earliest disc degeneration change appears. Also at this level the most advanced stages of disc aging are seen in later life. These observations would seem to indicate that the repeated wear and stress of this gliding movement is probably a factor in producing such degenerative changes with the resultant thinning and spur formation of the adjacent margins of the vertebral bodies.

———————————————————→

Fig. IV:11. General restriction of cervical spine movement in a woman of forty years. Radiograph A, made in attempted backward extension, shows the structure held straight and in the position of forward flexion. Film B, made approximately one year later, now reveals a normal backward curve of the cervical spine upon dorsal extension. This patient had completely recovered from spasm of the neck muscles during that interval.

SPRAINS

The apophyseal articulations of the neck, like the diarthrodial joints elsewhere, may sustain various degrees of sprain. As noted above the fixation of movement incidental to the resultant muscle spasm is clearly visualized upon the comparative flexion-extension studies (Figures IV:11, IV:12, IV:13 and IV:14).

ANGULATION

Forward angulation of the spine at one point occurs following injury to the stabilizing structures at a single level. It is extremely difficult to angulate the intact cadaver spine even by counter pressure at one point. It can be straightened or the curve reversed but angulation does not occur unless the specimen is damaged. This angulation can be accomplished, however, by incising the posterior interspinous ligament or by removing the anterior portion of an intervertebral disc (Figure IV:15).

Bilateral forward subluxation (incomplete dislocation) of the posterior joints in the mid-cervical region occurs at the point of angulation. It is usually possible to identify the upper articular surface of the joint where it has become displaced forward and upward upon the articular surface below. Also, the joint space is usually wider in back and narrower in front from the forward tipping of the uppermost vertebral body. The spinous processes are separated at the level of the forward angulation with increased distance between these structures (Figures IV:16 and IV:17). The

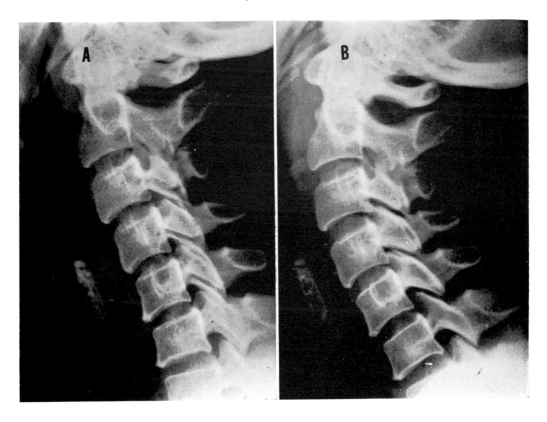

normal symmetrical curve of the neural arches as seen upon the lateral and oblique projections is distorted at the level of the angulation. If the subluxation is recent no bony bridging between vertebral bodies will have taken place. After about two months, calcification may be noted in the anterior longitudinal ligament if that structure has been avulsed. This bridge across the intervertebral space is an attempt to stabilize this weakened level of the spine (Figures IV:18, IV:19, IV:20 and IV:21).

In the mobile neck region adequate stabilization may result in a complete ankylosis of adjacent vertebral bodies. Angulation may result not only from subluxation but also from dislocation,

fracture and destructive disc or bone disease (Figures IV:22 and IV:23).

By balancing a group of cadaver skulls individually upon a swinging platform the center of gravity was found to lie on a line connecting the upper anterior-most attachments of the auricular appendages. With the skull in the upright position a vertical line from the center of gravity was found to pass through or closely adjacent to the occipital condyles. With forward angulation of the cervical spine from any cause, additional stresses are placed upon the supporting structure and its musculature in proportion to the displacement of the center of gravity from the normal weight-bearing axis (Figure IV:9).

SUBLUXATION (PARTIAL DISPLACEMENT) OF THE VERTEBRAL BODIES

Anterior or forward subluxation is the most frequent type of vertebral body displacement to be encountered in the cervical region (Figures IV:24, IV:25, and IV:26).

When backward subluxation of a vertebral body occurs the posterior margin of the upper vertebral body is seen behind the plane of the underlying vertebra. In this position the superior articular processes from the vertebra below thrust forward encroaching upon the intervertebral foramina. The anterior pos-

terior diameter of the spinal canal is decreased (Figure XIV:12).

A unilateral subluxation may result if the patient's head is turned in an unguarded moment at the time of a collision. Unilateral forward, rotary, subluxation may present radiographically one or more of the following features: (1) shift of the corresponding spinous process toward the side of the subluxation with the patient and film exactly centered; (2) slight increase in the size of the corresponding intervertebral fora-

---

Fig. IV:12. Lower cervical spine held in anterior flexion after trauma. This thirty-five-year-old woman was involved in an automobile accident causing ligamentous injury to the lower cervical region. The film made in flexion (F) shows the customary forward curve and separation of the spinous processes. However, in the attempted backward extension film (E), the lower cervical region, especially the fifth and sixth interspace levels, is still held angulated forward with the fifth and sixth, and seventh spinous processes widely separated. Only the upper cervical segments are able to flex backward in the normal manner. A reexamination film of this patient in attempted backward extension was made four years later (E4). This shows the lower cervical spine still held at the forward angulation position while the upper cervical area flexes backward normally. This patient is obviously the victim of permanent ligamentous injury to the lower cervical region.

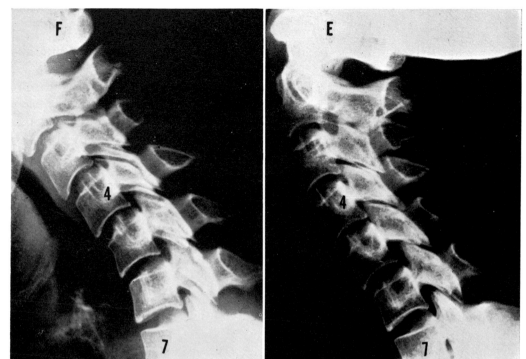
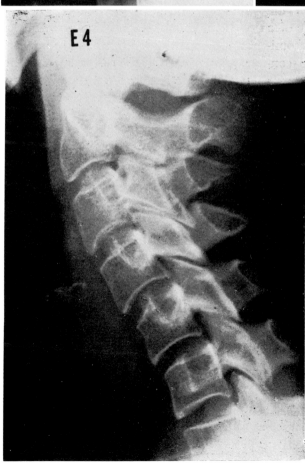

men; (3) encroachment of the opposite foramen; (4) displacement of the articular surfaces upon each other (5) because of the inclined plane of the posterior articulation, the side of the vertebra is elevated as it is carried forward. For that reason the disc appears thicker on the side of the unilateral forward subluxation (Figure IV:27).

With the uncommon unilateral subluxation posteriorly, the spinous process of the rotated vertebra shifts away from the side of the subluxation, the foramen is constricted and the disc does not become wedgeshaped.

DISPLACEMENT AT THE C$_1$-C$_2$ LEVELS

The capsules of the lateral joints between the atlas and axis are unusually lax to permit the rotary movement between these two structures. There is freedom for lateral movement of the odontoid in its pocket between the transverse ligament and the bony structure of the atlas (Figure IV:3). And lastly the two superior articular surfaces of the axis together constitute a segment of a sphere. Because of these three anatomical conditions there is normally a considerable amplitude of lateral movement at the atlanto-axial joint, especially in younger individuals. It is not unusual to visualize some asymmetry at this level in the absence of trauma. The lateral mass of the atlas may be nearer to the odontoid on one side than the other without any clinical significance whatsoever. By passive manipulation it is normally possible to slightly displace the atlas on the axis in a lateral direction. For a diagnosis of true lateral subluxation the radiographic findings must be supplemented by a history of injury, pain, and/or muscle spasm and the lateral displacement must remain fixed (Figures IV:28, IV:29 and IV:30, also XIV:-12 and V:8).

If unilateral dislocation occurs at the atlanto-axial joint the structure appears asymmetrical. On the dislocated side the lateral mass and the transverse process of the atlas are carried forward. The common articular surfaces of the altas and axis are convex and the joint capsule is loose. The head is carried with the chin rotated away from the subluxated joint and the patient has torticallis (Figure IV:31). The head cannot be easily rotated back toward the dislocated side

---

                                                                        ⟶

Fig. IV:13. Cervical spine of a fifty-five year old woman held in fixed dorsal extension eleven months after injury. A is the lateral projection during backward extension. However during attempted forward bending (B) the upper cervical arches separated in the normal manner but the lower cervical region remained flexed backward, apparently the result of injury to the lower cervical region. The relative positions of the occiput, atlas and axis indicate whether a certain examination is made in the backward extension or the forward bending position. At a previous examination (C) made eight years before, this patient had been able to bend the neck forward in a normal manner. (Compare the distances between the second and the sixth spinous processes of B and C.) Through the courtesy of Dr. F. J. O'Neill, Central Islip, N. Y. a reexamination (D) made eight years after A & B showed a recovery of the forward bending power. At the final examination the patient was again able to separate the spinous processes upon attempted anterior flexion. Compare the change in the texture of the bones (C at 47 years) and (D at 63 years of age).

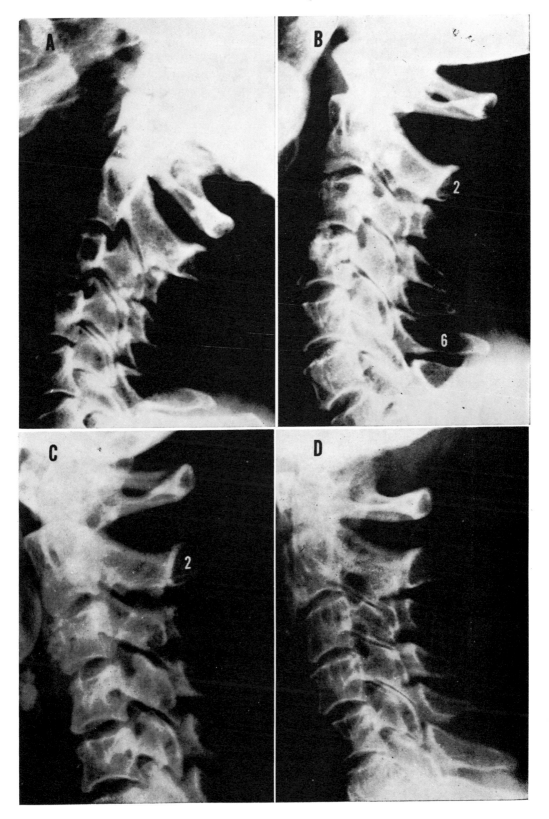

although anterior-posterior flexion between occiput and axis is possible. Meticulous care must be used in positioning the patient for this examination. Unilateral dislocation at the atlanto-axial articulation will show, in the A. P. view, the joint space more clearly on one side than the other with an asymmetry in the general appearance of the articular surfaces between atlas and axis. The forwardly displaced transverse process of the atlas may be palpable on the posterior pharyngeal wall if the patient is able to open the mouth.

Spontaneous subluxation at the C_1-C_2 level either unilateral or bilateral, is usually a sequel to an inflammatory process of the throat. It is more common in children, but may occur in adults and patients with spondylitis deformans or Paget's disease. There is a decalcification or erosion of the odontoid. Weakening of the ligaments and distension of the joint between the odontoid and the anterior arch may be additional features. The child may complain of painful torticollis, supporting his head with the hands. He should be carefully handled during the roentgenographic examination since death has resulted from careless movement of the head, causing pressure upon the medulla (Figures IV:32 and IV:33).

An increased amplitude of anterior-posterior movement between the upper cervical segments is normal in young children. It is painless and has no clinical significance. However it must not be mistaken for subluxation (Figure IV:7).

The subluxated atlas as well as a fractured odontoid process or the os odontoideum may be present with forward displacement of the atlas. When the atlas and the skull are carried forward the posterior arch of the atlas lies well anterior to the normal curved alignment of the arches below it. The distance between the ascending ramus of the jaw and the anterior surface of the spine is also greater than normal. In the case of subluxation there is a widened space between the anterior C_1 arch and the odontoid. Also the latter process preserves its normal alignment with the anterior surface of the centrum of the axis. The fractured odontoid and the os odontoidium, on the other hand, remain in contact with the anterior arch and assume a position in front of the anterior surface of the axis (Figures IV:35, IV:36, III:7, III:9, III:33, IX:7 and IX:13).

Fig. IV:14. A thirty-eight-year-old male was thrown from a motorcycle. Flexion extension studies showed no movement between C_2 and C_3 although posterior joint structures were present. A reexamination 23 years later (B) showed the fixation between C_2 and C_3 still present. The amplitude of A.P. movement measured between the occiput and C_5 decreased eleven degrees in twenty-three years. During this interval the patient had developed a large intercalary bone between C_5 and C_6. Despite this attempt at bony bridging the patient had retained some movement at this level. Compare the flexion-extension studies (B and C) at the white arrow. Some demineralization of the first neural arch occurred during this period (*black arrows in A and B*).

$\longrightarrow$

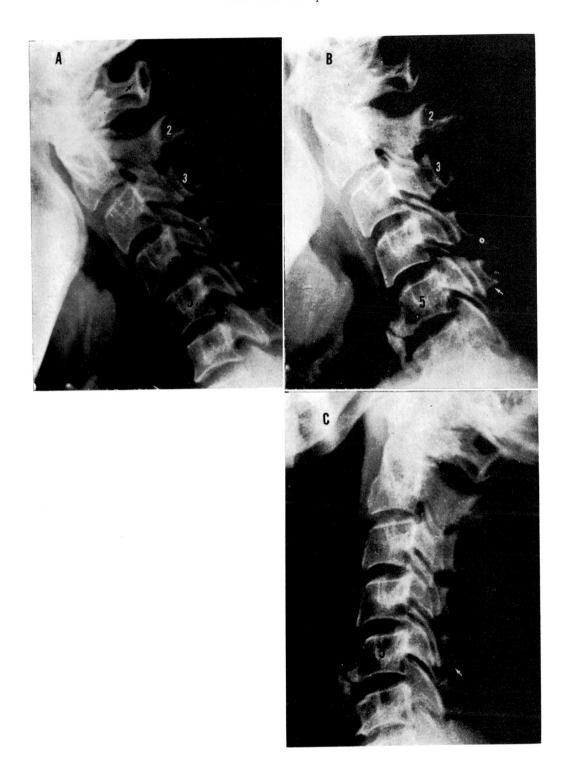

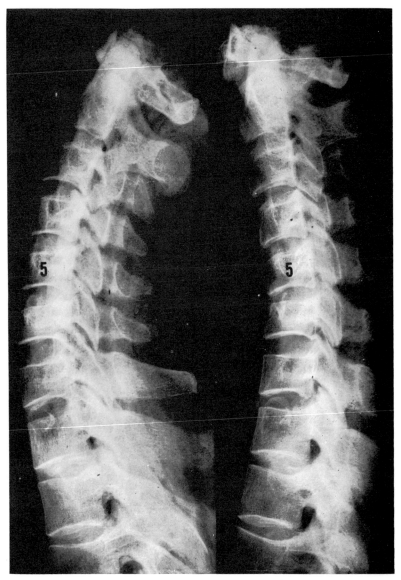

Fig. IV:15. A group of cadaver spines were studied by attaching a fifty-pound lead weight to the atlas and with the lower half of the specimen firmly lashed to the table. When the weight was attached, the spines became straight or assumed a symmetrical reversed curve forward. They did not angulate even when counter pressure was applied at one point. However, when either the anterior portion of a mid-cervical disc was curetted out or the interspinous ligament was cut, an angulation occurred at that level. Section of the capsules of the posterior articulations alone did not produce such an angulation. Neither could such a deformity be produced by curettment of a badly degenerated intervertebral disc. The radiograph on the left shows the preliminary condition of one of these specimens with its normal anterior curve. The film on the right was made after removing the anterior portion of the fifth disc, incising the fifth interspinous ligament and attaching the weight to the atlas. It would seem that the angulation of the cervical spine at one point indicates the level at which damage has occurred.

REFERENCES

Anatomy

Baeyer, E. V.: 1960, *Am. J. Roent., 84*:1037–1044.

Borden, A. G. B., *et al.*: 1960, *Rad., 74*:806–809.

Fielding, J. W., 1957, *J. Bone & Joint Surg., 39A*:1280–1288.

Morton, D. E., 1950, *Yale J. Biol. Med., 23*:126–146.

Schneider, R. C., 1956, *J. Bone & Joint Surg., 38A*:985–997.

Wholey, M. H., *et al.*: 1958, *Rad., 71*:350–356.

Dynamics

Bailey, D. K., 1952, *Rad., 59*:712–719, In children.

Dunlap, J. P., *et al.*: 1958, *J. Bone & Joint Surg., 40A*:681–686, In children.

Jacobson, G., *et al.*: 1959, *Am. J. Roent., 82*:471–472, In children.

Jirout, J., 1956, *Acta Rad., 46*:55–60.

Paul, L. W., *et al.*: 1949, *Am. J. Roent., 62*:519–524, Lateral.

Townsend, E. H., *et al.*: 1952, *Ped., 10*:567–573.

Spondylosis

Arnold, J. G., Jr.: 1955, *Ann. Surg., 141*:872–889.

Epstein, J. A., *et al.*: 1959, *Bull. N. Y. Acad. Med., 35*:370–386.

Friedenberg, Z. B., *et al.*: 1959, *J. Bone & Joint Surg., 41A*:61–70.

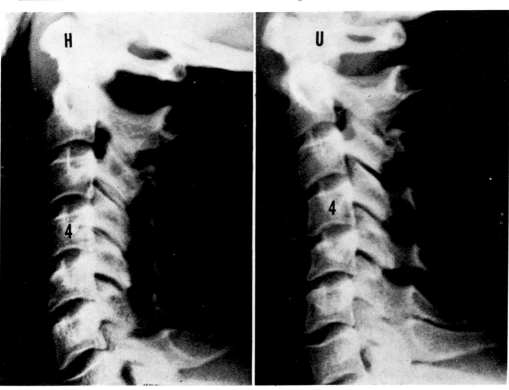

Fig. IV:16. Comparative studies to show the advantage of making the films with the patient sitting upright. This forty-two-year-old woman had fallen down stairs four years before. Radiographic examination at that time revealed an angulation at the fourth disc level. Her symptoms have persisted. Reexamination now lying in the horizontal position (H) shows very little. However when that examination is made with the patient sitting upright (U) it is seen that she has a persistent angulation at the fourth disc level. This should be considered a permanent injury.

Kuhns, J. G., 1956, *New Eng. J. Med., 254*:60–64.

Pallis, C., *et al.:* 1954, *Brain, 77*:274–289.

Spurling, R. G., *et al.:* 1953, *J.A.M.A., 151*:354–359.

Dysphagia from Spondylosis

Beahrs, O. H., *et al.:* 1959, *Ann. Surg., 149*:297–299.

Heck, C. V., 1956, *Surg. Gyn. Obst., 102*:657–660.

Kertzner, B., *et al.:* 1950, *Gastroenterology, 16:* 589–592.

Stephens, H., *et al.:* 1954, *Ann. Int. Med., 41:* 823–828.

Whiplash

Gay, J. R.: 1953, *J.A.M.A., 152*:1698–1704.

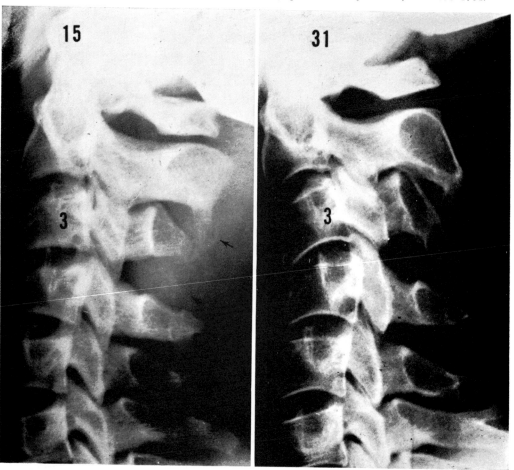

Fig. IV:17. This fifteen-year-old boy struck bottom bending his head forward when he dove into shallow water two weeks before his first examination. Angulation at the third disc was visualized on both the flexion and the extension films with distortion of the third disc and subluxation of the posterior articulations. Calcific material (*arrows*) was seen in the soft tissues between the second, third and fourth spinous processes. This calcification was diagnosed as evidence of ligamentous injury with haemorrhage in a young person two weeks after his accident. Through the courtesy of Dr. J. J. Fahey of Chicago, a reexamination of this patient was made at age thirty-one. It will be seen that the angulation is still present. During this sixteen year interval he has developed downward prolongations of the tips of the 2nd and 3rd spinous processes. One may assume that he sustained avulsions of the interspinous ligaments at these points with calcification in the resultant haemorrhage. Apparently healing occurred with the development of bony tissues in the calcific areas.

Myers, A., 1953, *Bull. Hosp. Joint Dis., 14:74*–85.

Zatzkin, H. R., *et al.:* 1960, *Rad., 75:577–583.*

Dislocation—Subluxation

Grogons, B. J. S., 1954, *J. Bone & Joint Surg., 36B:397–410.*

Jacobson, G., *et al.:* 1953, *Rad., 61:355–362.*

Jacobson, G., *et al.:* 1956, *Am. J. Ronet., 76:* 1081–1094.

Kovacs, A., 1955, *Acta Rad., 43:1–16.*

Rogers, Wm. A., 1957, *J. Bone & Joint Surg., 39A:341–376.*

Whitley, J. E., *et al.:* 1960, *Am. J. Roent., 83:* 633–644.

Wollin, D. G., *et al.:* 1958, *Am. J. Roent., 79:* 575–583.

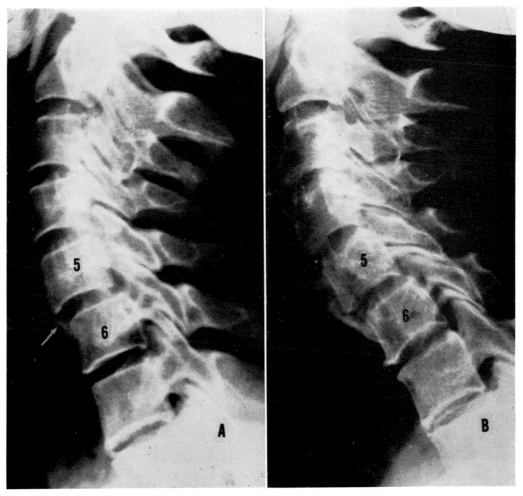

Fig. IV:18. Female, fifty-seven years of age. Patient's car was struck in rear by an oil truck. She complained of pain and muscle spasm in the cervical region.

A. Film made ten weeks after accident showing forward subluxation of C_5 on C_6 and beginning spur formation at the site of injury in the anterior longitudinal ligament (arrow). (Spinous processes and spur accentuated.)

B. Reexamination twenty-one months after injury. The subluxation has persisted. Stabilizing spur formation has developed during this one and one-half year interval, at the level of the avulsed anterior longitudinal ligament.

These studies indicate the length of time required for evidence of the healing process to appear in a patient of middle age.

Fracture of Odontoid

Amyes, E. W., 1956, *Arch. Surg., 72*:377–393.

Blackey, N. J., *et al.:* 1956, *J. Bone & Joint Surg., 38B*:794–817.

Nachemson, A., 1960, *Acta Ortho. Scand., 29*: 185–217.

Solovay, J., *et al.:* 1960, *Am. J. Roent., 83*:645–652.

Miscellaneous

Frykholm, R.: Cervical Nerve Root Compression Resulting from Disc Degeneration and Root-Sleeve Fibrosis, *Acta. Chir. Sand. Supp.* 160.

Kasabach, H. H., 1939, *Am. J. Roent., 42*:782–785, Technique.

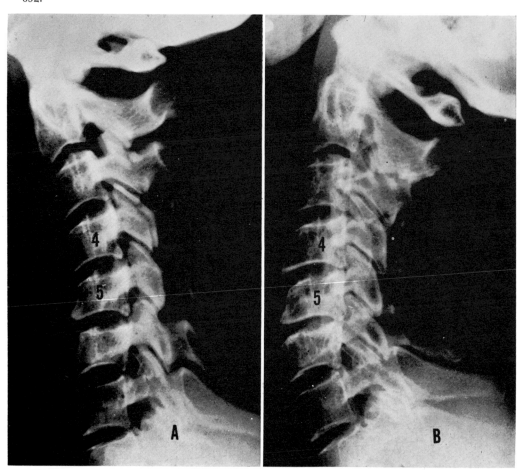

Fig. IV:19. Post traumatic angulation of the cervical spine in a woman of thirty-nine years with complete recovery. There was a history of recurrent attacks of pain and muscle spasm in the neck following an automobile accident six years before. Lateral radiograph A, made in attempted backward extension, shows a forward angulation at the C_{4-5} level. A reexamination of this patient, again in dorsal extension, B, made nineteen years later, failed to reveal angulation at the C_{4-5} level at that time. Apparently the patient had made a complete recovery during this interval. Note changes in bony texture incidental to the passage of time.

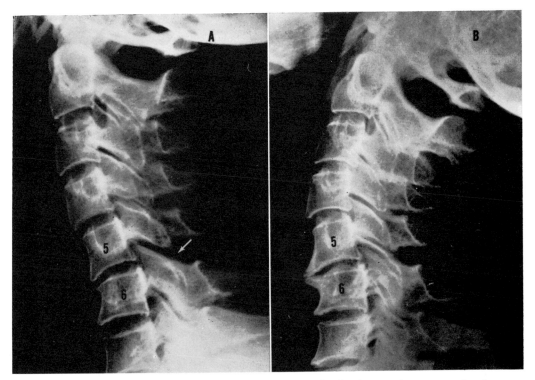

Fig. IV:20. Female, forty-four years of age. Fell down stairs the day previous to examination. There was some fixation of neck movement.

A. Radiograph made at the full limit of dorsal extension shows a forward angulation of C_5 on C_6 with subluxation of the corresponding posterior articulations and separation of the articular space posteriorly (*arrow*).

B. Reexamination twelve years later, courtesy of Dr. James T. McMillan of Des Moines, Iowa. Film in dorsal extension shows better flexibility of the upper cervical region than following the injury. At the fifth disc level, however, angulation has persisted, the dorsal spinous processes are separated and the degenerated disc is partially stabilized by a spur formation at its anterior margin.

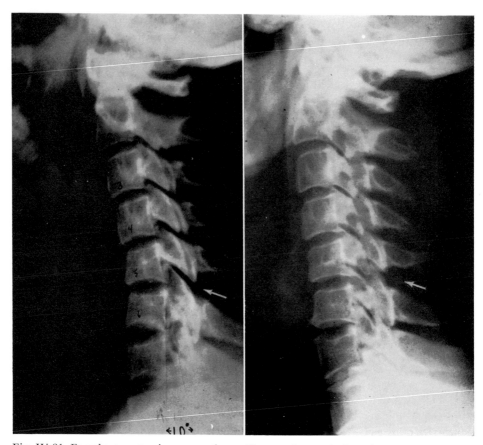

Fig. IV:21. Female, twenty-nine years of age. Traumatic angulation. Automobile accident five months previously. Pain, muscle spasm and limited neck movement. Subluxation of the C_{5-6} posterior articulations with 10 degrees forward angulation. Note separation of the corresponding spinous processes, displacement at the posterior articulations and widening of the articular space posteriorly (*arrow*).

The radiograph on the right was taken of the same patient nineteen years later, courtesy of Dr. J. M. Higgason of Chattanooga, Tennessee. The subluxation of the C_{5-6} posterior joints and the separation of the corresponding spinous process has become permanent. The angulation is now replaced by a straightening of the cervical spine. The patient, now age forty-eight, shows evidence of permanent anatomical change.

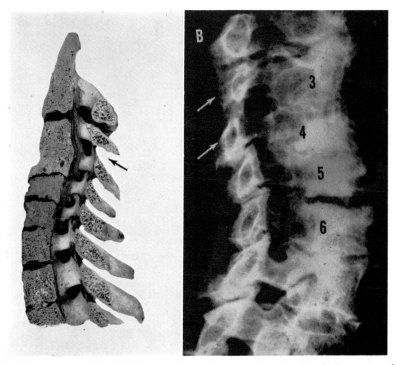

Fig. IV:22. Specimen anklosed in forward angulation at the C_{3-4} level. Compare with the next illustration. Note separation of the corresponding spinous processes (*black arrow*). In the oblique radiograph of this specimen (B) this separation is clearly shown between the neural arches with angulation of the customary symmetrical curve of these structures (*white arrows*). The foramen at this C_3 level is consequently larger than normal, while foramina 4, 5 and 6 are constricted by spurs from the covertebral joints. The seventh cervical foramen usually appears normal, because at the level where the anterior cervical curve is balanced by the posterior thoracic curve there is little tendency to encroachment of the intervertebral foramina.

$$\longrightarrow$$

Fig. IV:23. Female, forty-eight years of age. Automobile collision followed by angulation, pain and muscle spasm of the neck and with resultant changes developing during a quarter century.

A. Radiograph four and one-half months after accident reveals forward angulation at the fourth and fifth discs and subluxation of the corresponding posterior articulations.

B. Reexamination five and one-third years after injury. Complete bony bridging between the fourth, fifth and sixth cervical segments. Angulation is still present and the fourth disc is beginning to disappear. There is an arthrotic process involving the third posterior articulation (*arrow*). This spur impinges beneath the third transverse process.

C. Reexamination twenty-six years after injury. The neck is stiff and painful upon attempted movement. There is a demineralized, acquired block vertebra comprising the fourth, fifth and sixth segments. New bone has bridged along their anterior surfaces. The intervertebral discs and posterior articulations have been resorbed. Tubulization of the bodies and the articular processes, anteriorly and posteriorly has occurred.

D. Left oblique projection made twenty-six years after injury. Malalignment of the posterior arches has resulted from the angulation. One may note the normal curved alignment of the second, third and fourth neural arches but angulation has occurred between the fourth and fifth (*white arrows*). The third posterior joint shows advanced hypertrophic arthrotic changes with complete obliteration of the third foramen by a massive spur projecting anteriorly from the fourth superior articular process (*black arrows*). Since the lowermost four cervical segments are fused into a single block vertebra nearly all of the neck movement below C_2 occurs at the third joint level. This explains in part at least the advanced joint changes which developed at this point.

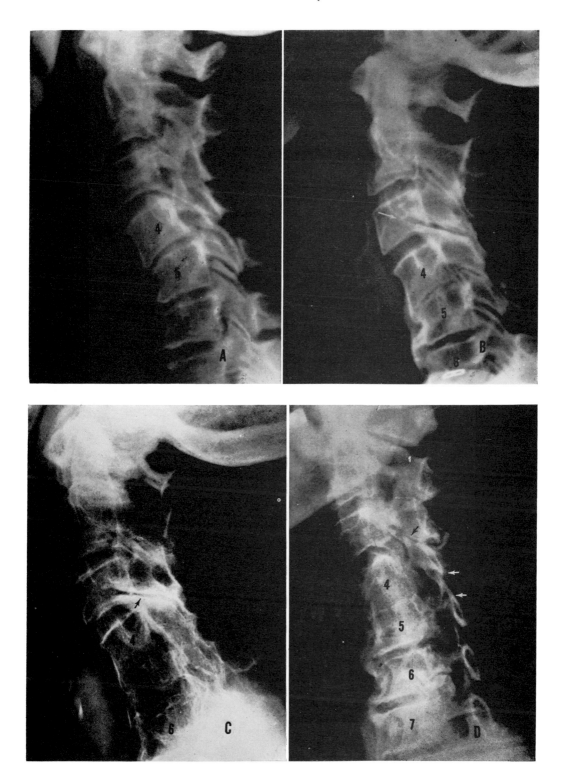

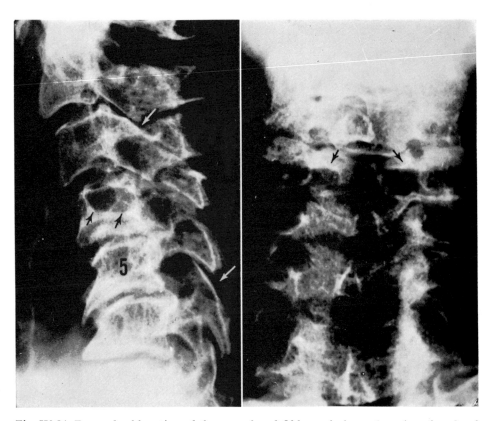

Fig. IV:24. Forward subluxation of the second and fifth cervical vertebrae in a female of sixty-six years. Note the positions of the posterior articular surfaces *(white arrows)*. C_5 is displaced anteriorly upon C_6 with its articular processes raised upward and forward. There was a history of a severe fall seven years before. Bone erosions circumscribed by white curvilinear lines of the type caused by vertebral artery tortuosities have involved both sides of the fourth vertebral body *(black arrows)* . See Chapter V.

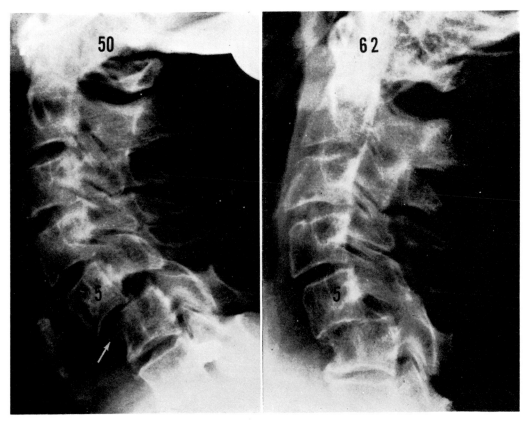

Fig. IV:25. This fifty-year-old man, involved in an automobile accident, sustained a fracture-dislocation at the C_{5-6} level. The right fifth inferior articular process was fractured and the vertebral body was dislocated forward fifteen weeks before the first examination. The anterior longitudinal ligament became avulsed and possibly the upper anterior margin of C_6 may have been fractured off. The original film shows filling in with bony tissue beneath the anterior longitudinal ligament at the angle between C_5 and C_6 (*white arrow*). A re-examination twelve years later by the courtesy of Doctor Nathan Kriss of Geneva, N. Y., showed a complete ankylosis of the posterior articulations and the vertebral bodies at the involved 5-6 level. The angles between C_5 and C_6 both anteriorly and posteriorly became filled in with bony tissue. Since the fifth neural arch was tilted upward, no encroachment of the spinal canal resulted.

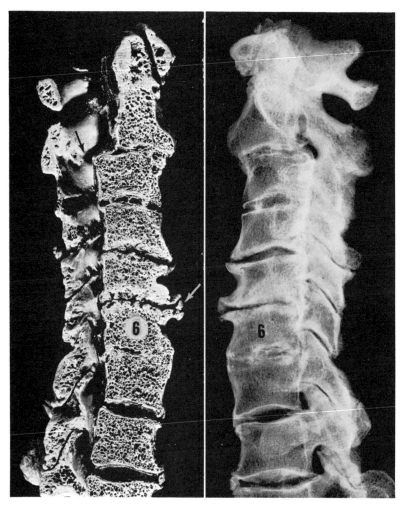

Fig. IV:26. Narrowing of the spinal canal by a subluxated axis. Specimen #539. Male, eighty-two years of age. Automobile accident fourteen years before death with multiple fractures (hand, rib and leg). C_2 is displaced forward on C_3 with the disc and posterior articulation ankylosed. The spinal canal is narrowed between the second arch and the third vertebral body (*black arrow*) but without intervertebral foramen encroachment. The man developed an acquired fusion at the 6-7 level with the posterior joint ankylosed but visualized upon the radiograph. An intercalary ossicle is present in the anterior portion of the fifth disc (*white arrow*). In contrast to Figure IV:25 the forward dislocation of C_2 in this individual produced a marked narrowing of the spinal canal because the second neural arch was carried forward with the vertebral body and not tilted upward.

Fig. IV:27. Male, twenty-two years of age. Traumatic subluxation, unilateral rotary anterior dislocation of C_2 on the right side. Automobile accident five days before. Spastic neck muscles with limited rotation and lateral bending. Anterior flexion is good but upon straightening up an undulating movement is noted; that is, the upper cervical region extends first to be followed by extension of the lower cervical spine. One is able to palpate the second cervical spinous process well to the right of the midline (see arrow in photograph)

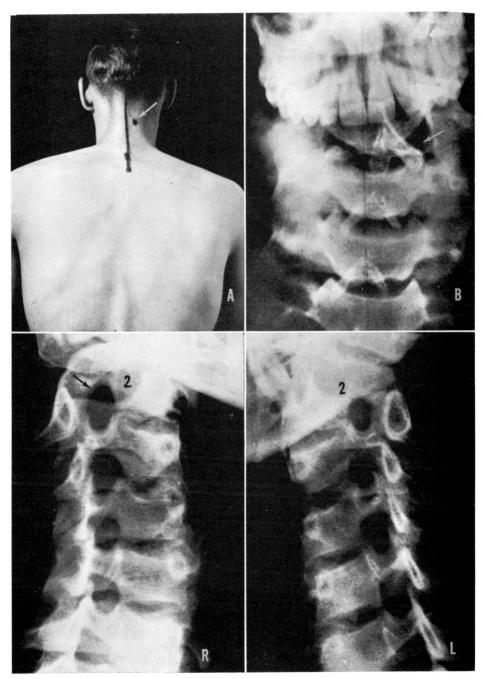

(A). The PA retouched radiograph (B) shows this spinous process displaced to the right of the normal position at the midline. Because of the inclined plane of the posterior articulations the rotation and forward subluxation of the second right posterior articulation has produced an elevation of the right side of C_2 and a consequent thickening of the disc on the right side (*white arrow*) together with enlargement of the second right foramen (*black arrow*) and slight constriction of the second left foramen. These latter are shown on the oblique films "R" and "L" respectively. No attempt was made to palpate in the posterior pharynx, the displaced right lateral mass of the second vertebra.

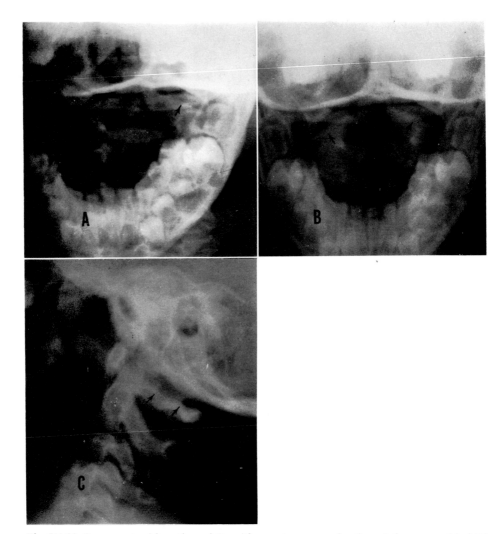

Fig. IV:28. Recurrent subluxation of C$_2$ with spontaneous reduction. A four-year-old child sustained an injury to the neck followed by recurrent attacks of muscle spasm and torticollis for the past eight months. These would become reduced spontaneously. When she was re-ferred for x-ray examination the child was obviously in distress with the chin rotated toward the right side. She was unable to turn the head back to its normal position. A, is a pre-liminary projection through the mouth and shows the chin rotated toward the right with a difference in the width of the two atlanto-axial joints (*arrows*). The articulation on the right appears much narrower because the lateral mass of the atlas on that side has dipped behind the articular surface of the axis. In the true lateral projection below, (C), the arrows indicate the posterior margins of the lateral masses on the two sides. These are not aligned because of the rotation of C$_1$. While the child was immobilized with sandbags, the spasm of the left sternomastoid became relaxed spontaneously and she announced, "my neck is all right now." Thereupon projection B was promptly made and reveals the joint spaces symme-trical on each side (*arrows*). In this case of course the atlas had rotated but never became displaced forward upon the axis.

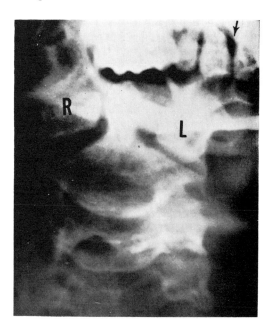

Fig. IV:29. Traumatic, unilateral C₁subluxation in a male eleven years of age following a football accident. Chin held to the left, rotation freely to the left but restricted to the right. No mass seen in posterior pharynx. Retouched radiograph shows asymmetry of the atlanto-axial joint and a difference in the widths of the atlanto-axial joint spaces on the two sides. Compare this with the following illustration. The chin is directed toward the left side and the lateral mass is close to the right side of the odontoid. The arrow indicates the space between the central incisors. This displacement toward the odontoid may normally be noted in early life without symptoms. It is also present in patients with congenital torticollis from a shortened sternomastoid muscle. Compare with Figure IV:31.

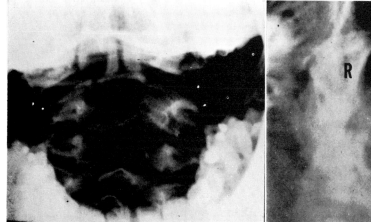
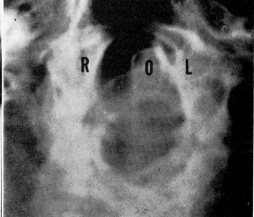

Fig. IV:30. Lateral displacement of the atlas on the axis in a child without AP subluxation. Male, eight years old injured during gymnasium exercises. The head was held tipped toward the right side. There was very minimal rotation. All neck movements were restricted. The left side of the neural arch and the spinous process of C₂ were easily palpable behind the left mastoid. In the A. P. projection the atlanto-axial joint spaces are equal in width. White dots have been placed on the lateral margins of the articular surfaces. These indicate the lateral displacement toward the right of C₁ upon C₂. In the base-vertex projection also the atlas is seen to be well displaced toward the right as judged by its relationship to the odontoid (O). This enabled the spinous process of the axis to be palpable behind the left mastoid. Lateral displacement of the atlas in a young person without asymmetry in the widths of the joint spaces and without other evidence of subluxation or injury has very little clinical significance. However in this instance the displacement followed trauma.

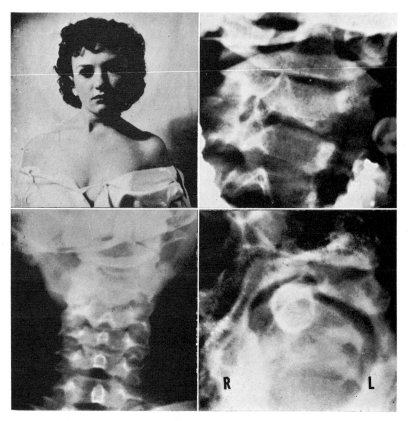

Fig. IV:31. In the photograph one may visualize the congenital tonic spasm of the right sternomastoid muscle with torticollis in a young woman of eighteen years. The atlas was rotated on the axis and displaced toward the right side *(lower right radiograph)*. The entire cervical spine was inclined toward the left side because of the shortened right sterno-mastoid muscle. The P.A. radiograph was retouched at the odontoid. The spastic muscle was later severed with an excellent cosmetic result. When this patient was seen twenty years later there was no evidence of torticollis and the operative scar along the clavical was barely discernible. She had normal movement of the head and neck. The sternomastoid was apparently absent but there was some compensatory hypertrophy of the platysma. See Figure IV:3C.

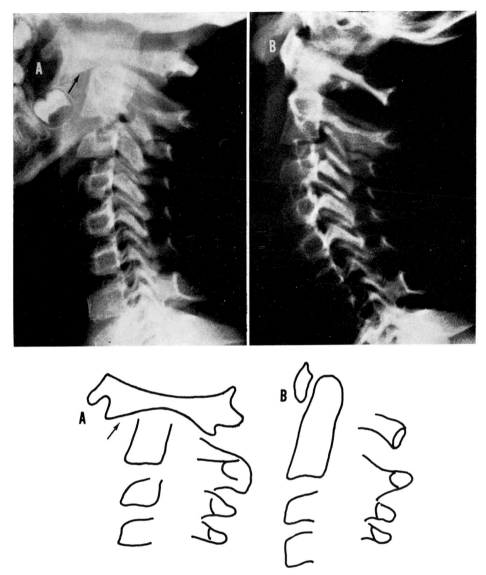

Fig. IV:32. Female, eight years of age. Spontaneous atlanto-axial rotation during hospitalization for massive exudate in the left hemithorax. Torticollis present, chin carried to the left.

A. Lateral film, shows extreme (nearly 60 degrees) rotation of atlas on the axis *(arrow)*. Traction halter was applied followed by a leather collar.

B. Lateral film made two months later shows the atlas now in normal position.

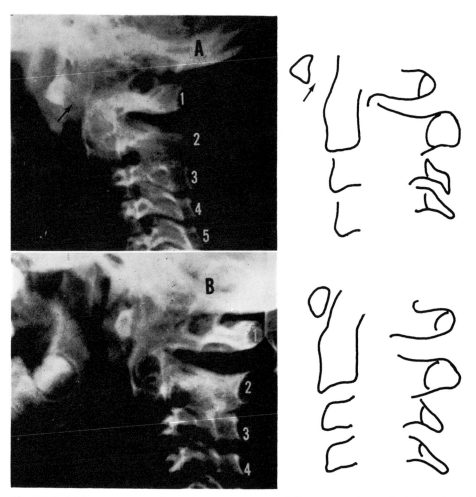

Fig. IV:33. Male, seven years of age. Spontaneous post-inflammatory forward subluxation of the atlas occurring while the child was hospitalized with cervical adenitis four months following scarlet fever. No trauma of any kind. Film of the cervical spine two months before showed no subluxation.

A. Atlas forward upon the axis. Demineralized odontoid poorly differentiated with increased space between it and the anterior neural arch of C_1 (*arrow*). Posteriorly the first neural arch is carried well anterior to the curved alignment of those arches below it. In this type of subluxation there is an encroachment upon the A. P. diameter of the spinal canal.

B. Same patient one month later following traction. Normal relationship between odontoid and the anterior arch of the atlas although there is still very minimal rotation of the atlas on the axis. The neural arch has returned to its normal alignment with the other posterior arches. When moving, these children attempt to immobilize the head by grasping it with the hands.

---

destroyed. The right superior articular surface of the axis (S) is clearly visualized. Compare with projection R (*above*) where the left postero-superior articular surface of the axis is entirely absent. (*arrow*)

These Kasabach studies demoinstrate the value of that position and of a critical comparison of details upon the two sides in differential diagnosis. This patient had undergone esophagectomy with gastric anastomosis for carcinoma eleven months before.

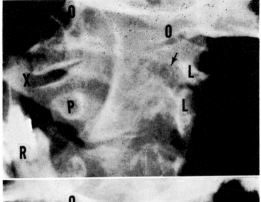

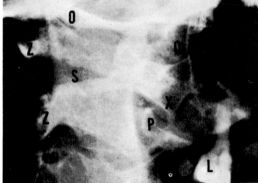

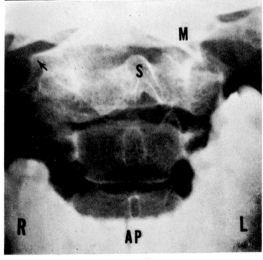

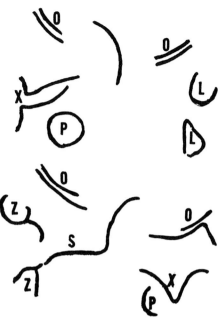

Fig. IV:34. Female, forty-seven years of age. Destruction posteriorly in the left lateral mass of C_2. Upon rotation of the face toward the left she experienced severe cervical and occipital pain with muscle spasm. The left occipital nerve was tender to pressure. The A.P. projection (below) shows the atlas displaced toward the right on the axis (arrow). The left lateral mass (M) of the atlas is depressed. Both inferior articular surfaces of the atlas are visualized but the left superior articular surface of the axis is poorly seen. Slight rotation of second spinous process (S) toward the left. This was at first thought to be only a posterior rotation of the atlas with subluxation toward the right side upon the axis with radiculitis.

The right and left comparative Kasabach oblique studies R and L show, however, a destruction of the superior articular surface of the axis on the left side (arrow). Compare the two oblique projections. Note the approximation of the first and second laminae on the left and their wide separation on the right; normal atlanto-occipital articulations on each side with the left one depressed.

R. Face turned to the right. Both atlanto-occipital joints are visualized (O). The atlanto-axial joint is visualized on the right (X) but not on the left. The arrow indicates the missing articular surface of C_2. The first and second left laminae are close together (L and L). The second right pedicle (P) is intact.

L. Face turned to the left. Both atlanto-occipital points are seen (O). There is no atlanto-axial joint on the left since the superior articular surface of the axis on that side is deficient and only the undersurface of the atlas is present (X). The first and second laminae are widely separated on the right side (Z and Z). The lateral and superior portions of the second left pedicle (P) are

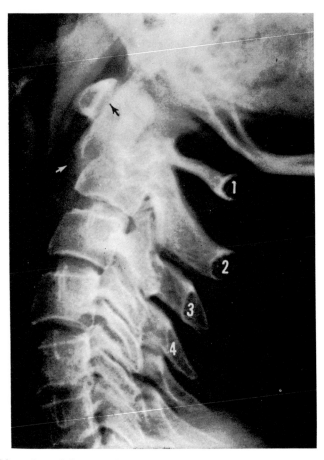

Fig. IV:35. Subluxation of the atlas forward with a fractured odontoid in a female, fifty-eight years old. The film reveals a fractured odontoid with forward displacement. Re-touched. One may note preservation of the normal relationship between the odontoid and the anterior arch of the atlas (*black arrow*) also the malalignment between the anterior surfaces of the odontoid and the second cervical vertebra (*white arrow*). The first neural arch is well anterior to the curved alignment of those below it. Compared with the spontaneous subluxation of the atlas forward (Figure IV:33). Also compare with the os odontoideum Figure III:7.

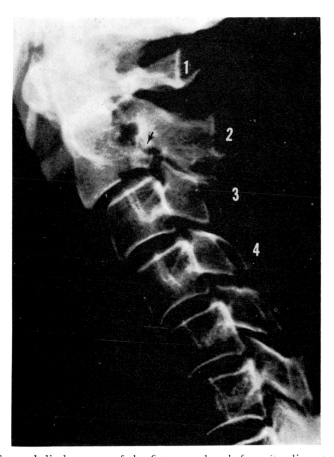

Fig. IV:36. Forward displacement of the first neural arch from its alignment with those below it because of fracture through the second arch in front of the posterior articulations.

Male, aged thirty-three, auto accident, head striking windshield, has pain and muscle spasm of the neck. The radiograph revealed a fracture through the pedicles of the axis (*arrow*). The posterior articulations and the second neural arch have maintained their normal relationship. However vertebral body number two has become displaced forward upon number three. This has carried with it the atlas and the skull. Again the forward displacement of C_1 has disturbed the normal alignment of the posterior arches, but since the atlas has maintained its normal relationship to the axis there has been no constriction of the spinal canal. Contrast this condition with that of other studies where such constriction did occur when the neural arch of the atlas became displaced forward. Compare Figures IX:7, IX:13, and IV:33 with Figures IV:35 IV:36, III:7, III:8, and III:9.

————————————————→

Fig. IV:37. Male, fifty-two years of age. A horse ran away fracturing this patient's cervical spine thirty-four years before. He was essentially asymptomatic until the past few years. There is now cervical muscle spasm with pain locally and referred to the arms and also paresthesia of the upper extremities. Radiographic studies reveal an old compression fracture of C_5 with angulation. The second, third, fourth and fifth vertebral bodies and their arches have become fused. The flexion-extension studies reveal practically all of the movement occurring between the sixth and the compressed fifth cervical segments. Upon anterior flexion (FLEX) the fifth vertebra glides forward upon the sixth segment and the posterior articular surfaces are in contact (*arrow*). Backward extension however (EXT) reverses this gliding movement of the segments while an extreme degree of subluxation and imbrication occurs with separation of the posterior articulations (*black arrows*). By this rocking movement the sixth superior articular processes becoming thrust upward and forward into the foramina. This encroachment upon the fifth left foramen is visualized in the oblique projection (*white arrow*). The fifth intervertebral foramina, like the second, third, and fourth, were probably not encroached upon at first. However most of the cervical movement for many years has necessarily occurred between the compressed fifth vertebra and the one below it. As a result one now visualizes the advanced arthrotic changes at the C_5-C_6 level with the posterior joint subluxation and foramen encroachment. The gradual development of this condition more recently probably explains why the patient has complained of local pain and radicular symptoms only in the past few years.

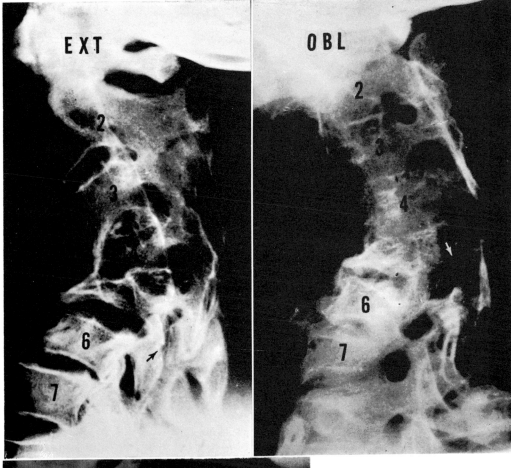
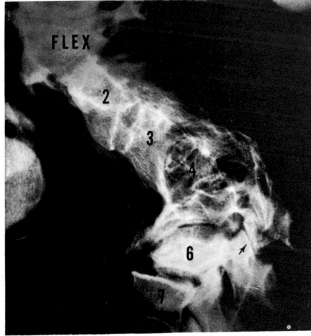

Chapter V

Vertebral Arteries

T HE VERTEBRAL artery arises from the subclavian and courses from the sixth vertebra upward as a captive vessel through the aligned foramina in the transverse processes (Figures I:16 and XIV:5). Sympathetic fibers lie posterior to the artery and it is surrounded by the posterior cervical sympathetic plexus. These structures pass upward through the foramen magnum and along the basilar artery to the circle of Willis.

In the lateral roentgenogram the neck seems much longer upon forward flexion than upon dorsal extension. However, since the artery lies in the central axis of movement between adjacent vertebrae, the distance from the inferior surface of the sixth to the upper surface of the second cervical transverse process measures the same in both positions (Figure IV:6). On the other hand, extremes of rotation and flexion occur at the upper cervical region. Four normal curves in the vertebral artery help to compensate for movements at this level. The lowermost curve is backward and laterally within the second transverse process before the vessel issues from its foramen. In its upward course between C_1 and C_2 there is a considerable laxity of the vessel to allow for the rotation occurring at this level. After passing through the first transverse process the artery turns sharply backward and after coursing along the upper surface of the first arch it finally encircles the posterior margin of the articular surface to enter the spinal canal opposite the medulla. As a result of arterial lengthening any of these curves may become exaggerated (Figure V:1 and V:2).

TORTUOSITY

Tortuosity or buckling of the carotid, subclavian and the innominate arteries have been described by various writers. Likewise tortuosity of the vertebral arteries with destructive bone changes merits serious consideration.

In a group of twenty-one cadavers aged forty-five to ninety-one years, four examples of tortuosity of the vertebral arteries with bone destruction were encountered. The vessels of the specimens shown in Figures V:3, V:4, XIV:3C, and IV:2 were tortuous and roentgenograms revealed various degrees of bone destruction. In each instance, sections of the vertebral artery showed degenerative changes in the vessel wall.

These anatomical observations have been repeatedly confirmed by the roentgenograms of patients showing the characteristic areas of bone erosion as visualized on the specimens. None of these have been confirmed by operation. Since the process develops slowly it is indicated on the film by a radiolucency surrounded by a fine white curvilinear line. The significance of the erosions produced by these tortuosities is the implication of vessel wall changes. There is a possibility that the erosions may be mistaken for the results of tumor pressure or other destructive processes involving bone.

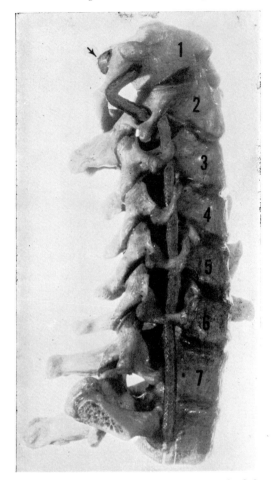

Fig. V:1. Specimen of a normal articulated adult cervical spine with a cord inserted in the foramina of the transverse processes to indicate the relative size, course and relationships of the normal vertebral artery. The vessel courses upward alongside the pedicles anterior to the cervical nerves from C_6 to C_2. In the lateral mass of the axis it makes a right angle turn to pass laterally and backward. Because of the extreme rotary mobility of the spine at this level there is a generous loop in the artery before it turns forward and upward to pass through the transverse process in the atlas. It then runs backward along the upper surface of the first cervical arch (*arrow*) and finally turns around the posterior margin of the articular surface of C_1 before it penetrates the dural sheath within the spinal canal.

When the vertebral bodies of the mid cervical region are involved the process may be visualized either by the oblique or the A.P. projection. Steroscopic studies are especially valuable and usually one of the stereo pair shows the condition somewhat better than its fellow. For some reason the mid cervical region shows a predilection for this process (Figures V:5, V:6, V:7 and IV:24).

An aneurism-like condition occurs not uncommonly within the cancellous lateral mass of the second cervical verte-

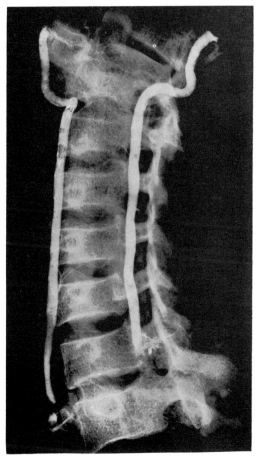

Fig. V:2. The vertebral arteries of a specimen injected with radiopaque material. Note the normal tortuosity above and the indentations on the postero-lateral surface of the vessel where the intervertebral nerves, issuing from the foramina pass outward in close proximity to the artery.

bra. At this point the artery makes a right angle turn backwards before proceeding laterally through the foramen in the transverse process. Within C_2 the tortuosity is visualized in both the A.P. and lateral projections. In the former the erosion may appear closely beneath the superior articular surface of the axis (Figures V:8 and V:9). Occasionally in the lateral projection the round shadow of the C_2 foramen transversarium may overlie that of the tortuosity. However the circular shadow of the tortuosity is larger than the foramen (Figure V:10).

DEFLECTION

Various authors have described vertebral artery deflection and the symptoms resulting from pressure upon this vessel.

In its course upward the vessel may be deflected by the adjacent spinal nerves, by bony spurs from covertebral

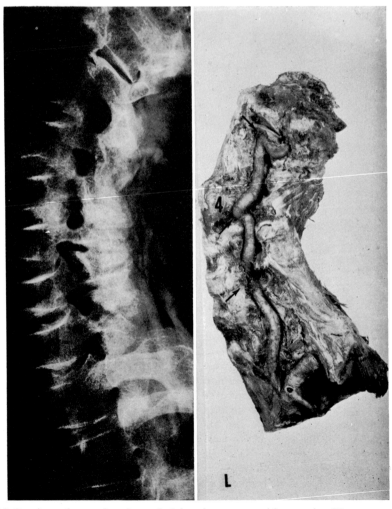

Fig. V:3. Specimen from a female aged eighty-three years with negative Wasserman. Photograph and roentgenogram of the left side showing pressure destruction with tortuosities at the C_2, C_4, and C_6 levels (*black arrows*). The right side was involved at the C_2 and C_6 levels. (Courtesy of the *American Journal of Roentgenology*.)

joints or by grossly hyperplastic arthrotic posterior vertebral articulations. Dorsal extension of the cervical spine allows the tip of the superior articular process of the posterior joint to glide forward and upward. If sufficiently hyperplastic it may encroach upon the vertebral artery or the intervertebral foramen. This deflection of the artery and any resulting symptoms are exaggerated by rotation and/or dorsal extension of the neck. As a result of pressure against the

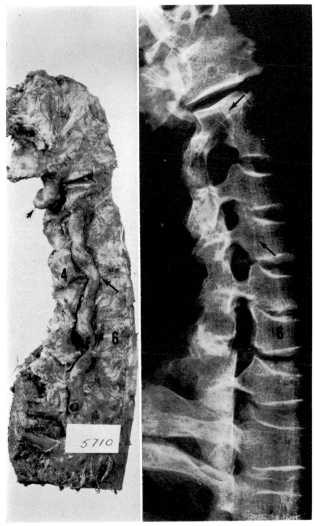

Fig. V:4. Dissection from a male, aged ninety-one. Sclerosis of peripheral vessels. Wasserman test negative. Mitral disease. Blood pressure 149/78. Section of the vertebral artery showed thinning of both the media and the intima. A pulsating tortuosity of the right vertebral artery has completely destroyed the sixth cervical pedicle. Curvilinear bone erosions from arterial pressure are also visualized on the posterior surface of the C_4 body and within the second transverse process (*arrows*). The latter was still incompletely uncovered when the photograph was made. The fourth posterior articulation displaces the artery forward (4). One may note a complete loop of the vertebral artery behind the altanto-axial joint (*small arrow head*). (Courtesy of the *American Journal of Roentgenology*.)

artery there may be temporary lessening in the volume of blood flow. Atheromatous changes may occur later in the vessel wall (Figures V:11, V:12, V:13, and XIV:2).

The vertebral artery is an important link in the collateral cerebral blood supply. Angiography is necessary to visualize pressure deflection or atheromata of this vessel. The symptoms of these changes are said to result from interference with the important circulation to the hind brain, and from pressure upon the sympathetic nerve and the plexus which surrounds this vessel. The symptoms constitute a most bizarre and confusing clinical picture, which has been described as the Barré-Lieou syndrome. They include: headache, vertigo, nausea, vomiting, nystagmus and suboccipital tenderness.

Lewis and Coburn studied a group of patients by vertebral angiography. They found that the symptoms were aggravated by dorsal extension of the neck. With the patient in this position they were able to visualize a partial blocking of one or both of the vertebral arteries.

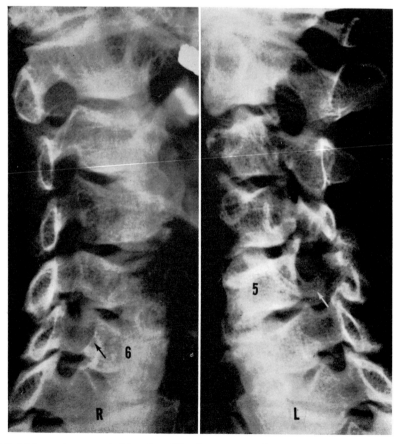

Fig. V:5. Male patient, aged thirty-five. Blood pressure 118/70. (L) This appears to be an example of tortuosity of the left vertebral artery with destruction of the fifth pedicle, similar to the condition seen in Figure V:4. The transverse process is clearly seen (*white arrow.*) The patient had bilateral involvement. There is partial destruction of the sixth vertebra on the right side (*black arrow*). Compare this with Figure V:3. (Courtesy of the *American Journal of Roentgenology.*)

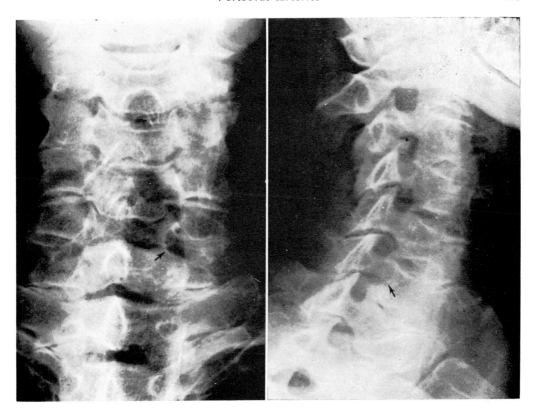

Fig. V:6. AP and left oblique radiographs of a male, sixty-three years of age. Blood pressure 140/80. This patient has an erosion involving the anterior portion of the left sixth transverse process and extending medially into the adjacent vertebral body *(arrows)*. Compare with Figures V:3 and V:4. Patients shown in Figures V:5 and V:6 had erosions in the mid and lower cervical regions similar to those present in the cadaver material. (Courtesy of Dr. G. P. Metzler, Syracuse, N.Y.)

On the other hand, Kovacs reported a group of patients with similar symptoms, aggravated by dorsal extension, who were relieved upon forward flexion and traction upon the neck (Figures V:14 and V:15).

REFERENCES

Boldrey, E., *et al.:* 1956, *J. Neurol., 13:*127–139.

Ecker, A.: 1951, *The Normal Cerebral Angrogram*, Charles C Thomas, Springfield, Ill.

Ford, F. R.: 1952, *Bull, John Hop. Hosp., 91:* 168–173, Artery obstruction.

Frykholm, R.: 1951, *Acta Chir. Scand., 101:*345.

Gayral, L., *et al.:* 1954, *New York State J. Med., 54:*1920–1926, Barré-Lieu.

Hadley, L. A.: 1957, *J. Bone J. Surg., 39A:*910–920, Covertebral articulations.

Hodges, F. J., and Holt, J. F.: *Year Book of Radiology*, Year Book Publishers, Inc., Chicago, 1956-1957, p 60.

Hoffman, H. H., *et al.:* 1957, *Arch. Surg., 74:* 430–437, Vertebral nerve.

Hutchinson, E. C., *et al.:* 1956, *Brain, 79:*319–331, Vertebral artery.

Hsu, I., *et al:* 1956, *Arch. Int. Med., 98:*712–719, Buckling vessels.

Kelley, A. B.: 1925, *J. Lar. & Otol., 40:*15–23, Tortuosity of carotid.

Kovacs, A.: 1955, *Acta Rad., 43:*1–16, Apophyseal joints.

Kovacs, A.: 1956, *Fortsch, a. d. Geb. d. Roent., 85:*142–153.

Lewis, R. C., *et al.:* 1956, *Missouri Med., 53:* 1059–1063, Vertebral artery.

Morris, L.: 1960, *Rad., 75:*785–787, Angioma upper cervical cord visualized by vertebral artery angiogram.

Namin, P.: 1954, *Jor. Neurosurg., 11:*442–457, Vertebral angiography.

Steinbach, H. L., *et al.:* 1952, *Rad., 59:*838–840, Absent pedicle.

Sugar, O., *et al.:* 1949, *Am. Jor. Roent., 61:*166–182, Vertebral angiography.

Sugar, O., *et al.:* 1954, *Jor. Neurosurg., 11:*607–615.

Tatlow, W. F. T., *et al.:* 1957, *Neurolog., 7:*331–340, Vertebral artery.

Virtama, P.: 1957, *Acta Rad., 48:*410–412, Covertebral spur impression upon vertebral artery.

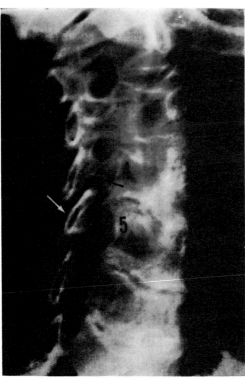

Fig. V:7. Right oblique projection showing distruction of the fifth right cervical pedicle in a female of seventy-seven years. The shadow faintly seen crossing the fifth foramen is the left side of the fifth neural arch, not the pedicle. The right fifth posterior articulation is displaced forward and upward into the fourth foramen (*black arrow*). There is advanced disc degeneration with thinning and marginal spur formation.

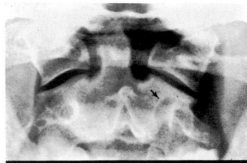

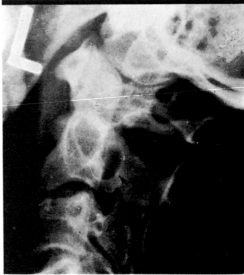

Fig. V:8. Male of forty years. Erosion within the left lateral mass of the axis (*arrows*). This was an incidental observation. There is some asymmetry of the atlanto-axial articulation following an automobile accident. (Courtesy of **Dr. J. H. Finley, Syracuse, N. Y.**)

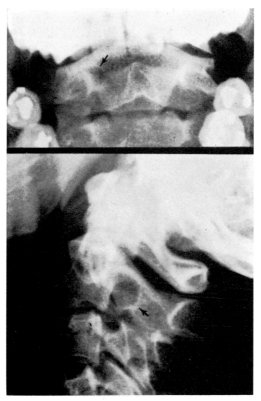

Fig. V:9. Female, with a large erosion in the right lateral mass of the axis. This patient was a relatively young woman of only twenty-eight years (*arrows*). Blood pressure 112/58. These erosions at a later age are not uncommon. Each case should be confirmed by the AP projection through the mouth. In some cases the erosion extends upward nearly to the articular surface. Figures V:8, V:9, and V:10 illustrate erosions in the upper cervical region. (Courtesy of Dr. E. G. Murphy, Syracuse, N. Y.)

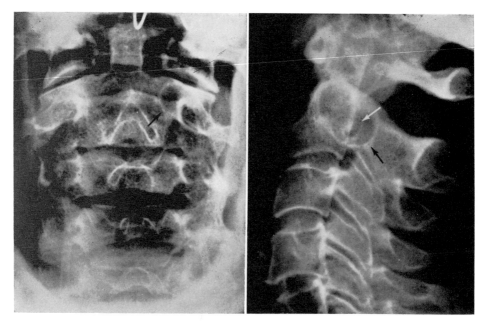

Fig. V:10. Female, aged fifty-six. Blood pressure 185/85. A curvilinear erosion (*black arrow*) is seen in the anteroposterior and lateral projecttions of the second cervical vertebra adjacent to the location of the vertebral artery. The appearance is similar to that in Figures V:3 and V:4. The C_2 left lateral mass and pedicle have been partially eroded, undoubtedly by a tortuosity of that vessel. The smaller, round, concentric shadow (*white arrow*) is cast by the foramen in the transverse process. Some confusion may arise when the plane of this foramen is more vertical than normal. The round shadow of the foramen, however, is always much smaller than that of an erosion caused by the vertebral artery. See also Figure VII 4b and c. (Courtesy of Dr. Samuel Gingold, Syracuse, N.Y., and the *American Journal of Roentgenology*.)

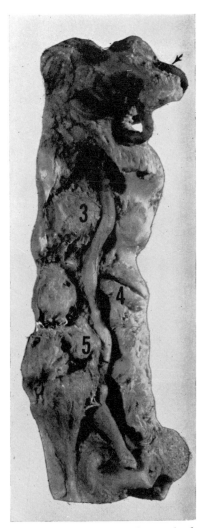

Fig. V:11. Dissection of the left vertebral artery showing deflections backward at the third and fifth disc levels and deflection forward by hyperplasia of the fourth posterior articulation. The loop at the atlanto-axial joint is clearly seen as well as the artery where it courses along the upper surface of the first neural arch arrow.

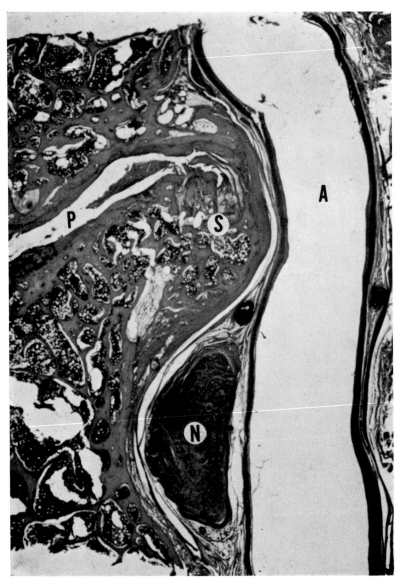

Fig. V:12. Photomicrograph (X10) showing a posterior cervical articulation (P) **with** a bony spur formation (S) deflecting the vertebral artery (A). Below is seen the somewhat distorted nerve (N) as it lies in close approximation to the artery.

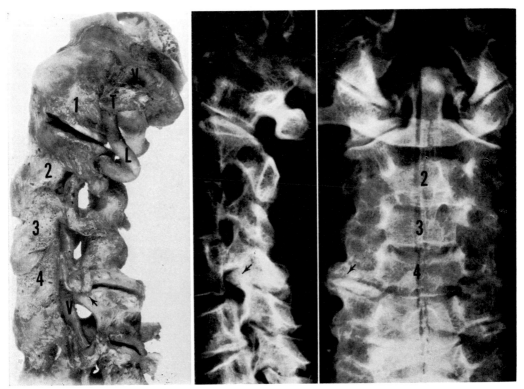

Fig. V:13. Photograph with PA and lateral radiographs of a specimen showing chronic advanced hyperplastic arthrotic changes involving the left fourth posterior cervical articulation *(arrows)*. On the PA projection compare with the articulation at the same level on the opposite side. The sclerotic bony spur has extended forward to impinge beneath the under surface of the fourth pedicle. Not only does it encroach upon the 4th intervertebral foramen but it also causes pressure against the vertebral artery (V), especially upon dorsal extension of the cervical spine. The artery at this point is a captive structure. Note the large loop behind the atlantoaxial joint (L) before the artery passes upward through the foramen in the first transverse process - here seen beneath the letter (T). The vessel is seen again (V) as it courses along the top of the first neural arch.

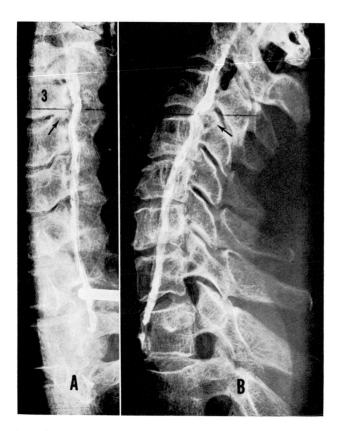

Fig. V:14. Specimen from a female, aged seventy-two. Arteriosclerosis. Wasserman test negative. Left of cervical spine. Angiogram of vertebral artery. (A) : The postero-anterior projection shows a covertebral spur below C_3 producing lateral deflection of the artery (*arrow*). (B) : The lateral roentgenogram made at full limit of dorsal extension shows the third posterior joint deflecting the artery forward (*arrow*) as described by Kovacs. This did not occur with the specimen in the neutral or anteflexed positions and corroborates the observations of Lewis and Coburn. These authors reported 11 patients showing angiographic evidence of interference with vertebral artery circulation upon extension of the neck. (Courtesy of the *American Journal of Roentgenology*.)

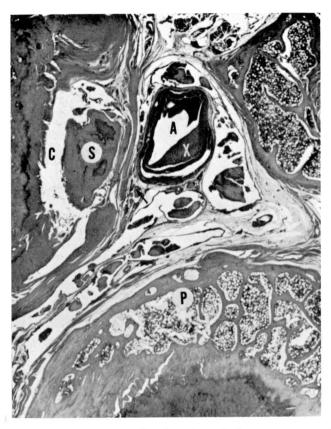

Fig. V:15. The transverse section, X8, is taken through the artery, covertebral spur and posterior articulation at the plane indicated by the lines on the roentgenograms in Figure V:14. C indicates the covertebral joint space between C_3 and C_4. The rectangular shaped artery (A) is grossly distorted by the covertebral spur (S) and the posterior articulation (P). The vertebral artery sections from other cadaver specimens were usually round or slightly oval. This one contains an organized atheromatous plaque (X) partially separated from the wall of the vessel, a condition described by Hutchinson and Yates. The arrow indicates the site of three sectioned sympathetic nerves. Even in the presence of deflecting pressure as observed in this and other specimens, the vertebral sympathetic continues to follow the artery, usually on its posterior surface. Hoffman and Kuntz state that the vertebral nerve with its inconstant ganglia may extend to the first or the second cervical root and then the vertebral sympathetic plexus becomes continuous with the intracranial basilar plexus above. The vertebral artery is accompanied by a rich network of veins. (Courtesy of the *American Journal of Roentgenology*.)

Chapter VI

The Posterior Spinal Articulations
with Innervation Studies

T HE CAUSAL relationship between the posterior joints and local back pain has been studied by Keller and by Kellgren. Like any diathrodial joint with its articular surfaces, synovia, capsule, ligaments and nerves, the apophyseal joint is subjected to sprain, dislocation and degeneration or pathological changes.

WIDENING OF THE POSTERIOR JOINTS

This not uncommon condition is visualized clearly in patients by studies made with the sagittal plane at 45 degrees to that of the film. Normally there is only a minimal variation in the width of the posterior joints. However, joint widening from disc degeneration, the interposition of soft tissue, spasm or other cause is easily demonstrated (Figures VI:1, VI:2, II:13 and XIII:30).

There is a group of patients who exhibit a separation of the joint surfaces incidental to trauma of the back. The joint displacement of a sprain may thus be visualized by the roentgenogram (Figure VI:3 and XIII:34).

The patient is usually aware of the exact time when the condition occurred and may describe a sensation of sudden instability or "catch." He may say that "something slipped." This may be at the time of some accident or even merely upon straightening up from a prolonged stooped position. The patient presents with back pain, muscle spasm and limitation of motion. The back may be held in some asymmetrical position. Figure VI:4 demonstrates this condition.

ANATOMICAL STUDIES

Longitudinal sections of the posterior joints show the normal articular surfaces covered with hyaline cartilage of varying thickness but unbroken continuity (Figures VI:5 and VI:6). The joint capsule is not attached to the joint margins. Rather, it is reflected around and attached to the outer surfaces of the articular processes. The articular cartilage likewise may extend well beyond the limits of bony contact, especially at the lower lumbar level. The joint space is actually continued around on to the posterior surface of the articular process (Figure II:9). This part of the smooth, rounded articular cartilage thus makes contact with the inside of the redundant capsule, thereby opposing the sidewise thrust of the joint. Functionally, this type of joint structure also increases the possible amplitude of movement, a mobility that is further increased by the laxity of the capsule at the lower margin of the joint (Figure VI:7).

Anatomically, the lower element of the posterior articulation, i.e., the superior articular process from below presents a concave, cylindrical articular surface

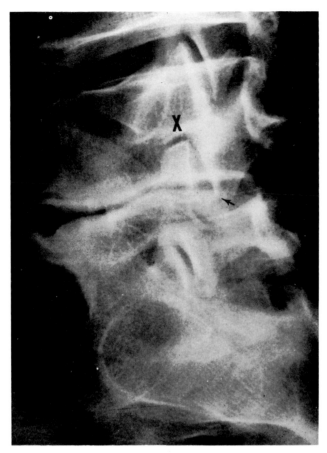

Fig. VI:1. Male of fifty-two years. Left oblique roentgenogram showing separation of the lower margin of the L₄ apophyseal articulation (*arrow*). Degeneration of the fourth disc had allowed telescoping of the posterior joints. The resultant impingement at X served as a fulcrum allowing the vertebral body to tip forward. This caused the separation below and placed a stress upon the joint capsule.

directed backward and medially. The corresponding articular surface of the upper element is somewhat biconvex (Figure VI:8).

DEGENERATIVE CHANGES OF THE POSTERIOR JOINTS

Macroscopically, the articular surfaces are at first smooth and glistening. Later, the degenerative changes may first appear as a velvety texture overlying the joint surface. Subsequently, the cartilage gradually disappears, leaving, in the late stages, only the bare bone. Other degenerative changes were noted, such as fissures of or adhesions between joint surfaces. In some cases fibrous tissue or bony masses were visualized completely occupying the joint space. Rarely, sulci were present dividing the joint into separate bearing surfaces. Pannus formation may be encountered. Bony spur formation at the articular margins and ossification within the capsular structure are a part of the later compensatory stabilizing process (Figures VI:9 and VI:10).

IMBRICATION—IMPINGEMENT—EBURNATION—EROSION

Thinning of the intervertebral disc, either as a result of a degenerative process or a loss of disc substance, results in a telescoping or imbrication of the posterior articulations (Figure IX:2R). The articular surfaces no longer register exactly opposite of each other. A pulling stress is placed upon the capsule. The intervertebral foramen may become encroached upon by the anterior inferior element of the joint becoming displaced upward into that opening. At times this may be sufficient to produce pressure upon the nerve root (Figure XIV:34B). If the plane of the articulation is inclined with its upper edge forward a backward subluxation of the uppermost vertebra will result.

If imbrication is excessive, painful bony impingements occur between the tips of the articular processes and the adjacent portion of the neural arch (Figure VI:1). A fibrocartilage pad or bumper may develop on the tip of the impinging articular process. A sclerosis or eburnation of the bony structure at the point of contact serves to counter the localized pressure stress (Figure VI:11). However, if the stress continues an actual bony erosion occurs as a result of the pressure. Harris and Macnab point out the relationship of symptoms to the posterior joint changes secondary to intervertebral disc degeneration.

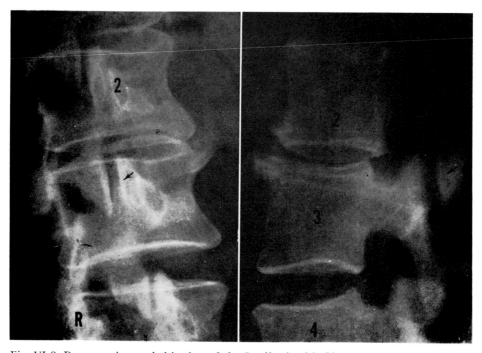

Fig. VI:2. Degeneration and thinning of the L_2 disc in this fifty-seven year old male has resulted in a backward displacement of L_2 and widening of the posterior joints with consequent capsule disturbance (*arrows*). Compare the discs, foramina and the posterior articulations at the 2-3 and 3-4 levels.

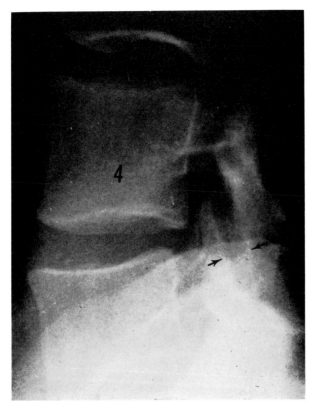

Fig. VI:3. This thirty-eight year old woman was involved in a head-on automobile collision in which she was thrown forcibly backward dislocating the 4th lumbar body posteriorly and spraining the apophyseal articulations. Arrows indicate the joint widening. The disc is normal in thickness.

THE SYNOVIA

Since the articular surfaces are not completely in contact, there are meniscus-like tabs of synovial tissue projecting inward from the capsule between these joint surfaces. Some of these tabs appear ragged or lobulated and may be quite long and thin, especially at the upper and lower joint margins. They consist of fibrous tissue, fibrocartilage, fat cells and many blood vessels. If there is a wider space between the articular processes, it is filled in with a thicker fleshy fat pad (Figures VI:12 - VI:13 - VI:14 - VI:15 and VI:16).

Sections of the joint capsule tissue and synovia prepared by a special nerve stain method reveal a rich supply of sensory nerve fibers in the capsule (Figures VI:17 - VI:18 and VI:19). No nerve fibers were observed in the synovia. Kellgren in studying the articular capsules of both animals and humans found a paucity of sensory fibers in the synovia. However he observed a rich plexus of sensory nerves in the fibrous ligaments of the joint capsule.

LIGAMENT AND NERVE STUDIES

Sections of the anterior and posterior longitudinal ligaments were cut in both the transverse and longitudinal direc-tions. These included the superficial layers of the annulus fibrosus wherever the disc was encountered. The material,

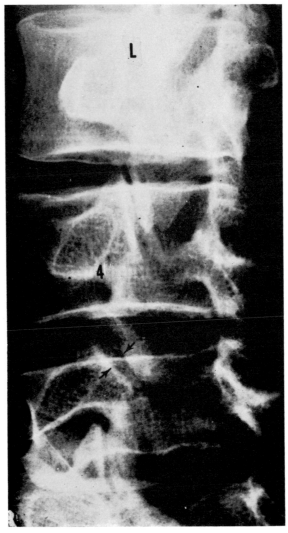

Fig. IV:4. After working in a stooped position this thirty-three year old male suddenly ex-perienced low back pain as he attempted to straighten up. The patient stood with a list toward the right side with the weight carried on the right foot. He was unable to bend at all toward the left. The roentgenogram shows a widening of the 4th left posterior articulation (*arrows*). Compare with those joints above and below. Sprain of the apopyseal articulations with widening of the space between the joint surfaces is not infrequent. Like other diarthro-dical articulations these structures may be subjected to trauma or disease. Also the sudden onset of pain upon straightening up from the stooped position is even more commonly en-countered. It would seem that the impingement of soft tissue between the articular sur-faces is a distinct possibility (See Figure VI:15.)

mounted in paraffin, was stained by a modified Bodian and Ungewitter silver nerve stain.

The anterior longitudinal ligament, closely attached to the vertebral bony surface, is made up of loosely arranged bundles of longitudinal fibers occasionally bound together by firm slender transverse bands of fibrous tissue. Where the anterior longitudinal ligament passes over the disc it is firmer and of much greater density, apparently adding some degree of support to that structure. Also it remains more or less separate from the annulus fibrosus and there may be small nerves between them. Upon the anterior surface of the ligament is an abundant supply of blood vessels and many nerves both large and small as well as the sympathetic chain. The nerve bundles, surrounded by the perineurium, contain many large alpha fibers some with well visualized myeline sheaths. Coursing with these are countless numbers of smaller gamma fibers and unmyelinated nerve elements. The nerves and the blood vessels penetrate the anterior ligament at certain points and their branches run in all directions between the bundles of longitudinal fibers (Figures VI:20, VI:21 and VI:22).

The posterior longitudinal ligament, on the other hand, is entirely detached from the vertebral body (Figures I:7 and

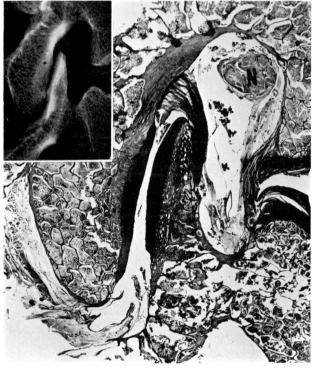

Fig. VI:5. Longitudinal section of a normal 5th posterior lumbar articulation from a male of fifty-seven years. The capsule above, formed from the ligamentum flavum, separates the joint from the normal sized intervertebral foramen. Note the relative diameter of the nerve (N) which in the lumbar region occupies the upper portion of the foramen, is no more than one-fifth the size of the opening which normally transmits it. The articular cartilage on both sides shows a normal thickness and smooth surface. The customary weakness of the capsule below is clearly seen. Insert is a radiograph of this joint before section.

VIII:6). Between this ligament and the posterior surface of the bone, occurs a rich plexus of nerves and blood vessels lying in fatty tissue. The posterior longitudinal ligament, unlike its counterpart in front, is dense, narrow, and very firm in structure. It does not pass separately over the annulus fibrosus like the anterior longitudinal ligament but fans out and blends with the fibers of the disc. Along the posterior, more dense, longitudinal ligament the nerve fibers tended to remain more upon the surface of the structure (Figure VI:23).

At no point, either in front or posteriorly, was I able to find any nerve structures within or between the fibers of the annulus. This corresponds to the observations of Jung and Brunschwig.

Of considerable functional significance was the observation of bare nerve filaments coursing between and actually within the bundles of the posterior ligament (Figure VI:24). I did not find any nerve terminations. Stilwell and Gardner have both observed sensory nerve endings within the fibrous structures of the tendons and joint capsules. These workers

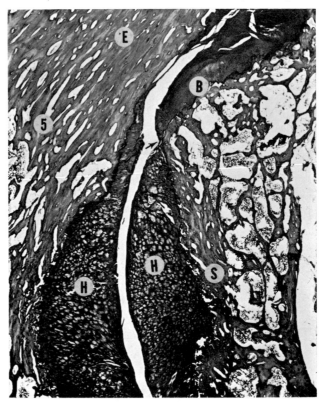

Fig. IV:6. Longitudinal section of the upper portion of a fifth lumbar articulation X9 to show the bumper formation of fibrocartilage (B) which develops between two points of bony pressure; in this case the superior articular process of the sacrum on the right and the inferior articular process of the fifth vertebra on the left. Compensatory eburnation (E) has occurred in the latter at the point of greatest pressure. The arrow indicates the nodal point between the fibrocartilage bumper above and the normal hyaline articular cartilage of the joint (H). There is some imbrication of the articular surfaces, the right side is higher, and fibrocartilage to counter this pressure is beginning to develop on the left side about opposite the arrow (Figure IX:4).

observed that twisting or stretching of these structures stimulated the pain endings. The capsule was found to be more sensitive than the synovia. Gardner reported that severe joint pain induced a reflex muscle spasm and if this was prolonged an atrophy resulted. The research of Jung and Brunschwig, studying the innervation of the vertebral articulations, is a classic. They were able to demonstate free sensory terminations in the ligamentous structures. They believed that the proprioceptive stimuli for balance and position of the spine arise in these afferent terminations and also that the origin of pain and reflex spasm occurs there. In the clinic of Leriche, muscle spasm was treated by anesthetizing the adjacent ligamentous structure. Jung and Brunschwig, working under Leriche, anesthetized the spinal ligaments of a patient suffering from tuberculosis of the spine. The spasm was relieved, only to recur when the anaesthetic was gone. They concluded from their studies that the sensory innervation of the vertebral articulations was located in the ligamentous structures.

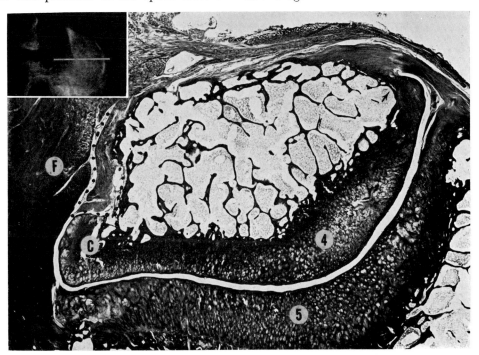

Fig. VI:7. Transverse section of the 4th left posterior lumbar articulation X10 at the plane indicated by the white line on the radiograph. The articular surface of the lower element from the 5th vertebral below and in front is concave and covered with hyaline cartilage (5). This opposes the convex catilaginous surface of the upper element (4). The ligamentum flavum (F) constitutes the capsule on the medial side of the joint. The arrow points above indicate the reflection of the capsule from the bone on each side. Note that the joint space on the left extends backward beneath the medial side of the capsule for a distance about equal to one-third of that between the articular surface themselves. The dotted lines enclose a tab of synovial membrane. C is a cushion of fibrocartilage attached to the medial border of the articular surface. It forms a bearing between the bone and the tough capsule structure and opposes the sidewise thrust of the joint. This section is seen from above with the posterior surface of the joint at the top of the illustration.

The importance of the apophyseal joints has merited our attention. It has been held that localized back pain, for the most part, arises in the posterior spinal articulations. Anatomical dissections and microscopic studies of these structures seem to confirm this observation. There is a laxity of the capsules.

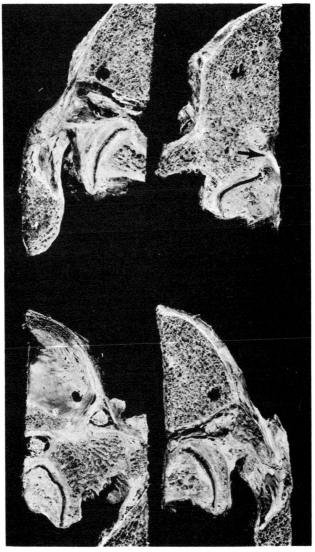

Fig. VI:8. A group of transverse sections through the posterior articulation. Note the intimate relationship between the nerve and the capsule of the joint. Some ossification in the ligamentum flavum is indicated by the arrow. The upper articulations have retained their cartilage and appear to be essentially normal. The lower left specimen shows erosion of the articular cartilage, pitting of the articular surface and bony spur formation at the posterior articular margin. The process from the lumbar vertebra above is always posterior to and/or medial to the process from the vertebra below. In the thoracic region the planes of the apophyseal articulations are nearly transverse (Figure XIV:17). Elsewhere the inclination of these curved planes varies considerably, not only at the different levels of the spine but between the two sides at the same level.

Back movements produce a gliding of one articular surface upon its fellow with some separation of the joint margins. Pinching of soft tissue structures between the articular surfaces would seem to be a factor in producing the "sudden catch," spontaneous type of localized back pain.

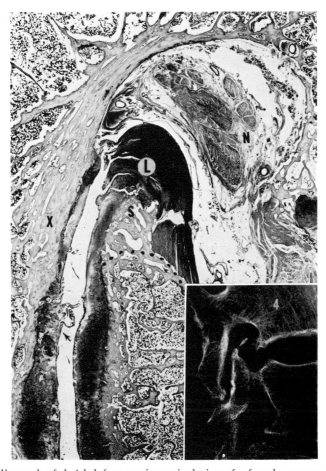

Fig. VI:9. Radiograph of th 4th left posterior articulation of a female seventy-three, shows a dense spur formation at the upper tip of the 5th superior articular process *(white arrow)*. The section (X7) shows that the spur has displaced the ligamentum flavum (L) upward the forward encroaching upon the intervertebral foramen and distorting the shape of the nerve root (N). Bony growth is occurring at the tip of the spur (S) which incidentally is devoid of marrow cells. The dotted line indicates the original position of the tip of the articular process. The black arrow in the joint space points to an area of cartilage fibrillation or early destruction. Immediately above the arrow is a partially detached fragment of cartilage which seems to have eroded the opposite surface. Such fragments of cartilage, when detached, become loose bodies within the joint. Normal cartilage covers the opposite articular surface below this level. The bony tissue of the upper element in back has developed an ivory-like density where pressure of the spur occurred (X). The radiograph shows impingement by a spur on the tip of the 4th inferior articular process against the isthmus of the fifth arch. A fibrocartilage bumper had developed at this point.

REFERENCES

Gardner, E.: 1960, *Bull, Hosp. Joint Dis., 21:* 153–161, Joint nerve supply.

Hadley, L. A.: 1961, *Am. Jor. Roent., 86:*270–276, Posterior joints.

Harris, R. I., and Macnob, I.: 1954, *J. Bone J. Surg., 36B:*304–322, Structure of discs.

Hasner, E., *et al.:* 1952, *Acta Rad., 37:*141–149, Movement.

Horwitz, T., *et al.:* 1940, *Am. Jor. Roent, 43:* 173–186, Arthritic.

Jirout, J.: 1956, *Acta Rad., 46:*55–60, Movements.

Jung, A., and Brunschwig, A.: 1932, *Press Med., 40:*316–317 L'innervation des articulations des corps vertébraux. Innervation of the vertebral body articulations.

Kellgren, J. H., *et al.:* 1950, *J. Bone J. Surg., 32B:*84–92, Innervation of capsule.

Keller, G.: 1953, *Zeitschrift fur Orthopadie und ihre Grenzgebiete, 83 BD., 4:*517–547, Die Bedeutung der Veranderungen an den kleinen Wirbelgelenken als Ursache des lokalen Ruckenschmerzes. Significance of the changes in the small vertebral joints as causes of localized back pain.

Keller, G.: 1959, *Zeitschrift fur Orthopadie und ihre Grenzgebiete, 91BD., 4:*538–550, Die Arthrose der Wirbelgelenke in ihrer Beziehung zum Ruckenschmerz. Significance of Arthrosis of the spinal joint in back pain.

Leriche, R.: 1930, *Press Med., 38:*417–418, L'innervation sensative des articulations. Sensory innervation of the articulations.

Lippmann, R. K.: 1953, *J. Bone J. Surg., 35A:* 967–979, Arthropathy.

Monger, F. P.: 1957, *J. Bone J. Surg., 39B:*6–22, Movements.

Schalimtzek, M.: 1959, *Acta Orth. Scand., 28:* 316–319, Movements.

Stilwell, D. L.: 1957, *Am. Jor. Anat., 100:*289–318, Innervation tendons.

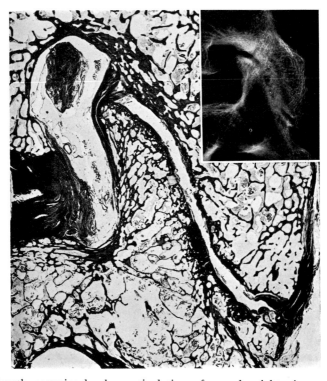

Fig. IV:10. Fourth posterior lumbar articulation of a male eighty-six years old X3.5. There is complete destruction of joint cartilage. Since there is no loss of intervertebral disc space, the foramen and nerve root are not encroached upon. Inset is a radiograph of the specimen before section. Compare with Figure VI:5.

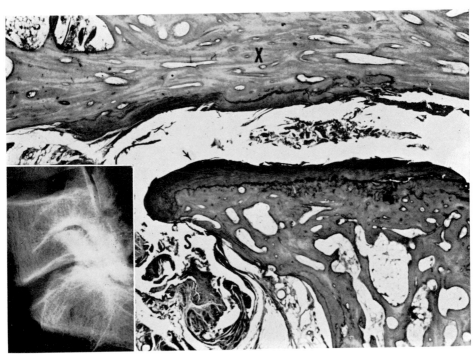

Fig. VI:11. Longitudinal section of the fifth lumbar articulation of a seventy-nine year old female. Imbrication and bony spur formation has progressed until extensive impingement has occurred beneath the fifth pedicle with eburnation of the latter. A fibrocartilage bumper at the point of contact has developed on the tip of the sacral articular process (*arrow*). The insert is a roentgenogram showing the telescoping and the sclerotic change in the bony structure of the joint. The photomicrograph (X18) of the tip of the sacral articular process shows the fibrocartilage bumper, a completely anomalous structure which has developed at the point of pressure. This is not the hyaline type of cartilage which normally covers the articular surfaces, as seen in Figure VI:7. The opposing sclerotic bone of the pedicle (X) is also protected by a slightly thinner coat of fibrocartilage. These cartilage bumpers are separated from the underlying bone by a narrow zone of darkly staining active cells. See Figure VI:6. Tabs of highly vascularized synovial tissue (S) are noted between the joint and the intervertebral foramen. (Courtesy of the *American Journal of Roentgenology*.)

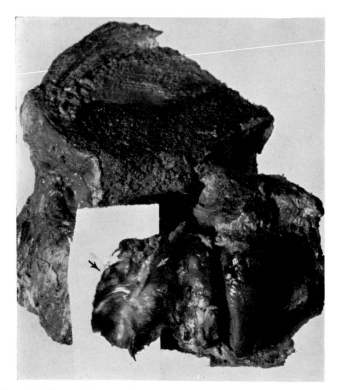

Fig. VI:12. Capsule dissected from the posterior surface of the 5th left posterior lumbar articulation from a female of sixty-five years. The capsule (*black arrow*) has been everted over a white background to show its smooth inner surface and the synovial tab (*white arrow*) which projected inward between the articular surfaces. The articular cartilage covers the edges of the articular processes and even the posterior surface of the one from L_5 on the right. This extends the joint space even behind the articular process and gives much greater mobility to the structure.

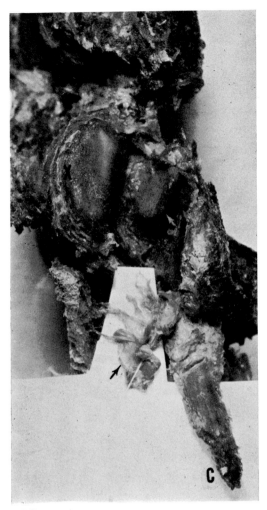

Fig. VI:13. The right third lumbar articulation from a male of sixty-nine years, laid open to show the articular surfaces and the synovial menisci. The capsule (C) was detached from the posterior surface of the upper element at X and reflected downward and to the right. It bears a long, thin, ragged fibrous synovial tab or meniscus. This was removed from between the articular surfaces and reflected to the left (*black arrow*). A thick, fleshy meniscus of fatty tissue is seen attached to the upper portion of the capsule but displaced slightly downward (*white arrow*). The thick meniscus was present above, because the upper margins of the joint were widely separated. The darker, concave, lower element of the joint beneath the fat pad was roughened by early degenerative change. One notes also roughening of the posterior edge of the upper element just to the right of X.

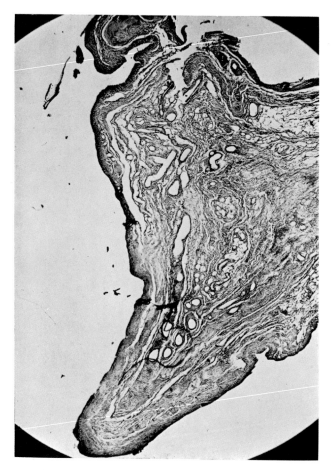

Fig. VI:14. Section of a synovial tab meniscus X40 with lobulation above. The structure is made up largely of fibrous tissue richly supplied with blood vessels and few fat cells. Other sections revealed a predominence of fatty tissue. I was unable to find evidence of nerve elements.

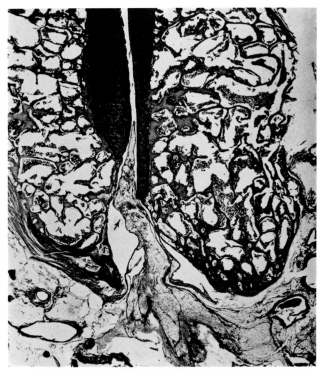

Fig. VI:15. Photomicrograph (X6) showing a large synovial tab (*arrow*) projecting upward between the articular surfaces. This originates from the inferior, loose portion of the capsule. The structure in this instance is largely composed of fatty tissue. The articular cartilage on the right side is partially worn down but the hyaline cartilage is of normal thickness on the left. This synovial tab might conceivably become pinched between the bony structures. (Courtesy of the *American Journal of Roentgenology.*)

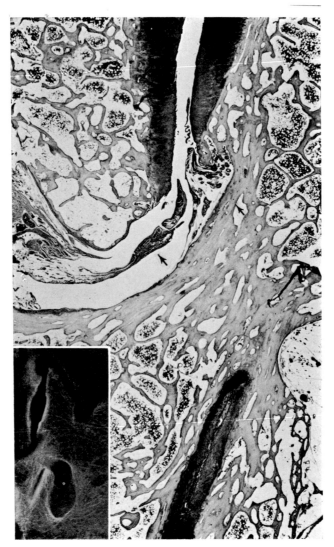

Fig. VI:16. Posterior articulations from a male of seventy-three years. The radiograph shows ankylosis of the 5th joint and a telescoping of the 4th articulation. The cartilages of the latter do not register exactly opposite of each other. The section X6 shows a long synovial tab as well as synovial tissue rich in blood vessels projecting into the 4th joint space from below (*arrows*). Articular cartilage and synovial elements remain entrapped within the ankylosed 5th joint below which is surrounded by sclerotic bone.

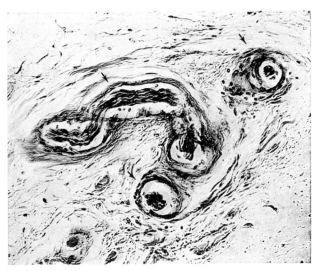

Fig. VI:17. Section from a posterior joint capsule X75 showing a group of nonmyelinated nerves *(arrows)*. These were stained by a modified Bodian and Ungewitter silver nerve stain.

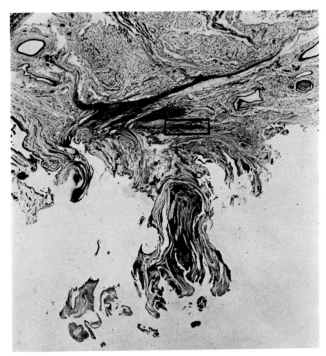

Fig. VI:18. A somewhat ragged synovial tab is seen projecting from the surface of the posterior joint capsule (X12). Note the sensory nerve *(in rectangle)* at the edge of the capsular tissue.

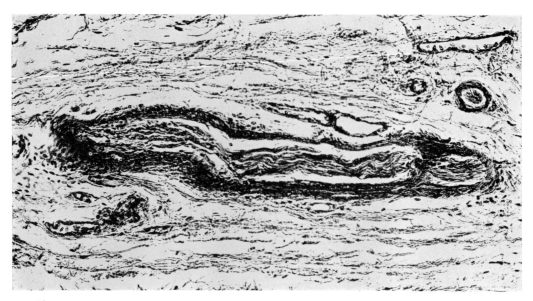

Fig. VI:19. Magnification X230 to show the unmyelinated sensory nerve fibers shown in Figure VI:18. They were stained by a silver nerve stain method. These three sections illustrate the excellent sensory nerve supply to the posterior joint capsule and their proximity to some of the synovial structures.

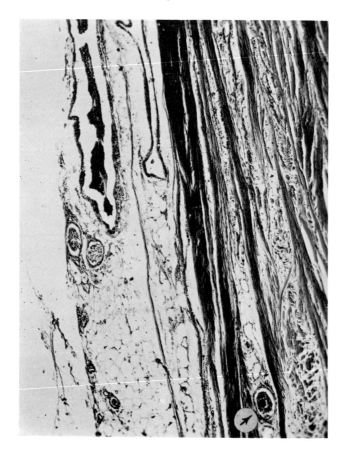

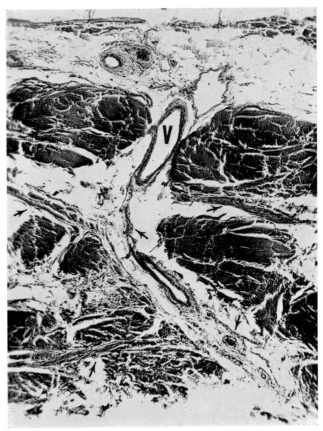

Fig. VI:21. In this section X175 the anterior longitudinal ligament is cut crosswise with its ventral surface above. The dark masses are the fiber bundles which make up the ligament here seen in cross section. The structure is penetrated at this point by a blood vessel (V) accompanied by a nerve. Many more nerves are visualized (four in this section) within the anterior longitudinal ligament *(arrows)* than within the posterior longitudinal ligament (Figure VI:23). Perhaps this is because the posterior longitudinal ligament is more dense. When the nerve happens to be cut in a longitudinal direction it is difficult to identify its fibers in the black and white reproduction. However in the original sections prepared by the Bodian-Ungewitter silver stain method, the nerve fibers are beautifully visualized as black filaments on a brown or yellow background.

Fig. VI:20. Sagittal section X175 of the anterior longitudinal ligament from the lumbar region. The fiber bundles are loosely arranged with open spaces between them through which course the nerves in various directions *(arrow)*. The fatty tissue on the ventral surface of this ligament is seen on the left. Within this are many nerves of different sizes as well as the blood vessels.

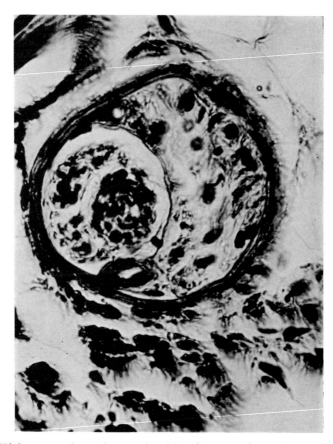

Fig. VI:22. High power photomicrograph X795 of a nerve from the same section as Fig. VI:21. This shows an intraneural blood vessel as well as both small fibers and large alpha fibers, some of them myelinated.

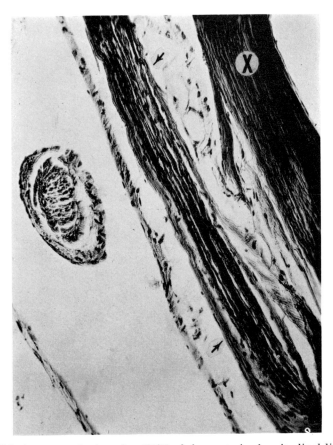

Fig. VI:23. This shows a sagittal section X175 of the posterior longitudinal ligament crossing the upper right hand corner (X). It is noticeable that the posterior ligament is much smaller and more dense in structure than the anterior. In the fat tissue on the ventral surface of this ligament is a nerve cut in a longitudinal direction (*arrows*).

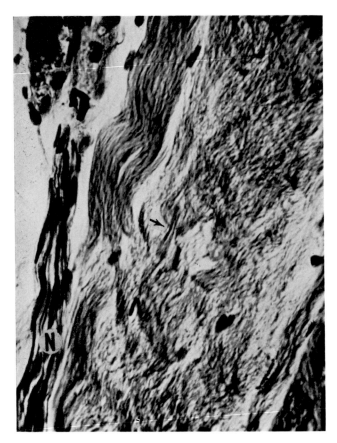

Fig. VI:24. In this high power photomicrograph X705 of the posterior longitudinal ligament a nerve (N) is seen penetrating the structure on the left side. Two isolated nerve fibers (*arrow*) were definitely identified on the stained section within the bundle although they are not distinctive in the reproduction. These studies confirm the observations of Jung and Brunschwig that the ligamentous structures of the spine are generously supplied with a sensory innervation.

Chapter VII

Changes in Bone Texture

THE NORMAL metabolism of bone tissue depends upon a balance between the constant anabolic and catabolic processes that are occurring therein at all times. When the anabolic or building up process predominates, the vertebra will present a dense, patchy or ivory-like appearance. On the other hand, a demineralized vertebral body with too little calcified bone may be caused by bone replacement, inadequate bone formation or by too much bone resorp-tion. Albright and Reifenstein have supplied the following classification for "too little calcified bone:"

1. Inadequate bone formation:
   a. Defect in matrix formation; osteoporosis.
   b. Defect in matrix calcification; osteomalacia.
2. Too much bone resorbed:
   a. Hyperparathyroidism.
   b. Chronic acidosis.

INADEQUATE FORMATION

A demineralization will gradually result unless there is a "maintenance growth," i.e., A replacement of the bone which is normally destroyed. A defect of matrix formation from diminished osteoblastic activity with its resultant osteoporosis may be caused by disuse. Inadequate protein from which to build the matrix may result from starvation, gastrectomy or liver disease. Deficient matrix production is responsible for the osteoporosis of old age incidental to atrophy and the lowered metabolic activity of that period (Figure VII:1). Post menopausal osteoporosis is said to result from a deficient stimulation by the estrogen hormone (Figure VII:2). Cushing's Syndrome results from an excessive adrenocortical hormone or prolonged administration of cortisone. This depresses the matrix formation (Figure VII:4). From these various causes osteoid matrix formation is deficient and osteoporosis results. In this condition the serum calcium, serum phosphorous and alkaline phosphatase are all within normal limits.

Osteoporosis also results from lessened osteoblastic activity in laying down adequate osteoid tissue in such conditions as osteogenesis imperfecta, hypophosphatasia and scurvy from lack of vitamin C (Figure VII:8). Biopsy studies show little evidence of osteoblastic activity.

In osteoporotic bone the hemopoietic marrow becomes replaced by fat (Figure VII:9). Replacement of the osteoporotic bone by normal tissue does not occur even when the cause of the condition has been removed. Innaccone *et al.*, also Albright and Reifenstein have shown in growing children the persistence of osteoporotic bone encased within normally forming bone. This occurred after cure of the adrenal disease. The resultant picture was similar to that of osteopetrosis (Figure XV:17).

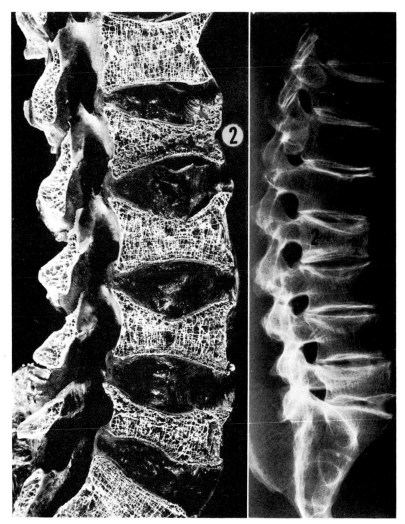

Fig. VII:1. Photo and radiograph of a cadaver specimen with osteoporosis showing delicate trabeculae formation. There was an old compression fracture of L_2 with minimal kyphosis. The ballooning discs bulge into the vertebral bodies somewhat more than seen on the film but in most cases the cartilage plates did not break. Ballooning occurs in the lumbar region of patients with osteoporosis but when the condition involves the thoracic spine the vertebrae become flattened or wedge shaped and the patient developes a kyphosis.

Osteomalacia in adults and rickets in childhood exhibit deficient ossified bone even though uncalcified osteoid tissue is adequate. In this case the biopsy may even show an excessive amount of osteoid matrix but it is not calcified properly because of a lack of vitamin D. Vitamin D promotes absorption of calcium from the intestine. The weakness of the bones stimulates an excessive activity of the osteoblasts in laying down new osteoid tissue so that in osteomalacia there is an increase of the alkaline phosphatase in contrast to Cushing's disease and osteoporosis.

Contrasting rickets and scurvy, in the

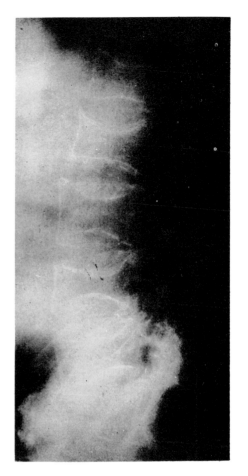

Fig. VII:2. Advanced endocrine demineralization in a woman of sixty years. So-called "fish vertebrae." The vertical trabeculae are not strong enough to withstand the pressure of the plates and as the former give away the discs bulge into the vertebral bodies. The cylindrical surface of the vertebra remains intact.

former the osteoid tissue is formed but does not calcify, while in scurvy, from lack of vitamin C, the osteoid tissue does not form. Normal bone formation is shown in Figure XV:1.

Deficient serum calcium may result from a low calcium threshold in the kidney. Sprue and steatorrhoea likewise may result in demineralization either because of loss of protein and/or calcium or because of loss of the fat soluble vitamin D.

We have now seen how bone may be deficient in amount because of not being formed in adequate quantities. Hyperparathyroidism on the other hand may induce a resorption of the bone tissue that is already formed.

HYPERPARATHYROIDISM

Generalized osteitis fibrosa cystica is a metabolic disease characterized by an osteoporosis involving the entire body. The primary form is caused by adenomas or hyperplasia of the parathyroid glands.

These structures elaborate a secretion, parathormone, which regulates calcium metabolism and the activity of the osteoclasts. In the presence of parathyroid adenomas an increased amount of parathormone is produced thus mobolizing an excessive amount of calcium from the bones leaving the skeletal structures partially demineralized. As a result the amounts of calcium in the blood and urine are both increased; while phosphorous, if the kidney is permeable to that substance, is decreased in the blood but increased in the urine. As a result the laboratory examination will show an increase of serum calcium and a decrease of phosphorous while both substances are increased in the urine. Because the bones are weakened, osteoid production is stimulated with the result that here as in osteomalacia the serum alkaline phosphatase value is elevated. A gradual loss of bone substance from the entire skeleton occurs. This progressive demineralization is relentless and eventually results in the death of the patient unless the parathyroid tumor is removed. Prompt relief of symptoms with eventual replacement of the bone deficiencies may be expected following surgery.

A secondary form of hyperparathyroidism may develop as a defense against the low serum calcium of pregnancy, lactation or incidental to chronic renal disease. With renal insufficiency and acidosis the kidneys excrete increasing amounts of calcium. This results in the development of nephrocalcinosis and nephrolithiasis. Acidosis is also increased by the retention of waste products incidental to the impaired excretion.

Since low blood calcium stimulates parathyroid activity, renal osteodystrophy establishes a vicious cycle with progressive renal damage, acidosis, loss of serum calcium, nephrocalcinosis and

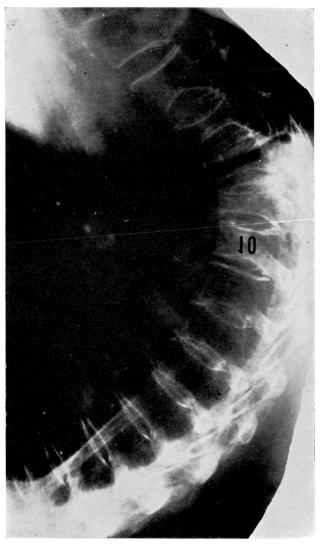

Fig. VII:3. Osteoporosis with kyphosis at the T-L level in a woman of eighty-five years. The localized compression of the lower thoracic vertebrae had resulted from an injury five years before.

hyperparathyroidism. There is a gradual replacement of the bone by proliferative connective tissue and uncalcified osteoid, giving rise to the term osteitis fibrosa cystica. Biopsy shows the marrow spaces filled with fibrous tissue. The osteoclasts are increased and there are many osteoblasts laying down osteoid tissue.

The demineralized vertebral bodies may fracture or show biconcave deformity, wedging or flattening. A differential point of considerable value is the pres-

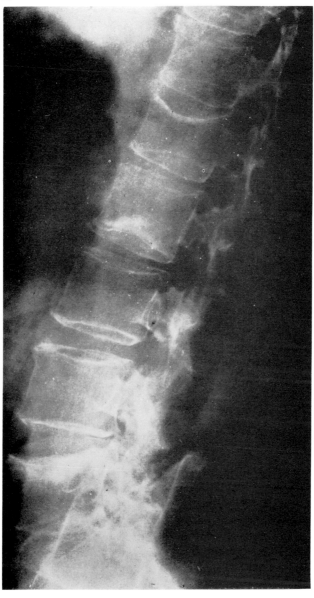

Fig. VII:4. Cushing's syndrome in an obese patient of fifty years following prolonged steroid therapy. She had suffered multiple exaccerbations and remissions of rheumatoid arthritis over a period of three years. There was generalized loss of ossified bone and the characteristic ground glass appearance together with infractions of L_1 - L_2 and L_5. (Courtesy of the University Hospital.)

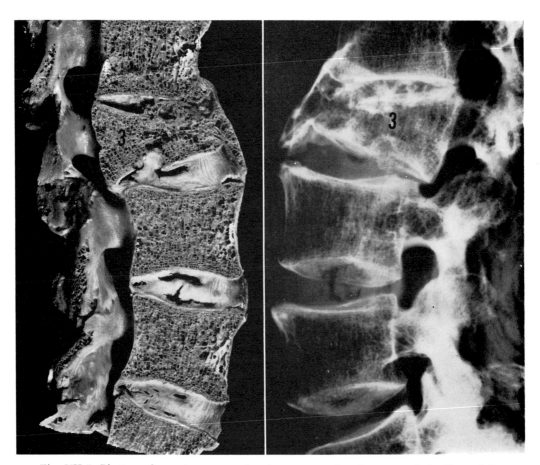

Fig. VII:5. Photo and roentgenogram showing compression fractures of the L_2 and L_3 vertebrae. There has been some backward displacement and kyphosis. A portion of the 3rd disc has become herniated upward into the fragmented 3rd body. At various levels in this specimen and in Figures VII:1 and VII:17 note the horizontal trabeculae adjacent to and parallel with the vertebral end plates. This is a condition dating from the adolescent growth period. See Figure VIII:20.

Fig. VII:6. Photo and roentgenogram of a specimen showing a compression fracture of T_{12} in a male of seventy-four years. There is evidence of healing and some kyphosis with the anterior portion of the vertebra collapsed. The compression has caused this vertebra to be more dense than the adjacent osteoporotic bodies. The section (S) of the central portion of this vertebra X9 shows bulging of the cartilage plates (*arrows*). These plates have each broken near the apex of the bulge. The osteoporotic trabeculae are quite slender. The marrow substance of the vertebral body is seen to be invading the upper disc on the left side at X.

---------->

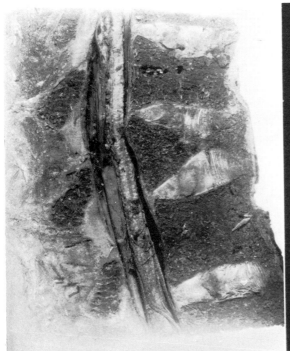
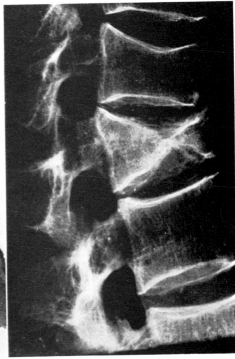

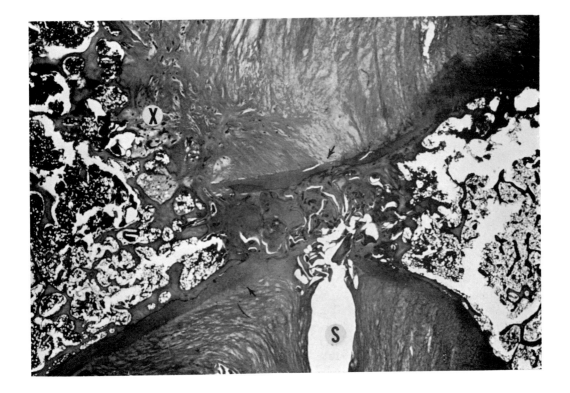

ence in hyperparathyroidism of subperiosteal areas of cortical resorption. These appear in the hands or the lateral ends of the clavicles and are not seen in osteomalacia or osteoporosis (Figure VII:13). The term "renal rickets" is a misnomer for this disease since rickets is a delayed calcification of osteoid tissue but renal osteodystrophy is a breaking down of bone already formed.

Hyperparathyroidism and chronic renal failure with osteosclerosis have been reported by various authors (see under references) rather than the usual demineralization. These observers have reported such cases of increased bone density involving the spine. Bands of dense bone formation adjacent to the discs may resemble those seen in osteopetrosis, Figure XV:17. In other cases

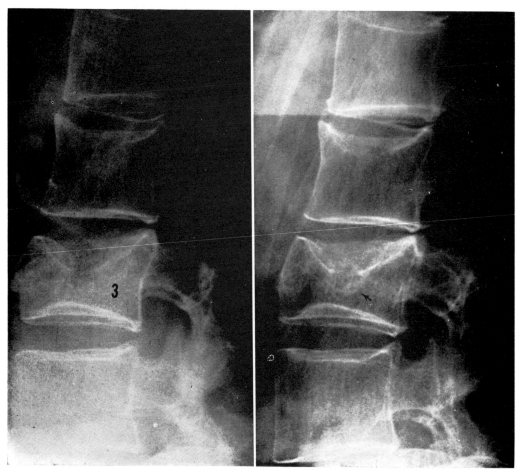

Fig. VII:7. Generalized osteoporosis probably of endocrine origin in a woman of fifty-six years, who developed compression fracture following minimal trauma. Sudden pain in the lower back referred to the left leg had occurred after lifting a heavy piece of furniture three months before. She had suffered less pain recently. Radiograph on the left shows a compression fracture of L_3 with the anterior fragment rotated on a transverse axis and with the disc above bulging downward into the vertebra. The film on the right, made fifteen months later, reveals healing of the fracture and increased density of bone surrounding the herniated disc (*arrow*). There was obviously bulging of disc substance downward into the osteoporotic second vertebra also.

the typical os in os formation may be seen wherein a small core of denser bone appears in the center of each vertebral body. Biopsy of these has shown thick heavy dense trabeculae with osteoid on their surfaces. On these coarse trabeculae the osteoblastic activity exceeds the osteoclastic, thus resulting in bone of increased density (Figure VII:12 and VII:13).

Certain of the collagen diseases as well as chronic renal failure, produce a demineralization of the skeletal structures. Nephrocalcinosis, renal calculi or calcific deposits in the soft tissues may occur as a result of this resorption (Figure VII:14).

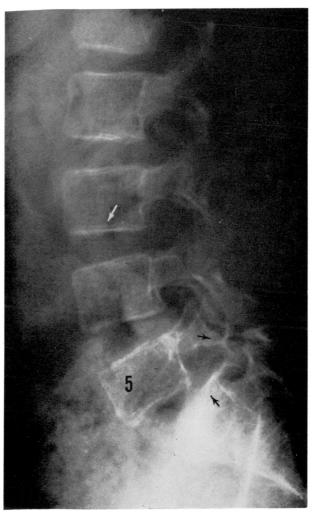

Fig. VII:8. Female of nine years with osteogenesis imperfecta. The child has blue sclera, and has sustained repeated fractures after minor traumata. There is a break in the 5th neural arch with a first degree spondylolisthesis *(black arrows)*. Osteoporosis of this type is caused by inadequate osteoblastic activity. Note the lines of increased density parallel to the epiphyseal plates *(white arrow)*. These correspond to the previous locations of the growth lines at times of temporarily arrested growth. (Courtesy of the Children's Hospital Home of Utica, N. Y.)

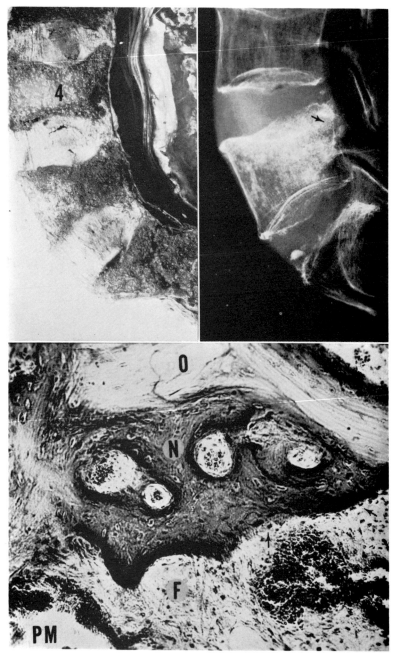

Fig. VII:9. Advanced osteoporosis in a female of eighty-six years. The trabeculae are slender. Fat marrow occupies the central portion of the 4th vertebra, giving it a yellow color. An infraction has occurred in the posterior portion of L₅ (*arrow*). The increased density seen on the roentgenogram and low power section (S) of L₅ is cast by layers of newly formed cellular bone tissue laid down upon the surface of the old trabeculae. In the photomicrograph (PM) X100 the old laminated trabeculae (O) are covered by layers of new bone (N) formed by the osteoblasts (*arrows*) in the fibrous tissue (F). In the low power (S) section X9 the new bone trabeculae (T) are seen along the healed fracture line.

OTHER CAUSES OF LESSENED BONE SUBSTANCE

Replacement of the normal bone tissue in the vertebral bodies may occur from a variety of different causes, the most common of which is malignancy. This may be either primary or metastatic, and at one or multiple levels.

Hemangiomas which are cavernous spaces lined with a single layer of cells and filled with blood were found by Schmorl in 10 per cent of the specimens examined. Many of these are too small to be visualized upon the roentgenogram. They are characterized by areas of radiolucency interspersed with coarse trabeculae arranged in a longitudinal axis. The neural arch may be involved. There may be pain and muscle spasm but they are usually asymptomatic un-

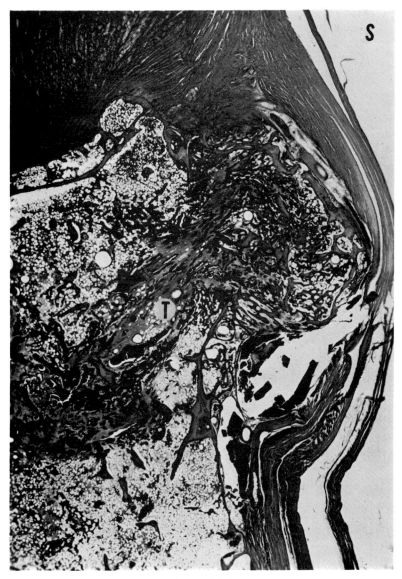

Fig. VII:9 A

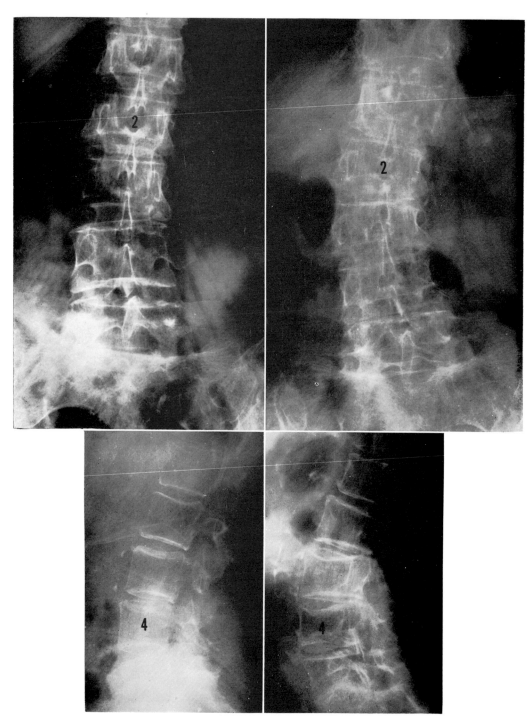

Fig. VII:10. Osteomalacia developing in a woman over a period of eight years. Radiographs on the left were made at age sixty-four because of low back pain referred down the left leg. These show some demineralization. During the following eight years the patient developed Looser's "umbauzonen," lines of decreased density in the ribs with stress fractures and a compression fracture of L_2 on the left side with a resultant scoliosis. On the later films at age seventy-two in addition to the scoliosis one may note compression of L_4, increased calcification of the abdominal aorta and calcific deposits in the region of the left kidney, probably indicative of chronic renal disease with acidosis.

less the spinal canal is invaded. Bell has reported myelopathy as a result of collapse and compression (Figures VII:15, VII:16 and VII:17).

Leukemic cell infiltration of the vertebral bodies, as in the long bone, is characterized by a band of radiolucency adjacent to the zone of provisional calcification (Figure VII:18). In the Cooley's anaemia and also the sickle cell type, there may be a diffuse infiltration with generalized demineralization of the entire vertebral body. The replacement of the marrow by the leukemic cells causes a disruption of the cancellous bone structure. Later myelosclerosis may occur.

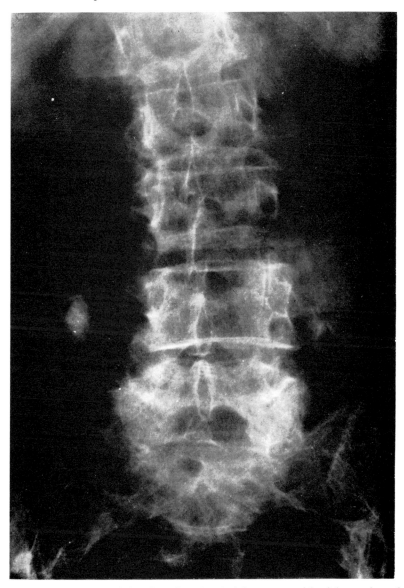

Fig. VII:11. Hyperparathyroidism in a female of eighty years with right nephrocalcinosis in a nonfunctioning kidney. There was also a right ureteral calculus. The roentgenograms revealed a spotty demineralization, especially in the pelvic bones. (Courtesy of the University Hospital.)

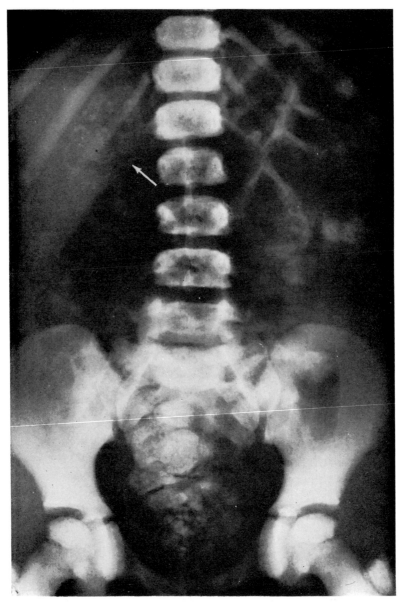

Fig. VII:12. This nine year old female in chronic renal failure developed progressive osteo-sclerosis of the spine. Earlier at the age of six the bones had showed a demineralization. At that time there was a decreased renal function and nephrocalcinosis. Two years later, how-ever the bones had begun to show diffuse sclerotic changes, a condition which gradually in-creased throughout the remainder of her life. Cortical sclerosis encroached upon the medul-lary cavities. In addition to the nephrocalcinosis (*white arrow*) there were calcific deposits in various vessels and soft tissues of the body. Note the sclerosis at the base of the skull as well as the cervical spine. All of the vertebral bodies as well as the ilia and the femurs were sclerotic. This child suffered loss of bone calcium in the beginning but later with the development or renal failure as reported by Vaughan and by Templeton an unusual type of secondary hyperparathyroidism occurred with osteosclerosis. (Courtesy of the Syra-cuse Memorial Hospital.)

Thyrotoxicosis with increased metabolism from hyperthyroid disease results in osteoporosis because of increased calcium excretion and lessened matrix formation.

FIBROUS DYSPLASIA

This is a condition of the bones characterized by radiolucent areas which appear to be like cysts, but upon biopsy they are found to be filled with fibrous tissue. The etiology is unknown. The disease occurs in childhood or early life; over seventy per cent of the cases appearing before the twentieth year. The ultimate prognosis is good.

As the fibrous tissue gradually replaces bone the medullary canals become widened and the cortex thinned. The bones become weakened and pathological fractures are common. The skull may show sclerotic involvement simulating Paget's disease or punched out areas like xanthomatosis. Rarely there is an osteoporosis of the vertebrae with biconvex discs, collapse, angulation or kyphoscoliosis. The condition is frequently unilateral and may then be confused with enchondromatosis.

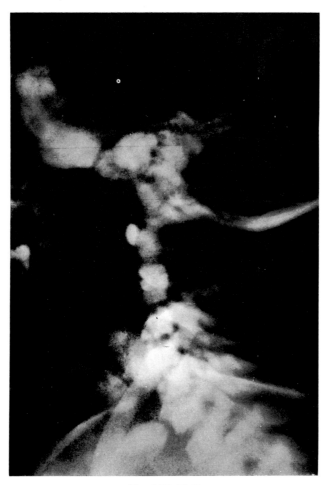

Fig. VII:12 B

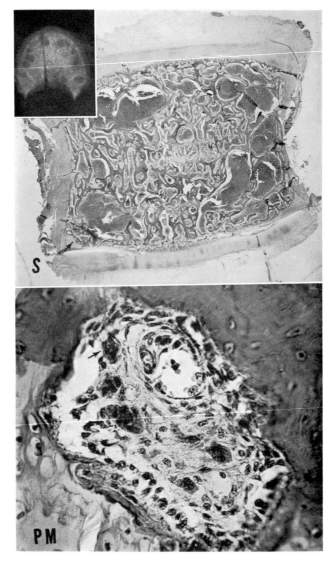

Fig. VII:13. Renal osteodystrophy with acidosis and secondary hyperparathyroidism in a female infant with bilateral polycystic kidneys. The pyelogram made at four weeks reveals left utero-pelvic stenosis. Each vertebral body at that time showed a dense core and a radiolucent zone adjacent to each epiphyseal plate. In these zones normal ossification was already deficient. The roentgenogram made at nineteen months reveals in each vertebra the central more dense core (*arrows*) with radiolucent zones on each side. The core has been described as the so-called "os in os," a condition wherein the core is a smaller replica of the larger bone in which it lies. A forearm study of the patient at 24 months shows deficient epiphyseal development and the inability of those structures to produce normal bone. Note the subperiosteal erosion of the cortex at the upper end of the radius (*arrow*). This is a differential point indicative of hyperathyroidism. Kidney failure developed and the child succumbed at three years. At autopsy cystic disease was found to have involved both kidneys with the right one completely destroyed. Section of a lumbar vertebra (S) X5 shows a dense mid portion with thickened trabeculae constituting the core. There are small marrow

$\longrightarrow$

Fibrous dysplasia is not confined entirely to the skeletal structures. Albright and associates have reported its occurrence with skin pigmentation and precocious puberty in young girls. The cause of this endocrine disturbance occurring in the more florid cases remains unexplained.

The disease is a metaplasia of fibrous tissue which is somewhat avascular. It may contain islets of cartilage which tend to ossify. The lesions may eventually stabilize but do not heal completely. Surgery has proved to be of questionable value. Early closure of the epiphyses in these children frequently results in dwarfism.

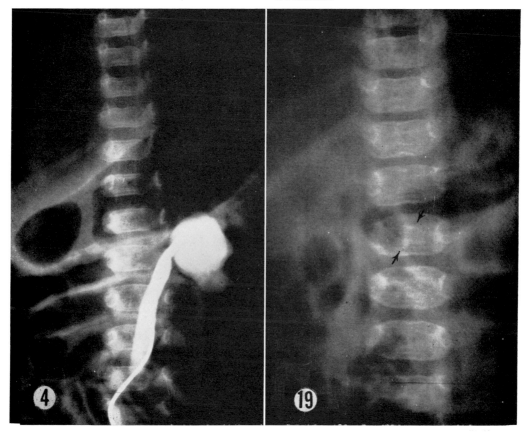

spaces in the central dense portion, many of them containing fibrous tissue. Ranged about the periphery are large spaces filled with normal appearing bone marrow. Enchondral bone formation along the cartilage plates is somewhat more restricted than usual. The inset is a roentgenogram of the adjacent vertebral body showing the peripheral marrow spaces. These zones of radiolucency are frequently seen in the dysplasias of growing bones but are occupied by bone trabeculae when the bone is normal. The photomicrograph (PM) X390 shows a lacuna taken from the extreme lower left corner of the section (tip of arrow on S above). Bordering the lacuna above and on the right is a darker zone of osteoid tissue. The lighter area in the lower left corner is poorly differentiated cartilage plate in which the enchondral bone production is deficient. Within the lacuna are five large, dark staining, multinucleated, osteoclasts *(arrow)*. Osteoblasts are ranged about the border of the space and with a blood vessel in its upper portion. This picture is well compatible with hyperparathyroidism. (Courtesy of the Memorial Hospital.)

Before roentgenographic visualization is possible, at least 1cc. of tissue must be missing from the vertebra if the bone is normal. If the structure is demineralized at least 60 per cent of the total calcium must be lacking before the change can be detected radiographically.

The characteristic picture of demineralization of the vertebra is well known. The ground glass appearance of the body with the sharply delineated cortex or the coarsened vertical trabeculae and loss of the horizontal trabeculae are all quite significant. Secondary changes, such as dorsal wedging, lumbar biconcavity, flattening or compression fracture occur somewhat later (Figure VII:19).

No attempt has been made to offer a complete discussion of the various conditions which may result in too little calcified bone. Certain bone conditions may present both osteolytic and osteosclerotic phases of activity. A definitive diagnosis cannot be made from the films alone.

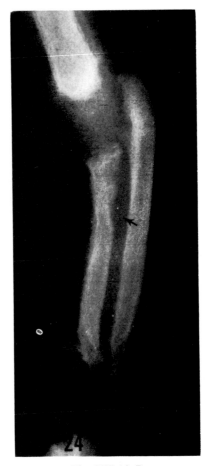

Fig. VII:13 B

INCREASED DENSITY OF BONE

The physiological eburnation of bone tissue subjected to pressure is a compensatory adaptation reaction. The trabeculae become shorter and thickened while the marrow spaces become smaller or disappear entirely (Figure VII:21). Points of contact between bony surfaces may become cushioned by newly formed bumpers of fibrous cartilage (Figure IX:4).

TRANSVERSE LINES

On the roentgenogram of a growing vertebra the white line adjacent to the vertebral disc is cast, not by bone, but rather by the calcified cartilage matrix in the zone of provisional calcification. This is the growth zone and has been called the epiphyseal line. (For the following immediate discussion see Figure XV:1). In the adult, the white line adjacent to the disc represents the perforated bony end plate of the vertebra.

During skeletal growth the cartilage production at the epiphyseal line may be temporarily halted by illness, fever or lack of adequate protein building materials. Whereupon the osteoblasts, unable to continue growth in a longitudinal direction, spread out laterally beneath the cartilage plate and deposit a layer of bone upon the undersurface of the calcified matrix already formed. This produces a network of bony trabeculae the thickness of which depends upon the rate of growth and the length of illness. This layer is seen on the roentgenogram as a white line parallel to the end of the bone and is left behind in the shaft when growth is resumed. In a slow growing bone like the vertebral body the stratum appears later as a line parallel to and near the cartilage surface (Figures VII:1, VII:8 and VII:17).

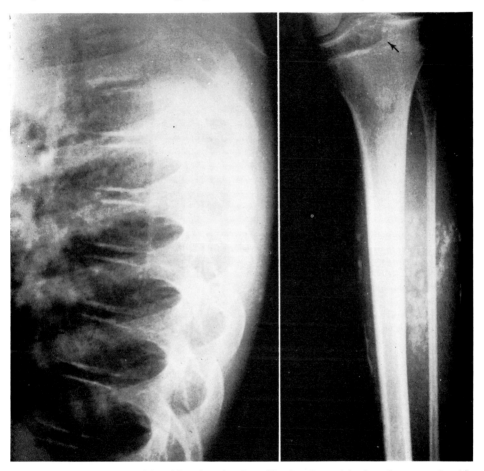

Fig. VII:14. Dermatomyositis with spine demineralization in a girl of twelve years. In this type of collagen disease the thickened bundles of collagen materal infiltrate the walls of the blood vessels. The demineralization and calcinosis here visualized result from vascular changes in the kidneys. Dermatomyositis, in addition to demineralization and calcinosis, is characterized by mottled erythematous skin and boggy, thickened, indurated subcutaneous tissue. The patient had arthritic changes with flexion deformities and myositis with tight painful muscles. Calcification was noted in the muscles and fascial planes and she developed a popliteal abscess which extruded cheesy, calcific material. This can be seen on the roentgenogram lying behind the upper end of the tibia (*arrow*). Dermatomyositis somewhat resembles another collagen disturbance scleroderma, but it is differentiated by facial edema, light sensitive skin and thickened brawny subcutaneous induration. These conditions have been well described by Talbott and Ferrandis. (Courtesy of The Memorial Hospital.)

We have seen how illness and malnutrition may alter the structure of growing bones. Other conditions such as congenital syphilis, vitamin deficiency and certain poisons may likewise leave their autographs.

Vitamin C (ascorbic acid in fruit juice) promotes osteoid (collagen) growth. In scurvy (lack of vitamin C) an adequate calcified matrix is produced but osteoid production is deficient. The spine may be osteoporotic as a result. This failure of osteoblasts to lay down bony tissue on the surface of calcified cartilage matrix is also a feature of congenital syphilis as well as lead and bismuth poisoning. These last two exhibit zones of increased bone density.

Phosphorous and fluoride poisoning stimulate the activity of osteoblasts to lay down thick heavy trabeculae of bone resulting in dense cancellous tissue with small marrow spaces. The roentgenographic picture is similar to that of osteopetrosis (Figure XV:16) or metastases from prostatic carcinoma (Figure VII:-23).

The reaction of bone to metastases from breast and prostate cancer has been ably studied by Sharpe *et al.* These authors found that about 97 per cent of breast cancer metastases were of the lytic type and about the same percentage of metastases from prostate cancer were bone producing. Emboli in the blood vessels become the source of infarcts of carcinoma cells.

In those metastases, principally from the breast, which exhibited the lytic type reaction, there were large masses of cancer cells but only very little fibrous tissue was to be found. Few osteoclasts were observed by Sharpe altho rapid destruction of bone was obviously occurring. Masses of tumor cells in direct contact

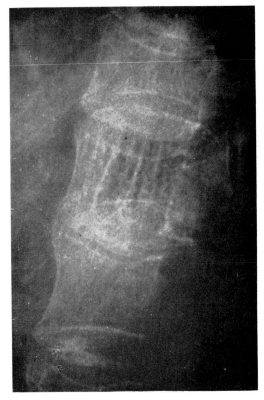

Fig. VII:15. Hemangioma of T_{12} in a woman of seventy-five years. This illustrates the pillar-like formation of the coarse trabeculae. These structures develop within the weakened vertebra along those longitudinal lines of stress perpendicular to the vertebral plates.

with the bone appeared to have the faculty of eroding that tissue and were acting as osteoclasts. Destruction of both spongy and cortical bone may also take place in the presence of osteoclastic activity as seen in Figure VII:20.

Osteosclerotic metastases, largely from prostatic cancer, were found by Sharpe *et al* to be characterized by few islands of cancer cells but consisted principally of fibrous tissue and osteoid. These authors believed that there was a transition of fibroblasts to osteoblasts and that prostate tumor cells were able to stimulate endosteal and subperiosteal osteoblasts to activity. Islands of osteoid within the fibrous tissue were seen to be surrounded by large active osteoblasts. Apparently the dense bone of "ivory" vertebrae such as seen in certain metastases, various poisonings, Hodgkin's disease and other conditions, results from a stimulation of fibrous tissue hyperplasia and its transition into bone forming elements (Figures VII:24 and VII:-25).

MYELOSCLEROSIS

In connection with various leukemias, anaemias and polycythemia vera there is at first a hyperplasia of the bone marrow elements. At this stage the roentgenogram of the vertebral bodies may present them as somewhat demineralized structures. Later as myelofibromatosis develops there is a replacement of the marrow by fibrous tissue with some transformation to osteoblastic cells. The condition gradually progresses and osteosclerosis of the vertebra occurs, with coarse bone trabeculae of increased width and number. With the diminution in size of the marrow spaces, extramedullary hemopoiesis is established. There is a compensatory enlargement of the liver and spleen. In myelosclerosis the vertebral bodies show an increased density of a patchy or homogeneous char-

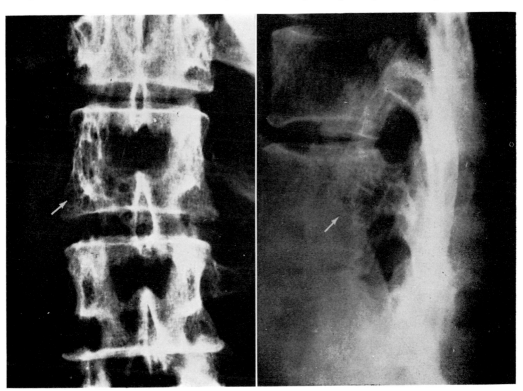

Fig. VII:16. Hemangioma of the left side of the arch in a female of thirty-four years. There was a history of chronic pain in the lower left dorsal region. The roentgenogram shows the lesion involving the left half of the neural arch and limited anteriorly at about the neuro-central junction (*white arrows*). Radiation to a total dosage of 2000r units was administered. Reexamination twelve years later showed the size of the involvement unchanged. At that time the patient complained of discomfort only upon fatigue.

acter and the patient presents with hepatosplenomegaly. Splenectomy and radiation therapy are both said to be contraindicated.

Apparently there are numerous conditions affecting the bone marrow some of them primarily osteolytic in character which may terminate as myelosclerosis. As indicated earlier, increased density of the vertebra may be secondary to metastatic malignancy, Hodgkins and marrow toxins such as benzol, phosphorous and flouride (Figure VII:25). Rarely multiple myeloma as reported by Engles *et al.*, and by Odelberg-Johnson may cause a myelosclerosis.

Osteosclerosis may also be encountered in urticaria pigmentosa (Figure VII:26) as well as vitamin A poisoning, the hypercalcemia of infancy and the atypical type of osteomalacia reported by Frame *et al.* For the early and late changes of myelosclerosis see Figures VII:27 and VII:28.

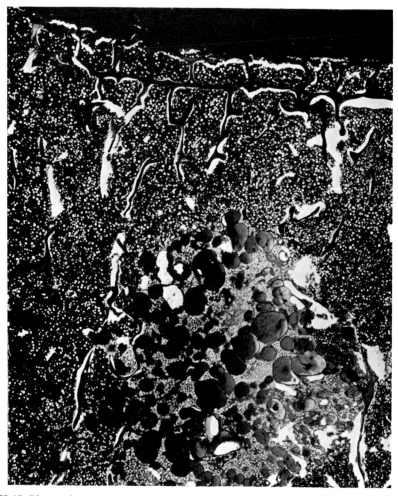

Fig. VII:17. Photomicropraph X12 from the vertebral body of a man eighty-three years old. This hemangioma was too small to be visualized upon the roentgenogram. It consists of dilated blood spaces which have replaced the trabeculae. In this osteoporotic vertebra the trabeculae are quite slender. Note the two parallel trabeculae underlying the cartilage plate of the disc at the top of the illustration similar to the condition seen in VII:9.

The response of the vertebrae to various influences may at times be paradoxical as we have seen in lytic bone marrow disease and the hyperparathyroidism which eventuates in osteosclerosis. This type of response is probably another compensatory phenomenon. Vertebral bodies which are being destroyed by a malignant process on one side may present a supporting bone column on the other (Figures XVI:5 and XVI:11).

In this chapter it has been possible to study only a few of the conditions which cause either a decrease or an increase of the vertebral bone density and to present the morphological changes responsible in some cases.

Publications

Albright, F., and Reifenstein, E. C., Jr., Parathyroid Glands and Metabolic Bone Disease, Williams & Wilkins Co., Baltimore, 1948.

Caffey, J., Pediatric X-ray Diagnosis, 4th Edition 1961, Year Book Medical Publishers, Inc., Chicago.

Epstein, B. S., The Spine, Lea & Febiger, Philadelphia, 1962.

Follis, R. H., Deficiency Disease 1958, C. C. Thomas, Springfield, Ill.

Geschickter, C. F., and Copeland, M. M., Tumors of Bone, J. B. Lippincott, Philadelphia.

Harris, H. A., Bone Growth in Health and Disease, Oxford University Press, London, 1933.

Schmorl, G. and Junghanns, H., The Human Spine in Health and Disease, Grune & Stratton, New York, 1959.

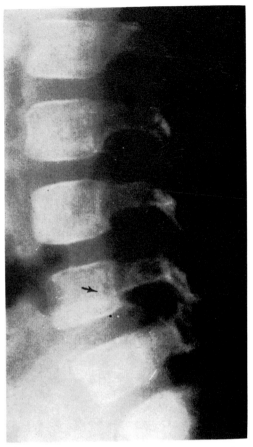

Fig. VII:18. Acute lymphatic leukemia in a boy of two years. Note the zone of radiolucency adjacent to the epiphyseal line similar to that visualized in the long bones.

Stowens, D., Pediatric Pathology, Williams & Wilkins, Baltimore, 1959.

Talbott, J. H., & Ferrandis, R. M., Collagen Diseases, Grune & Stratton, New York, 1956.

REFERENCES

Baker, S. L., *et al.*: 1954, *Brit. Jor. Rad., 27*:604–629, Symposium Osteoporosis.

Boland, E. W.: 1952, *J.A.M.A., 150*:1281–1288, Cortisone.

Chute, A. L., *et al.*: 1949, *Jor. Ped., 34*:20–39.

Cushing, H.: 1932, *Bull. John Hop. Hosp., 50*: 137–195, Hypophyseal, basophile adenoma.

Innaccone, A., *et al.*: 1960, *Ann. Int. Med., 52*: 570–586, Cushing's.

Jackson, W. P. U.: 1958, *J. Bone J. Surg., 40B*: 420–441, Osteoporosis.

Moldawer, M.: 1958, *J. Clin. Endocrin. Metabol., 18*:1028–1029, Permanent vertebral porosis.

Reiss, O., *et al.*: 1932, *Am. J. Dis. Child., 43*:365–386, Platyspondyle by Goucher cells.

Sherman, Mary: 1950, *J. Bone J. Surg., 32A*:193–206, Osteomalacia.

Sissons, H. A.: 1956, *J. Bone J. Surg., 38*:418–433, Cushing's.

Smith, R. W., *et al.*: 1960, *Ann. Int. Med., 52*: 773–781, Senile osteoporosis.

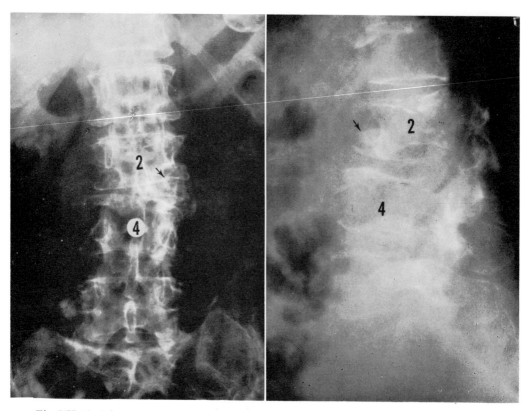

Fig. VII:19. Advanced osteolytic process (plasma cell myeloma) in a female of fifty-seven years. Replacement of the trabeculae has left only the outlines and ground glass texture to the vertebral bodies. There has been an infraction of L_2 and almost complete destruction of L_3, a small remnant of which is still seen in front of L_2 and paravertebrally on the left (*arrows*). There is a posterior displacement of L_2 with kyphotic angulation. The ring shadow at the top is an aneurism of the splenic artery. (Courtesy of the Memorial Hospital.)

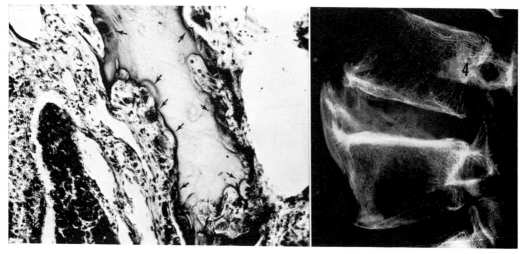

Fig. VII:20. Specimen showing metastatic carcinoma of the lytic type involving the fourth lumbar vertebra of a female sixty-six years old. The marrow of the vertebra was replaced by tumor tissue. The few remaining trabeculae presented a moth-eaten, eroded appearance. The photomicrograph X160 shows multiple lacunae along the surface of the bone and there are many darkly staining multinucleated osteoclasts present (*arrows*).

Osteoporosis—Lack of Protein Material

Baird, I. McL., *et al:* 1957, *Gastero. 33*:284–292, Gastrectomy.

Levin, E. J.: 1956, *Rad., 67*:714–722, Biliary atresia.

Melick, R. A., *et al:* 1959, *New Eng. J. Med., 260*:976–978, Gastrectomy.

Miyakawa, G., *et al:* 1942, *J. Bone J. Surg., 24:* 429–437, Steatorrhoea.

Pyrah, L. N., *et al:* 1956, *Lancet., 1*:935–937, Steatorrhoea.

Teng, C. T., *et al:* 1961, *Jor. Ped., 59*:684–702, Liver disease.

Hyperparathyroidism-Renal Osteodystrophy

Albright, F., *et al:* 1937, *Bull. John Hop. Hosp., 60*:337–399, Biopsy.

Borrelli, F. J., *et al:* 1945, *Urol. & Cut. Review, 49*:213–216.

Brockman, E. P.: 1927, *Brit. J. Surg., 14*:634–645.

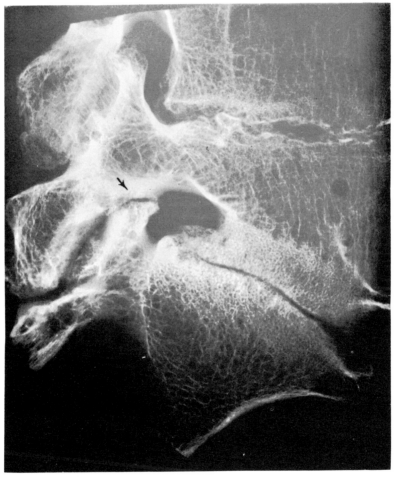

Fig. VII:21. Roentgenogram X2 of the specimen, Figure XIV:33Y. This contrasts the normal structure of the vertebral body with the greatly increased numbers of trabeculae and small marrow spaces within an area of bony sclerosis. Attrition of the S_1 articular process and disturbed relations of the fifth posterior articulation has allowed forward slipping of L_5. With telescoping of the posterior articulation an impingement of the remainder of the S_1 articular process has occurred beneath the fifth pedicle *(arrow)*. The resultant eburnation consists of very dense bone almost devoid of trabecular structure.

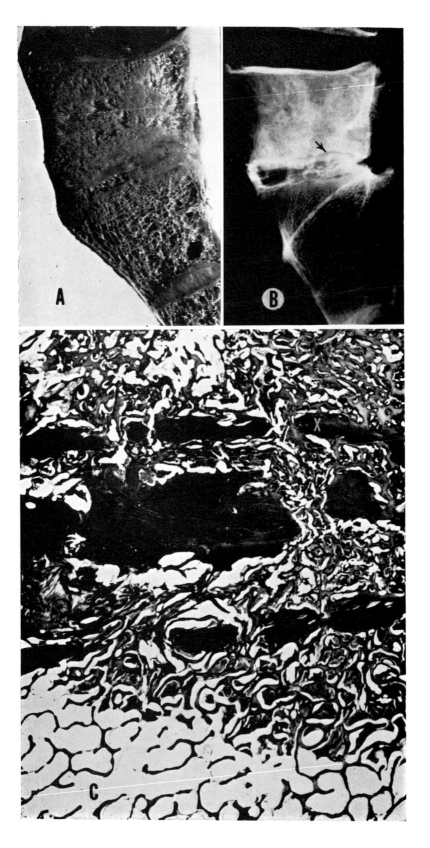

Cancelmo, J. J., and Neuhauser, E. B. D.: 1951, *Am. Jor. Roent.*, *65*:889–915, In children.

Dresken, E. A., *et al:* 1950, *Arch. Int. Med.*, *86:* 533–557, Sections.

Feinberg, S. B., *et al:* 1958, *Am. Jor. Roent.*, *80:* 468–474, Infancy.

Jackson, A., *et al:* 1950, *Arch. Int. Med.*, *85:*11–26.

McCune, D. T., *et al:* 1943, *Am. J. Dis. Child.*, *65:*81–146, Fanconi Syndrome.

Moehlig, R. C.: 1943, *Am. Jor. Roent.*, *50:*582–601.

Pugh, D. G.: 1951, *Am. Jor. Roent.*, *66:*577–586, Subperiosteal cortical resorption.

Rule, C., *et al:* 1944, *Ann. Int. Med.*, *20:*63–74.

Teng, C. T., *et al:* 1960, *Am. Jor. Roent.*, *83:* 716–731.

Hyperparathyroidism with Osteosclerosis

Crawford, T., *et al:* 1954, *Lancet.*, *2:*981–988, Renal disease.

Folles, R. H., *et al:* 1952, *Am. Jor. Roent.*, *68:* 709–724.

Templeton, A. W., *et al:* 1962, *Rad.*, *78:*955–958.

Vaughan, B. F., *et al:* 1959, *Jor. Fac. Rad.*, *10:* 197–200.

Wolf, H. L., *et al:* 1958, *Am. Jor. Med. Scien.*, *235:*33–42, Renal disease.

Haemangioma of the Vertebra

Bell, R. L.: 1955, *Jor. Neurosurg.*, *12:*570–576, Collapse and cord pressure.

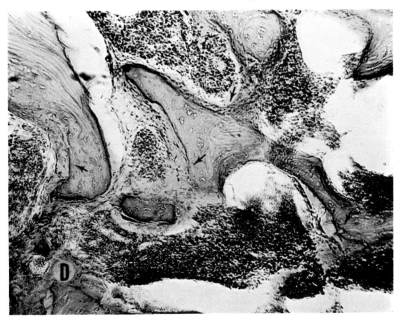

Fig. 22 D

Fig. VII:22. Photo, roentgenogram and sections from the lumbo-sacral level of a seventy-five year old man with sclerotic L$_5$ "ivory" vertebra (B). S$_1$ shows normal bony trabeculae except in its upper posterior portion. The photomicrograph (C) X9 shows the dense trabeculae and sclerotic tissue penetrating various breaks in the cartilages of the posterior portion of the intervertebral disc. These fragments of residual disc cartilage are visualized in both A and B *(arrow)*. The trabeculae of L$_5$ as seen in section C are thickened and close together, compared with the normal ones of S$_1$ at the lower margin of the section. The high power section (D) X130 was taken just above the break in the cartilage (X figure C). This section shows osteoid tissue being applied to the surfaces of the closely placed thickened trabeculae *(arrows)*. There are masses of marrow cells but relatively little fibrous tissue. The cause of this myelosclerosis is unknown although the roentgenogram resembles that of Figure VII:23.

Bucy, P. C., *et al:* 1930, *Am. Jor. Roent., 23:*1–33.

Ferber, L., *et al:* 1942, *Arch. Neurol. & Psy., 47:* 19–29.

Foster, D. B., *et al:* 1947, *Am. Jor. Roent., 57:* 556–561.

Ghormley, R. K., *et al:* 1941, *J. Bone J. Surg., 23:*887–895.

Lindquist, I.: 1951, *Acta Rad., 35:*400–405.

Manning, H. J.: 1951, *Rad., 56:*58–65.

Sherman, R. S., *et al:* 1961, *Am. Jor. Roent., 86:* 1146–1159.

Thomas, A.: 1942, *Surg. Gyn. Obst., 74:*777–795.

Bone Changes in Leukemia

Baty, J. M., *et al:* 1935, *Am. Jor. Roent., 34:*310–313.

Epstein, B. S.: 1957, *Rad., 68:*65–69.

Hilbish, T. F., *et al:* 1959, *Arch. Int. Med., 104:* 741–747.

Jaffe, H.: 1952, *Bull. Hosp. Joint Dis., 13:*217–238, Leukemia in Hodgkins.

Silverman, F. N.: 1948, *Am. Jor. Roent., 59:*819–843.

Demineralization—Anaemias

Barton, C. J., *et al:* 1962, *Am. Jor. Roent., 88:* 523–532, Sickle cell.

Becker, J. A.: 1962, *Am. Jor. Roent., 88:*503–511, Sickle cell.

Caffey, J.: 1957, *Am. Jor. Roent., 78:*381–391, Cooley's Anaemia.

Mosley, J. E.: 1953, *Rad., 60:*656–665, Sickle cell.

Reich, R. S., *et al:* 1953, *J. Bone J. Surg., 35A:* 894–904, Hemolytic.

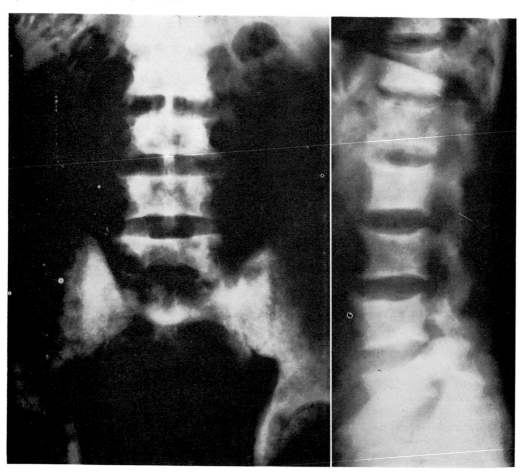

Fig. VII:23. Osteosclerotic type of generalized metastatic involvement from carcinoma of the prostate. The vertebrae show an ivory-like density but the discs seem to have remained essentially normal in thickness. (Courtesy of the V. A. Hospital.)

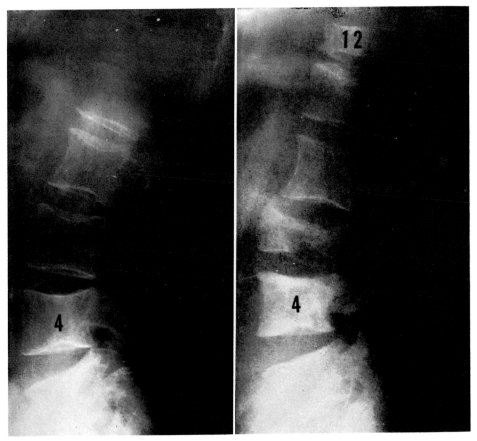

Fig. VII:24. A combination of both the lytic and the sclerotic types of spinal metastases from carcinoma of the breast in a female of fifty-nine years. The film on the left, made seven months following mastectomy showed demineralization of L_3 and the beginning sclerosis of L_4. The film on the right made two years subsequently reveals collapse of T_{12} and L_3. There has been considerable increase in the osteosclerosis of L_4 during this interval. Apparently cells from the same primary lesion are capable, both of stimulating fibrosis with bone production, and of acting as osteoclasts to destroy bone. (Courtesy of the Memorial Hospital.)

Fibrous Dysplasia

Albright, F., *et al:* 1937, *New Eng., J. Med., 216:* 727–746.

Coleman, M.: 1939, *Brit. J. Surg., 26:*705–713.

Dockerty, M. B., *et al:* 1945, *Arch. Int. Med., 75:* 357–375.

Furst, N. J., *et al:* 1943, *Rad., 40:*501–515.

Kornblum, K.: 1941, *Am. Jor. Roent., 46:*145–159.

Lichtenstein, H., and Jaffe, H. L.: 1942, *Arch. Path., 33:*777–816.

Wells, P. O.: 1949, *Rad., 52:*642–653.

Growth Lines—Poisoning

Caffey, J.: 1937, *Am. J. Dis. Child., 53:*56–78, Bismuth.

Eliot, M. M., *et al:* 1927, *Bull. John Hop. Hosp., 41:*364–388.

Holm, O. F.: 1942, *Acta Rad., 23:*549–651, Phosphorous.

Jackson, D., *et al:* 1935, *Jor. Ped., 7:*741–753, Scurvy.

Jaffe, N.: 1961, *Brit. J. Roent., 34:*429–437, Scurvy.

Park, E. A.: 1931, *Am. J. Dis. Child., 41:*485–499, Lead.

Park, E. A., *et al:* 1933, *Jor. Ped., 3:*265–298, Growth Lines.

Siegling, J. A.: 1941, *J. Bone J. Surg., 23:*23–36, Phosphorous.

Sontag, L. W.: 1938, *Am. J. Dis. Child., 56:*114–118, Phosphorous.

Wolf, H. G., *et al:* 1954, *Fort. a. d. G. d. Roent., 80:*141–153.

Abst.: *A. J. R., 73:*163 and *Rad., 63:*900.

Fluoride Osteosclerosis

Bishop, P. A.: 1936, *Am. Jor. Roent., 35:*577–585.

Kilborn, L. G., *et al:* 1950, *Canad. Med. A. Jor., 62:*135–141.

Linsman, J. F., *et al:* 1943, *Rad., 40:*474–484.

Moller, P. F., and Gudjonsson, S. V.: 1932, *Acta Rad., 13:*269–294.

Stevenston, C. A., *et al:* 1957, *Am. Jor. Roent., 78:*13–18.

Reaction of Bone to Metastases

Brunschwig, A.: 1936, *Surg. Gyn. Obst., 63:*273–282.

Sharpe, W. S., *et al:* 1942, *Arch. Path., 33:*312–325.

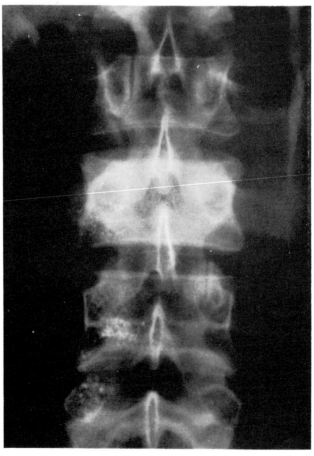

Fig. VII:25. Sclerotic type of Hodgkins disease involving the third lumbar vertebra in a male patient of thirty-two years. The patient has mediastinal, abdominal, pelvic and cervical distribution of his disease as well as the spinal process. A positive scalene node biopsy was obtained four years before. Some minimal evidence of beginning sclerosis was visualized in L$_3$ seven months before this roentgenogram. The fine motteling seen below remains from the lymphangiographic examination. (Courtesy of the Syracuse V. A. Hospital.)

Osteosclerosis

Fucilla, I. S., *et al:* 1961, *Rad.,* 77:53–60, Hodgkins.

Gerber, A., *et al:* 1954, *Am. Jor. Med.,* 16:729–745, Vitamin A poisoning.

Schiers, J. A., Neuhauser, E. B. D., *et al:* 1957, *Am. Jor. Roent.,* 78:19–29, Hypercalcemia.

Vieta, J. O., *et al:* 1942, *Rad.,* 39:1–15, Hodgkin's vs Lymphoma bone.

Young, J. M., *et al:* 1953, *J. Bone J. Surg., 35A:* 55–64, Sclerotic Hodgkin's.

Myelofibrosis-Myelosclerosis

Bersack, S. R., *et al:* 1946, *Am. Jor. Roent., 56:* 470–479.

Engles, E. P., *et al:* 1960, *Rad.,* 75:242–247.

Frame, B., *et al:* 1961, *Ann. Int. Med.,* 55:632–639.

Jacobson, H. G., *et al:* 1959, *Rad.,* 72:716–725.

Leigh, T. F., *et al:* 1959, *Am. Jor. Roent.,* 82: 183–193.

Mulcahy, F.: 1957, *Proc. Roy. Soc. Med.,* 50: 100–103.

Rosenthal, N., *et al:* 1943, *Arch. Int. Med.,* 71: 793–813.

Sussman, M. L.: 1947, *Am. Jor. Roent.,* 57:313–320.

Swenson, P. C., *et al:* 1938, *Rad.,* 31:333–339.

Windholz, F., *et al:* 1949, *Am. Jor. Roent.,* 61: 61–76.

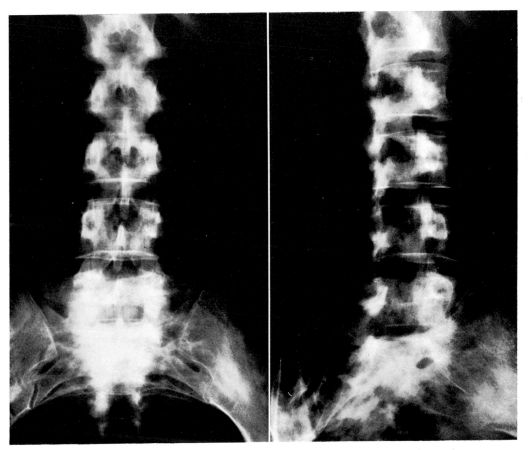

Fig. VII:26. Sclerotic changes involving the neural arches of the lumbar spine and sacrum in a female of forty years. The condition had been diagnosed as urticaria pigmentosa on the basis of raised nodular reddish brown papules. These are caused by intradermal infiltration with mast cells. Note that the sclerosis seems to be limited anteriorly at the neuro-central junctions both in the lumbar and the sacral areas. The bone changes are said to resemble closely the thickened trabeculae and increased density which is characteristic of fluoride poisoning and myelosclerosis. (Courtesy of the Syracuse Memorial Hospital.)

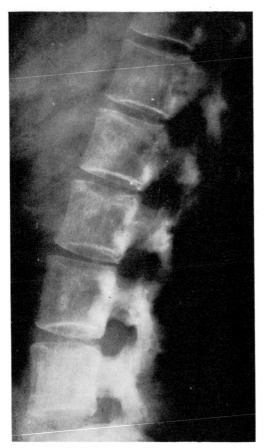

Fig. VII:26 A

Urticaria Pigmentosa

Jensen, W. N., *et al:* 1958, *Rad., 71*:826–832.

Zak, F. G., *et al:* 1957, *New Eng. J. Med., 256:* 56–59.

→

Fig. VII:27. Early changes of myelosclerosis in a male of fifty-nine years. There were at the time of this examination dense patchy areas of sclerosis in the vertebral bodies of both the thoracic and lumbar areas. The spleen (retouched) was enlarged downward nearly to the iliac crest (*arrow*). Seven years before, the patient was known to have hepatospleno-megaly but no increased density of bone structure was noted. At that time a biopsy sec-tion (S) from the iliac crest showed patchy areas of myelofibrosis replacing the bone marrow but there was no evidence of osteosclerosis. A curved area of fibrotic tissue (F) sweeps across the middle of the field with groups of marrow cells (M) above and below it. Other fields of bone marrow revealed "patchy areas of hyperplasia showing all types of blood cells." This section obviously indicated an early stage of myelofibromatosis. The patchy areas of bone sclerosis developed during the seven year interval. (Courtesy of Dr. John Hogan.)

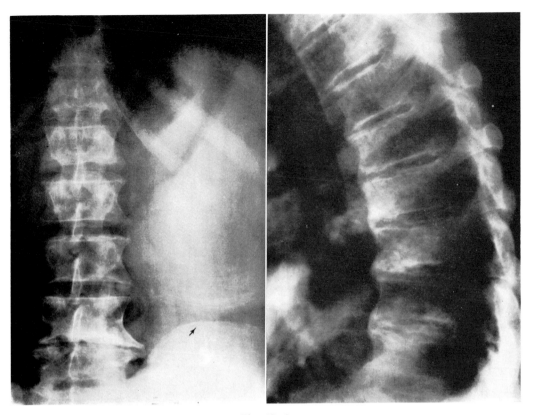

Fig. 27a-b

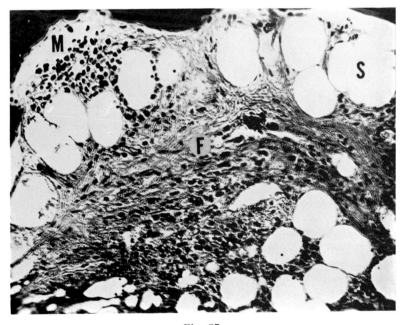

Fig. 27c

Fig. VII:28. Photo and roentgenogram showing late myelosclerosis in a male of eighty-four years. A section (S) X3 from C_4 shows the marrow cavity largely replaced by dense bony trabeculae (T). The central marrow spaces are partially preserved but there are only small spaces within the sclerotic trabeculae. The high magnification (HM) X160, shows a dense laminated trabecula (T) with fibrous tissue above (F) and a darker staining, S-shaped layer of osteoid (O) being laid down upon the surface of the bone. On the photograph the denser areas of the vertebrae are seen slightly lighter in color than the normal marrow (*arrows*). This section compared with that of Figure VII:27 reveals a late stage of myelo-sclerosis.

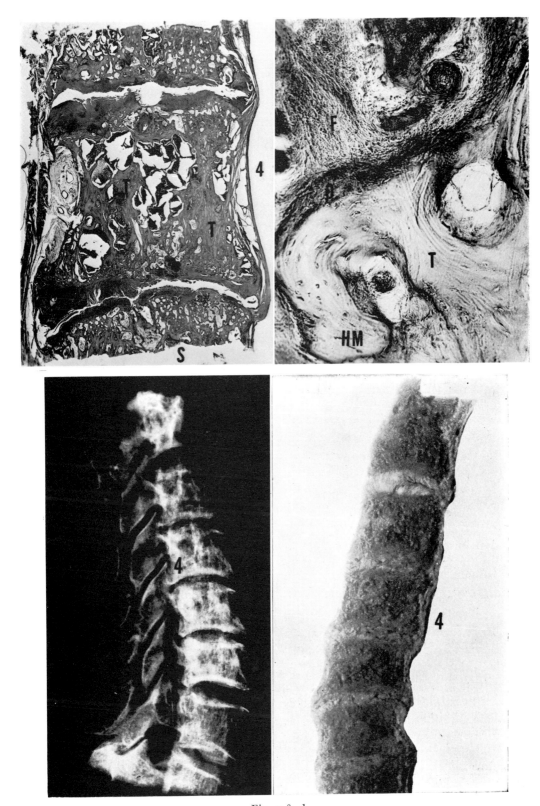

Fig. c & d

Chapter VIII

The Intervertebral Discs

As seen in Chapter I the discs develop from those dense cellular zones between the cartilaginous provertebrae. At about the tenth week of gestation the notochord becomes extruded from the vertebral body into the center of the disc tissue (Figures I:6 and I:7).

The center of the adult disc is occupied by the semigelatinous nucleus pulposus. This structure is bounded above and below by the cartilaginous plates adjacent to the vertebral bodies. Surrounding the nucleus is the dense annulus fibrosus. This is a very strong structure made up of interlacing cross fibers of collagen attached to the adjacent vertebral bodies in such a manner as to allow flexion, rotary and shearing movements. It is under elastic tension in the normal state and serves to contain the nucleus pulposus. This latter structure, high in water content, acts as a hydrostatic ball bearing, cushion and support for the superimposed weight. Its successful function depends upon the integrity of the surrounding annulus and the cartilage plates (Figure VIII:1).

Morphologically, as Hendry has shown, the nucleus pulposus is a lattice of collagen fibrils supporting a protein pollysaccharide gel complex. This colloid has the property, called imbibition, of taking up and holding body fluids even against substantial pressures. This makes the nucleus pulposus ideally suitable as a movable support of the superimposed body weight.

In the mid cervical region the disc serves somewhat as a cushion allowing the anterior-posterior gliding of the vertebrae upon each other (Figure IV:6). In the lumbar region however the normal A. P. movement is a rocking motion with the discs becoming somewhat wedge shaped upon extreme hyperextension (Figure XII:9). Since the hydrostatic pressure is equal throughout the disc and the edges of vertebrae are closer together at the narrow side of the wedge, the disc margins tend to bulge on the concave side of the curve (Figure VIII:2). The downward thrust of the superimposed body weight is transmitted centrifugally by the nucleus and balanced by the counter pressure of the elastic annulus fibrosus, thus creating a resilient cushion for weight bearing.

As a result of the natural ageing process the muco-protein gel deteriorates losing a part of its imbibition or affinity for taking up and holding fluids. Also some of the gel is replaced by coarse collagen fibrils. As the disc loses some of its water content, the intradiscal pressure becomes lessened allowing the cartilage plates to come closer together. This results in a bulging of the annulus fibrosus. In the lumbar region this lessened pressure within the disc permits an abnormal instability. As described by Knutsson, this very early evidence of disc ageing is indicated by a certain degree of backward-forward gliding of the vertebrae during flexion movements. This abnormal movement is somewhat analogous to the normal gliding movement in the more mobile cervical region. Instability is no longer present when the disc finally becomes sclerotic. Further inspissation of the nucleus and bulging of the annulus fibrosis changes entirely the dynamics of the disc. No longer is the body weight carried by the incompressible nucleus pulposus. With degeneration and disc thinning the weight becomes increasingly carried by the annulus fibrosus. This structure undergoes fissure formation and other degenerative changes (Figures VIII:3 and VIII:4 also VIII:26). Tension upon the longitudinal ligaments by

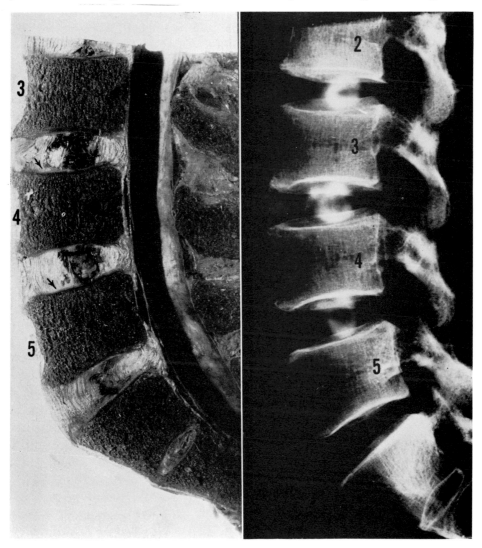

Fig. VIII:1. Lumbo-sacral area from a male of sixty-five years. The normal intervertebral discs have been injected with a colored radiopaque material. This reveals the nucleus pulposus as a roughly spherial mass occupying the central portion of the disc. The nucleus is surrounded peripherally by the dense annulus fibrosus while the cartilaginous plates (*arrows*) separate it from the vertebral bodies. The unbroken integrity of these structures is necessary for the normal dynamic function of the nucleus pulposus as a hydrostatic ball bearing. The L_2 disc, sectioned in a transverse direction, clearly shows the nucleus completely surrounded by the annulus fibrosus.

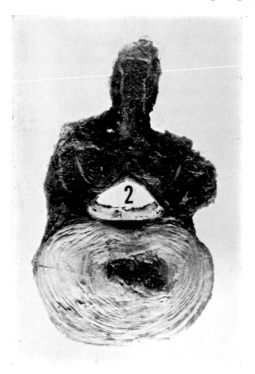

Fig. VIII:1 C.

the bulging disc substance stimulates the production of stabilizing spur formation.

Pressure upon the annulus is greatest at the concave side of any spinal curve. In the lumbar region this is likely to be posterior or postero-lateral (Figures VIII:5 and VIII:6). The nucleus pulposus under pressure can only escape from the disc thru a defect in the annulus fibrosus or one of the cartilage plates. Fissure formation of the annulus is a gradual wearing out process. It does not form by a single traumatic episode. Nachemson has shown experimentally, by the application of excessive stress, that it is impossible to rupture the disc without fracturing the vertebra. Since an outward herniation of disc substance must pass thru a break in the annulus fibrosus it is obvious that unless the annulus is detached a disc herniation cannot result from a single accident. Such herniation rather is the result of chronic attrition of the annulus fibrosus. It was also shown by stress experimentation that bone is more fragile than disc and that the end plate of the vertebral body is the weakest point. A sudden blow delivered longitudinally could fracture the central portion of the vertebral plate from a younger individual. In case the disc was partially degenerated the fracture was more likely to occur near the margin of the vertebra.

Upon lifting heavy objects the increased weight is necessarily borne by the intervertebral discs. If the lifting is done in a forward stooped position there is a tremendous leverage disadvantage not only to the discs but also to the sacrospinalis group of back muscles. Laborers who have developed massive lumbar osteophytes have thus increased the size and strength of their weight-supporting vertebral surfaces. In connection with weight-lifting in a stooped forward position it is interesting to note that if the diaphragm and the lateral abdominal wall muscles are held rigidly fixed, a substantial portion of the weight stress is transmitted directly to the pelvis by the abdominal organs and fluids without the interposition of the spinal structures at all. This can be corroborated by the sensation of increased intracranial pressure transmitted upward from within the abdomen during the effort.

DISC DEGENERATION

The ageing or degenerative changes may begin as early as the third decade. The nucleus loses much of its intercellular gelatinous material and becomes less hygroscopic. It gradually loses water in spite of the normal transfer of fluids across the cartilage plate in both directions. At the same time there is a gradual replacement of both nucleus pulposus and the annulus by fibrous elements and fibro cartilage. In this manner the normal resiliency of the disc is lost. The vertebral bodies rock backward and forward over the nucleus pulposus normally. However following disc degeneration the axis of movement becomes displaced backward into the posterior joints placing disruptive stresses upon these structures (Figures VIII:7 and VIII:8).

Disc degeneration has been termed a pressure atrophy. This is particularly true in the presence of scoliosis. Under these circumstances, the greatest degree of disc pressure occurs on the concave side of the curve. It is here that the more advanced degenerative changes and spur formation develop (Figures VIII:5 and XII:4).

SPUR FORMATION

Spurs or osteophyte growths are not pathological but rather they are a benign defense or compensatory provision. They supply support or immobilization to skeletal structures where needed. As we have seen, they serve on the concave side

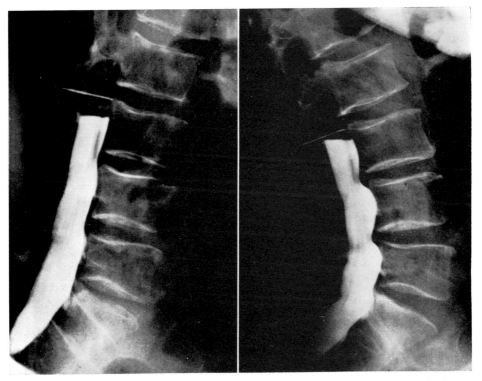

Fig. VIII:2. Lower lumbar myelograms made in flexion and hyperextension. In the latter the discs are wedge shaped. The margins of the vertebral bodies are closer together posteriorly than they are in front. This permits the normal backward bulging of the disc substance upon dorsal extension. During this movement the annulus fibrosus is compressed backward somewhat by the approximation of the margins of the vertebral bodies in back. Also note during hyperextension some infolding encroachment by the ligamentum flavum posteriorly. (Courtesy of Dr. Ivan M. Woolley, Portland, Oregon and Mr. William Cornwell, Rochester, N. Y.)

of spinal curves and at the margins of degenerated discs and arthrotic posterior joints. They strengthen bone weakened by age or disease and in certain cases supply a broadened support base to areas of increased dynamic stress.

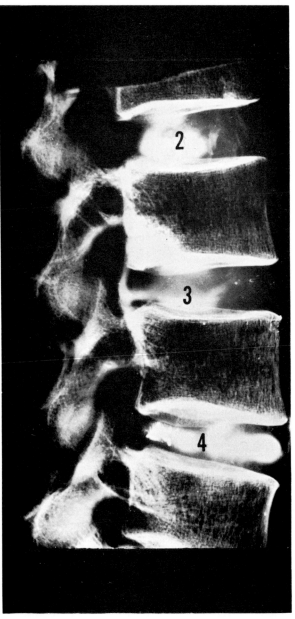

Fig. VIII:3. Radiograph and sections of a series of lumbar discs showing early degeneration. In L$_2$ the destructive process is widespread but has not broken thru the annulus fibrosus. The annulus of L$_3$ disc is destroyed posteriorly allowing the nucleus pulposus to break thru into the spinal canal beneath the posterior longitudinal ligament. The deficiencies as here noted in the 3rd and 4th discs allow herniation of disc material into the spinal canal. Of greater potential seriousness however are those radial defects extending in a postero-lateral direction toward the intervertebral foramina.

The development of these useful structures is initiated by pulling or shearing stresses upon the attachments of the longitudinal ligaments or joint capsules. Few spurs develop posteriorly because the stresses are partly borne by the posterior joints and arches and also because the posterior longitudinal ligaments attach only to the discs and are separated from the vertebral bodies by the venous plexus (Figure VIII:6). In the beginning osteophytes may be more or less sharp and directed outward, upward, or downward. There may still be a surprising degree of movement between the adjacent vertebral bodies (Figure IV:14). It is possible to identify a small tract of fibrous tissue extending from the disc outward to the point of the spur. If the vertebral column becomes rigid at that level the sharp lip-

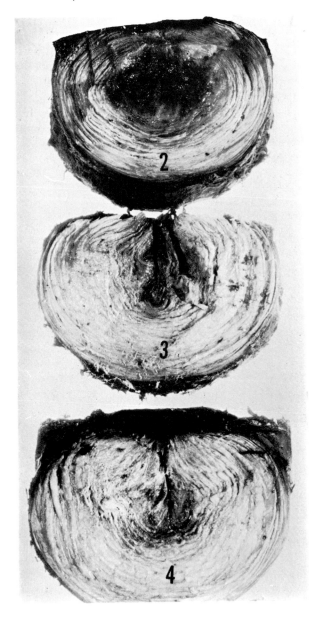

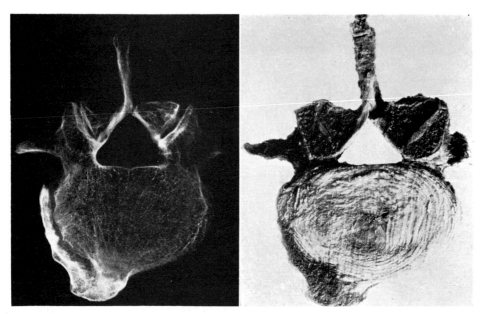

Fig. VIII:4. Transverse section thru a mid lumbar disc from a male of eighty-two years. The outer circular fibers of the annulus fibrosus on the right side in front have in some way become broken. As a result, disc material has escaped, migrating around to the right side of the vertebra beneath the longitudinal ligament. There is some asymmetry in the planes of the posterior articulations. The adjacent vertebrae were united by a massive spur formation.

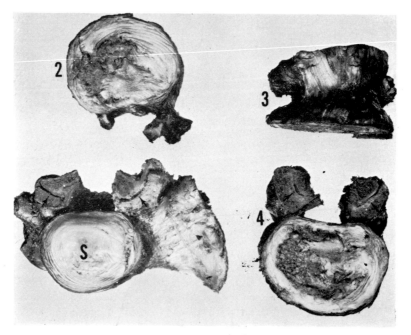

Fig. VIII:5. Vertebral bodies from an individual with lumbar scoliosis convex toward the left side with the apex at L_3. The lumbo-sacral disc is essentially normal. The undersurface of L_2 and the upper surface of L_4 reveal the second and third discs degenerated on the right side at the concavity of the curve. This has probably resulted from the asymmetrical pressure incidental to the scoliosis. Note the different planes of the posterior L_{3-4} and L_5-S_1 articulations (*arrows*).

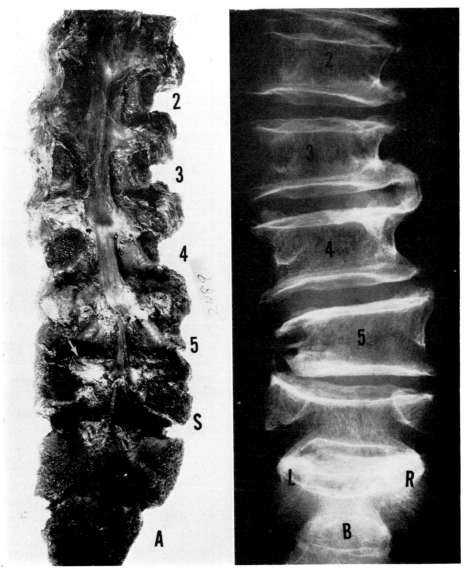

Fig. VIII:6. Dissection (A) showing the posterior surface of the lumbo-sacral spine of a male of seventy-nine years. There is a mild degree of scoliosis convex toward the left (B). The neural arches and spinal cord have been removed exposing the posterior longitudinal ligament which becomes narrowed below and ends at the first sacral segment. This ligament is not as wide as the canal. Unlike the anterior longitudinal ligament it does no attach to the bony substance of the vertebral bodies. It is attached only to the posterior surface of each intervertebral disc. Lying between it and each vertebral body is a plexus of blood vessels. The 5th disc was herniated backward and into the 5th left intervertebral foramen (*white arrow*). A lateral roentgenogram (C) shows the degenerated fifth disc and encroached foramen. The P. A. roentgenogram (B) reveals a lateral subluxation of L_5 toward the right side. The L_5 disc is wedge shaped and thinner on the left side. A photograph of the under surface of the fifth lumbar vertebra shows preservation of the normal annulus fibrosus on the right side but the disc is destroyed on the left side posteriorly where the herniation occurred (*arrow*). It is difficult to evaluate the exact relationship and chronology between the scoliosis, the lateral subluxation of L_5 and the disc herniation.

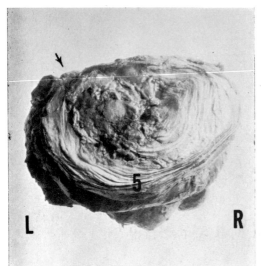

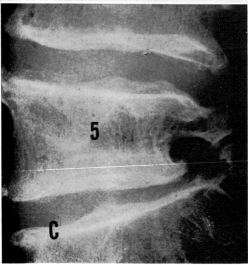

Fig. VIII:6C.

Bony spur formation may produce nerve root encroachment at the lumbosacral disc or within the intervertebral foramina of the lumbar or cervical region (see Chapter XIV). There have been numerous reports of dysphagia resulting from massive spur formation on the anterior surfaces of the cervical vertebrae and resultant esophageal puncture during instrumentation has been reported (Figure VIII:12). As outlined in Chapter V the vertebral arteries may be encroached upon by osteophytes developing at the covertebral joints or the posterior cervical articulations.

Spurs develop slowly. Following accident a legal question may arise as to the causal relation and the length of time required to develop osteophytes. When the periosteum or longitudinal ligament is suddenly torn from the surface of the vertebra, a calcium deposit may be visualized at the site of injury within four to ten weeks. At first this has a soft flocculent appearance. After a year or two the resulting osteophyte becomes dense and well organized (Figure IV:18).

The strong longitudinal ligament moulds and supports the intervertebral disc laterally and in front, also it covers any spur formations which may develop. The condition is somewhat different in ankylosing rheumatoid spondylitis wherein the final stage is an ossification of the posterior joint capsules, the longitudinal ligaments and other connective tissue structures of the spine (Figure IX:9)

ping and spurring becomes rounded off into a smooth solid bony bridging between the vertebral bodies. This constitutes a spontaneous arthrodesis (Figures VIII:9 and VIII:10).

LATE DEGENERATIVE DISC CHANGES

In the later stages of disc degeneration the cartilage plate which is a barrier between the nucleus and the vertebral body may become broken. As a result disc substance may herniate thru into the spongiosa while blood vessels and marrow elements penetrate into the disc. The latter becomes replaced by fibrous tissue and the cartilage plates are to some extent destroyed. Penetration of the disc

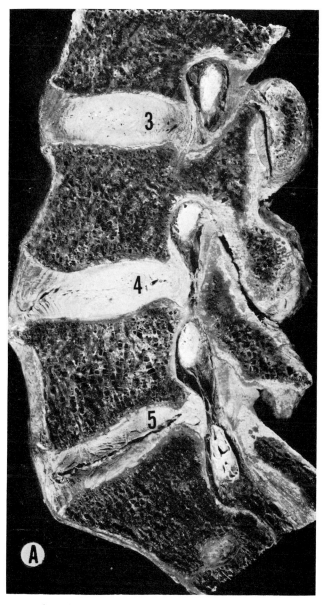

Fig. VIII:7. Photograph and roentgenogram of a lumbo-sacral specimen showing a normal third disc. There is early degeneration of L_4 with some thinning, fissure formation anteriorly, and beginning spur formation. Loss of intra disc pressure diminishes vertebral stability allowing some increased A. P. movement. This tends to promote spur formation and posterior joint stresses. There is some evidence of early posterior joint degeneration here at L_4. At L_5 the disc degeneration has progressed further with discoloration, additional thinning and fissure formation of the entire disc. Note the ample perineural space in each of the intervertebral foramina. The planes of the posterior articulations are nearly vertical above, but become somewhat more inclined in the lower lumbar region. (See also Figure XII:4.)

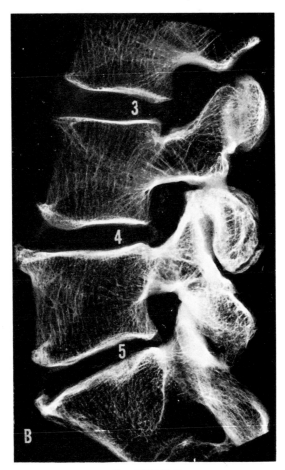

Fig. VIII:7 B

by blood vessels allows bone forming elements to be carried in. The structure may be partially or completely replaced by bony tissue. The intervertebral disc has no power to regenerate back to a normal condition (Figures VIII:13 and VIII:14). Since there are no sensory nerves in the disc these degenerative changes are not painful. Nerves have been demonstrated in longitudinal ligaments however, and the posterior joint capsules possess an adequate innervation (Chapter VI).

DISC HERNIATION

The semigelatinous nucleus pulposus, altho under pressure, remains within the center of the disc as long as its containing envelope is intact. A break in the annulus or one of the cartilage plates however allows some of the material to escape. Normally the cartilage plate, supported by the underlying bony plate of the vertebral body, is quite resistant to pressure. If some point of weakness is present in the cartilage plate, either a small fracture, a vessel scar or a prenatal defect from the notochord, the exploring nucleus may find its way thru into the substance of the vertebral body. Transmitted pressure from the disc causes the hernia to enlarge within the spongiosa for a time. It is not visualized roentgeno- graphically at first but later it may become walled off by a surrounding bony shell. Schmorl reported an incidence of 38% of such hernias in a series of some

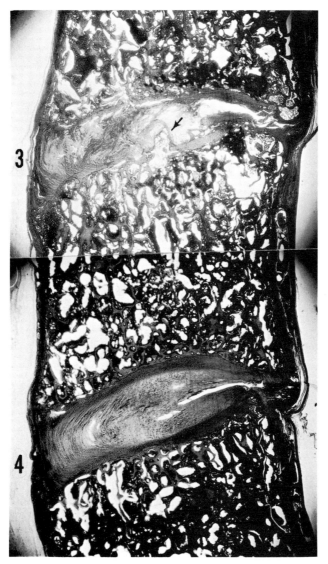

Fig. VIII:8. Sections of the 3rd and 4th cervical discs X3. In the 4th disc one may note above and below the hyaline cartilage plates in contact with the vertebral bodies and with the nucleus pulposus in the center between them. Anteriorly, to the left, the annulus fibrosus is intact. Posteriorly on the concave side of the cervical curve at the area of greatest compression, the annulus is beginning to show degenerative changes. These are incidental to pressure between the posterior margins of the vertebral bodies. The third disc shows more advanced degeneration. The cartilage plates are fragmented and the resilient disc substance has been replaced by fibrous tissue. A bony trabecula is seen growing from the vertebra upward into the disc substance (*arrow*). (Courtesy of *The American Journal of Roentgenology*.)

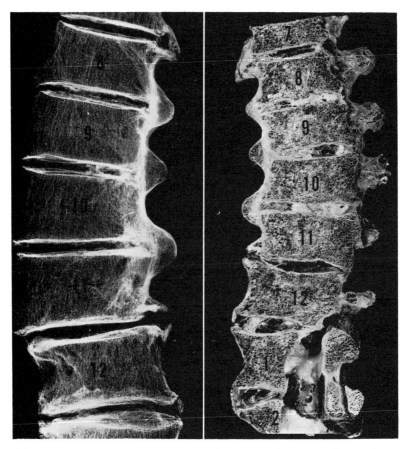

Fig. VIII:9. Photograph and roentgenogram of the opposite sides of a sectioned lower thoracic spine. A parrot-beak type of spur is visualized at T_7. The prolongation of fibrous tissue from the disc can be followed outward to the tip of the beak. No matter how long this sharp type of spur becomes the prolongation of fibrous tissue persists. The amplitude of movement at such a disc may remain surprisingly free (Figure IV:14).

Discs 8, 9, and 10 illustrate the solid type of bony bridging in which the prolongation of fibrous tissue no longer occurs. All movement at this level has ceased. At the disc margin the bone is sclerotic but the outer part of the bony bridge is trabeculated. The bridging occurred at the concavity of a scoliotic area. Note the rearrangement of supportive trabeculae within the vertebral body. The 11th disc shows the early parrot-beak type of spur formation. The spur is not developing from the corner of the vertebra at the disc margin. Rather it is arising slightly away from that point on the surface of the vertebra at the area of attachment for the longitudinal ligament. The spur formation, both here and at T_7, appears to be curving about and enclosing a mass of disc tissue which has been extruded from between the vertebral bodies. It would seem that the longitudinal ligament had been slightly stripped away from the vertebra by the pressure of this mass. The condition is somewhat similar to that noted in Figure IV:18.

In the anterior margin of the disc at T_{12} is a separate so-called intercalary ossicle (*arrows*). These consist of trabeculated bone that frequently develop within the disc substance. Following accident they should not be misdiagnosed as fractured spurs (Figures XII:20 and XIV:5B).

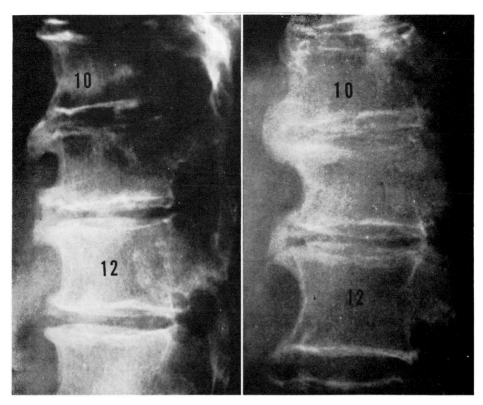

Fig. VIII:10. Female, age sixty-four, with degenerative spondylosis showing osteophytes in various stages of development. In the disc below T_{10} (arrow, left radiograph) it will be noted that the structure is somewhat pointed. The radiograph on the right shows the same area of this patient made ten years later. During this decade the spur at T_{10} had become a solid bony bridge with cortices and trabeculae firmly uniting the 10th and 11th vertebrae. This indicates that all movement between these two segments had ceased. Additional enlargement has occurred at most of the other spurs during this interval. At the T_9 level above, the sharp spur at sixty-four years had also become a solid bony bridge at seventy-four as shown by the roentgenogram on the right.

10,000 autopsies. These lesions are without clinical significance except as they may allow posterior joint stresses incidental to the disc thinning (Figures VIII:15, VIII:16 and VIII:17).

Of much greater importance than the Schmorl's nodes are those herniations of disc tissue which thrust their way thru deficiencies in the annulus fibrosus to appear in the spinal canal or especially within the intervertebral foramen (Figures XIV:34, XIV:38 and XIV:40). Posteriorly, in the lumbar region, the longitudinal ligament offers little or no impediment to the protrusion of these masses (Figure VII:6). Herniation of the intervertebral disc occurs thru a previously existent deficiency in the annulus fibrosus (Figures VIII:3 and VIII:18). Since a deficiency of this type is only the result of gradual attrition it has been held that herniation disc substance is not the result of a single trauma. This position is strengthened by the inability of the Swedish investigators to damage the annulus fibrosus experimentally by a single massive stress. It would seem however as an exception that a young person subjected to severe trauma might conceivably develop such a hernia of the disc substance if the annulus became detached (Figure VIII:19).

JUVENILE EPIPHYSITIS

Of some interest clinically is a group of adolescent male patients complaining of pain, backache and restricted movement whose roentgenograms show a defect at the upper anterior margin of one or more of the vertebral bodies. These correspond to the point where the epiphyseal plate curves over the edge of the vertebra (Figure I:18). These defects are surrounded by a zone of reaction within the bone and have been diagnosed as an epiphysitis beneath the ring epiphysis.

The clinical picture and the radiograph would seem to indicate a diagnosis of aseptic epiphysitis. That the ring escapes destruction is evidenced in certain follow-up studies by the development of normal appearing margins upon the vertebral plates. It has been stated that a herniation of disc substance occurs beneath the ring and into the involved area. This is confined by the strong anterior longitudinal ligament. The development of such a hernia would seem

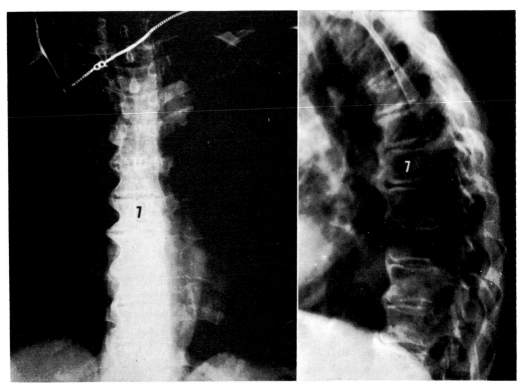

Fig. VIII:11. Sixty-six-year-old female with aortic sclerosis and advanced thoracic spondylosis. There is extensive bony bridging and spur formation upon the anterior and right lateral surfaces of the thoracic vertebrae. As reported by Culver and by Shapiro, pulsation of the descending aorta seems to have prevented the development of osteophytes on the left side. Those spurs on the anterior surfaces of the 6th and 7th discs do not come into contact with the aorta (see Figure IX:10).

tenable since in the case shown as Figure VIII:20, which was followed over a period of twenty-four years, the lesion finally appeared as a small area of decreased density surrounded by a bony shell somewhat resembling the Schmorl's nodes usually seen near center of the discs. Since the vertebra enlarges in diameter by subperiosteal bone growth, somewhat more rapidly anteriorly than posteriorly, the lesion appears to recede from the vertebral margin as growth progresses (Figure VIII:20). In certain cases the ring remains detached constituting the so-called limbus bone (Figure VIII:21). During the active inflammatory stage the vertebral body adjacent to the localized epiphysitis may proliferate more rapidly than elsewhere so that it bulges upward into the disc space. In one heavy sixteen-year-old patient, Figure VIII:22, the epiphyseal ring became asymmetrically dislocated. Upon reexamination nine years later the condition was found to be unchanged.

JUVENILE KYPHOSIS

Adolescent kyphosis or the juvenile epiphysitis described by the Danish orthopedist Scheuermann is characterized by deformity, pain, backache, restricted movement and reflex muscle spasm. Unlike the localized epiphysitis above described this condition involves essentially the entire epiphyseal plate. It is a dystrophy of the early teens wherein the enchondral bone growth of the mid

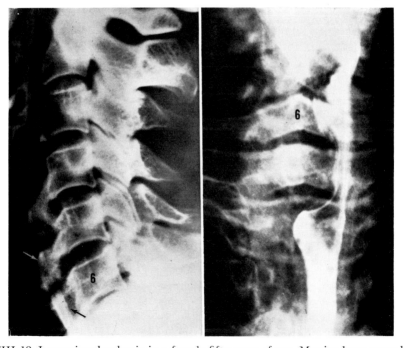

Fig. VIII:12. Increasing dysphagia in a female fifty years of age. Massive bony spurs bridge the anterior surfaces of the lower cervical bodies causing a deflection of the esophagus toward the left side. In the lateral projection the esophagus is seen lying alongside these bony masses (*arrows*). Puncture at esophagoscopy which has been reported in this condition suggests the desirability of a lateral roentgenogram before undertaking such an examination.

thoracic vertebrae is restricted. Enchondral bone proliferation in the growing vertebra occurs beneath the cartilaginous plates, (Figure I:18). It contributes to the height of the vertebral body. At the apex of the kyphotic curve the pressure upon the disc is increased by the mechanical disadvantage of the displaced center of gravity. Also the pressure is greater upon the anterior margin of the plate than upon its posterior margin. Since epiphyseal bone growth is restricted by pressure, the vertebral bodies at this level are either flattened, wedge shaped or both. Periosteal bone growth, increasing the diameter of the vertebra, is not restricted.

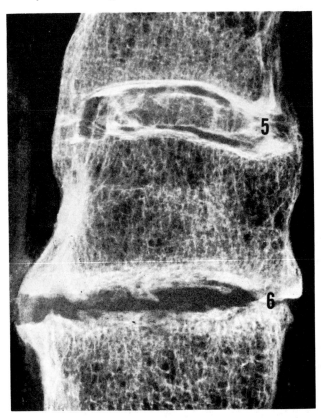

Fig. 13a

Fig. VIII:13. Roentgenogram and sections from the 5th and 6th cervical discs showing advanced intervertebral disc degeneration. The photomicrograph X5 of the fifth disc (*above*) shows the cartilage plates to have been largely preserved. The disc material between them has become replaced by bony trabeculae and marrow substance. The disc is ankylosed anteriorly by a solid bony bridge (*left side*). The sixth disc (*below*) shows the more typical advanced degenerative changes: (1) loss of the normal disc structure and its replacement by fibrous tissue, (2) fragmentation of the cartilage plates, (3) thinning of the disc, (4) eburnation of the adjacent bony surfaces and (5) osteophyte formation at the anterior margin of the disc. A higher power magnification (H) X150 of the area within the small rectangle shows the disorganized masses of fibrous tissue. The fragmented disc cartilage (*arrows*) is undergoing disintegration and resorption. Below is a group of small blood vessels. Even though some degree of movement may still occur at such a disc the structure can hardly be expected to possess a normal degree of resiliency and unrestricted movement.

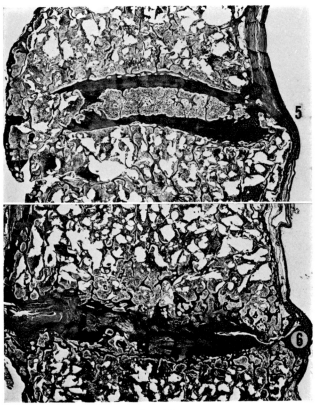

Fig. 13b

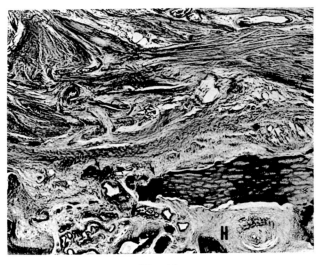

Fig. 13c

Four features characterize the roentgenographic picture of this condition: (1) kyphosis, (2) flattened or wedge-shaped vertebral bodies, (3) irregularity and waviness of the broken cartilage plates, and (4) a greater A. P. diameter of the involved vertebrae than those immediately below (Figure VIII:23). The condition must not be confused with tuberculosis or other infection of the spine.

The patients recover but retain their deformities and the uneven, fissured and partially destroyed cartilage plates. These late residuals are visualized in the specimen Figure VIII:24 from a male of 49 years.

Maudsley and other observers have reported epiphysitis of the spine as related to multiple epiphyseal dyplasia and coxae senilis.

CALCIFIED DISCS

Altho blood vessels are absent in the normal adult disc we have seen how degenerative defects in the cartilage plates allow a vascular penetration from the

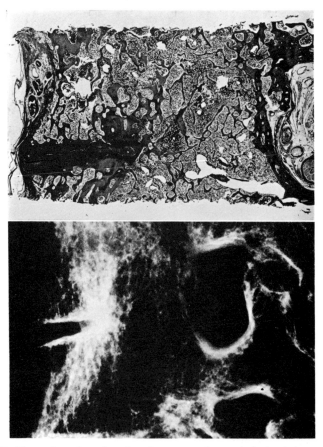

Fig. VIII:14. Radiograph and section showing a complete ankylosis of the posterior half of the 5th cervical disc from a male of eighty-five years. The photomicrograph X3 shows the ankylosis adjacent to the intervertebral foramen with the trabeculae continuous from one vertebra into the other. There is no residue of disc cartilage at that point, altho some of the remaining fibrotic disc material is visualized anteriorly. Just behind this the dense mass of sclerotic bone is seen connecting the two vertebrae.

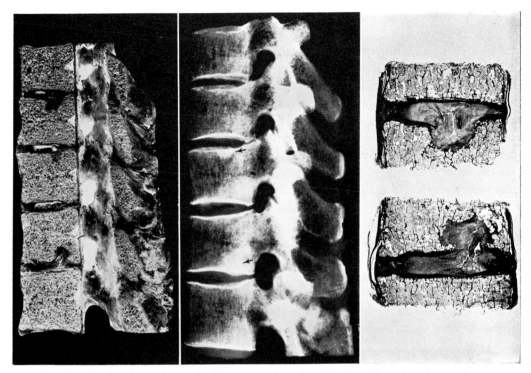

Fig. VIII:15. Specimen from the lower dorsal region showing three herniated discs or Schmorl's nodes. A roentgenogram of the specimen revealed only very minimal evidence of herniation (*arrows*) where sclerosis of the middle and lowermost lesions had occurred. Anatomical studies have repeatedly shown more extensive pathology than that visualized upon the radiographs. The sections, X2 were taken from the upper and lowermost of the Schmorl's nodes shown in the photograph. The cartilage plate (*dark band*) is broken on one side of each disc allowing disc substance to herniate thru and escape outward into the adjacent vertebral body. The transmitted pressure erodes for itself a pocket within the spongiosa.

marrow spaces into the cartilage substance. These blood vessels carry calcium and other bone forming elements. In childhood, blood vessels are still present within the disc substance as shown in Figure I:18 from a boy of eight years.

There have been various reports of calcification in the discs of children. In certain cases this calcification becomes resorbed.

Disc calcification may also occur as the result of metabolic disturbance.

ALKAPTONURIA-OCHRONOSIS

Alkaptonuria, or homogentisic acid in the urine is a hereditary disease caused by a congenital anomaly of metabolism. Alkaptons in the urine cause darkening upon standing or addition of alkali. Dark stains result from these substances in the perspiration. Pigment is deposited in the cartilage of the ears, nose and elsewhere. Pigment granules were described by Virchow as having a pale yellow ocher color, hence the term ochronosis as applied to this disease when the articular cartilage is involved. This is said to occur in about 50 per cent of the cases. Such cartilage becomes brittle and may undergo various degrees of disintegration and arthritic changes. The patients complain of backache and limitation of spinal movements or rigidity. Kyphosis may be present. The roentgenograms reveal extensive degeneration and increased density of the disc structures. While the organic ochronotic pigment material is deposited in the cartilage the radiograph may show this part of the disc free of any radiopaque material. Apparently the disc degeneration with probable calcification is a secondary response (Figures VIII:25 and VIII:26).

We have seen how the intervertebral disc is subject to attrition. As a natural process of ageing the structure gradually becomes worn out with the passage of time. As a result it develops certain defensive mechanisms. In Chapter XI is described the response of this structure to infection. The elasticity of the annulus and consequent resiliency of the entire disc enables it to adapt itself by counterpressure to the position and state of the adjacent vertebral bodies. Witness the change in shape incidental to the spinal movements.

When the lumbar vertebrae become osteoporotic the discs expand sufficiently to counterbalance the weakened bone support. This prevents the spinal canal, bridged by the neural arches, from becoming shortened. As a result of the imbibition power the compensating biconvex discs may be enlarged to more than double their normal thickness. The car-

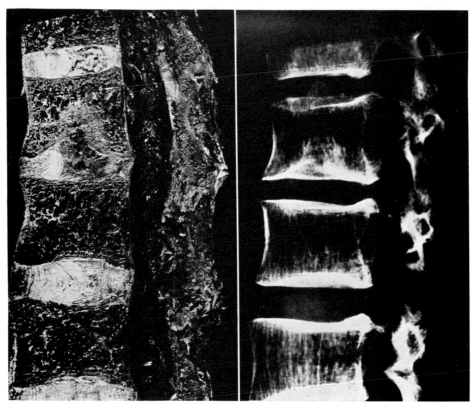

Fig. VIII:16. Specimen from a male of sixty years showing a large hernia upward into the lumbar vertebra above. The photograph shows numerous blood vessels within the mass which is somewhat larger than indicated by the roentgenogram.

tilage plates become bent and finally rupture if their limit of strength is passed (Figures VIII:27 and XV:14).

The elasticity of the disc enables it to resist pressure. This resiliency also prevents its destruction by pulsating tumors or aneurisms which may erode the adjacent bone (Figures XVI:7 and

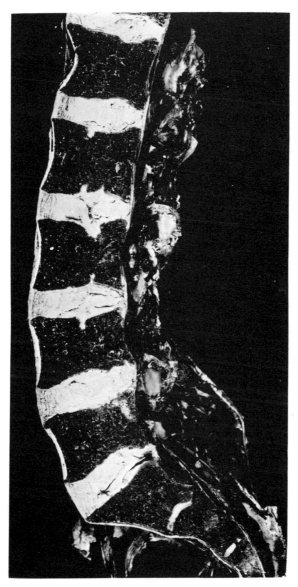

Fig. VIII:17. Sagittal section of a specimen showing small herniations of the lumbar discs. There are three Schmorl's nodes at the second disc with probable beginning backward disc herniation at the 4th and 5th levels. Herniation of disc substance into the spinal canal and especially the intervertebral foramen may have a definite clinical importance. Herniation into a vertebral body, i.e., the Schmorl's node, is usually entirely asymptomatic per se since the area is said to be without sensory innervation. Such herniation however may be a factor in disc degeneration, which together with posterior joint changes has a very definite clinical significance.

XVI:10). The cartilage plate of the disc also resists the extension of metastases which may invade the adjacent vertebra. Penetration of the disc substance itself occurs only after the cartilage plate has become broken (Figures VIII:28 and VII:22).

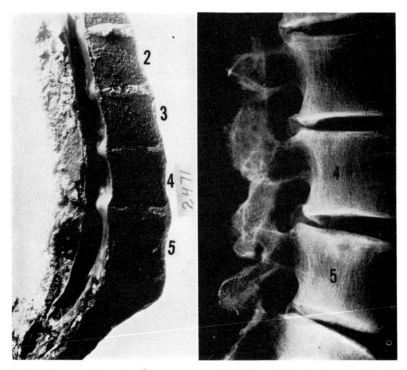

Fig. VIII:18. Photograph and roëntgenogram, left side of the lumbosacral level from a male of eighty-two years. There are posterior herniations into the canal of the 2nd, 3rd and 4th partially degenerated discs. The 5th disc which is completely destroyed shows no evidence of herniation whatsoever. Obviously the presence of some disc substance is necessary in order to have a herniation occur. The roentgenogram (herniations accentuated) reveals only minimal displacement into the 3rd and 4th foramina.

————————————————————→

Fig. VIII:19. Traumatic spondylosis at T_{10}. This patient developed a curve of the spine, weakness of the legs and loss of coordination after falling from an apple tree as a child. From the age of fifteen years she was spastic and unable to walk. She also suffered from dysfunction of the bladder and rectal sphincters. There was diminished sensation below T_{12}. The first lateral roentgenogram (A) was made at the age of thirty and showed some kyphosis, wedging and spur formation at the 10th disc. Lipiodol, ascending in the spinal canal was delayed at the T_{10} disc (C). At operation the cord was found to be displaced backward by the bulging disc substance and showed no transmitted pulsation. The disc was curretted but no fusion was attempted. The hemangioma of T_9 extending into the pedicles and spinous process was an incidental condition and without clinical significance. Upon radiographic reexamination two and one-half years later (B) the kyphosis had increased and the stabilizing spur at the tenth disc level had become larger. The neurological symptoms had not altered. In retrospect it would seem that a localized traumatic spondylosis and disc herniation with cord pressure had developed following injury 16 years before. The postoperative increased kyphosis resulted from removal of the interspinous ligaments and loss of disc substance.

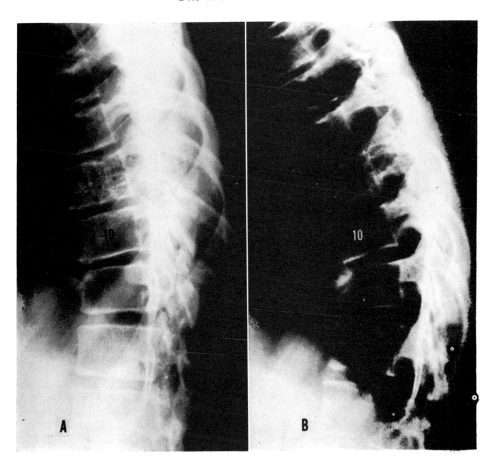

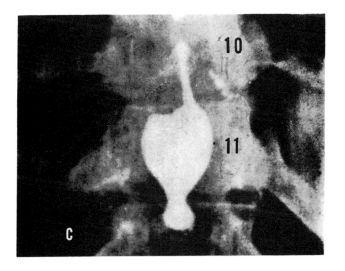

REFERENCES

Anatomical Studies

Beadle, O. A.: Medical Research Council, Sp. Report, Series #161, London.

Bick, E. M., and Copel, J. W.: 1950, *J. Bone J. Surg., 32A*:803–814.

Bick, E. M., et al: 1951, *J. Bone, J .Surg., 33A*: 783–787.

Coventry, M. B., et al: 1945, *J. Bone J. Surg., 27*: 105–112.

Editorial: *Rad., 71*:877.

Erlocher, P. R.: 1952, *J. Bone J. Surg., 34B*:204–210.

Hendry, N. G. C.: 1958, *J. Bone J. Surg., 40B*: 132–144.

Horwitz, T.: 1939, *Surg., 6*:410–425.

Keyes, D. C., and Compere, E. L.: 1932, *J. Bone J. Surg., 14*:897–938.

Roofe, P. G.: 1940, *Arch. Neuro. Psych., 44*:100–103.

Movement and Stress Studies

Brown, T., et al: 1957, *J. Bone J. Surg., 39A*: 1135–1165.

Knutsson, F.: 1944, *Acta Rad., 25*:593–609.

Nachemson, A.: *Acta Orth. Scan.,* Supp. 43.

Perey, O.: 1957, *Acta Ortho. Scand.,* Supp. 25.

Disc Degeneration

Bick, E. M., et al: 1952, *J. Bone J. Surg., 34A*: 110–114.

Bohatirchuk, F.: 1955, *Brit. Jor. Rad., 28*:389–404.

Coventry, M. B., et al: 1945, *J. Bone J. Surg., 27*: 233–247.

Friberg, S,: 1948, *Acta Orth. Scan., 17*:224–230.

Gershon-Cohen, et al: 1954, *Rad., 62*:383–387.

Hirsch, C.: 1959, *J. Bone J. Surg., 41B*:237–243.

Lindblom, K.: 1957, *J. Bone J. Surg., 39A*:933–945.

Lyon, E.: 1942, *J. Bone J. Surg., 24*:805–811.

Marr, J. T.: 1953, *Am. Jor. Roent., 70*:804–809.

Raines, J. R.: 1953, *Am. Jor. Roent., 70*:964–966.

Spur Formation

Bauer, F.: 1953, *Jor. Lar. & Otol., 67*:615–630.

Beahrs, O. H., et al: 1959, *Ann. Surg., 149*:297–299.

Culver, G. J., et al: 1956, *Am. Jor. Roent., 76*: 1157–1160.

Heck, C. V.: 1956, *Surg. Gyn. Obs., 102*:657–660.

Nathan, H.: 1962, *J. Bone J. Surg., 44A*:243–268.

Fig. VIII:20. Serial studies in the course of a vertebral epiphysitis followed over a period of twenty-four years. This boy was first examined at the age of fourteen. (The numerals indicate age of the patient at the time of examination.) He was complaining of lumbar pain, muscle spasm and limitation of movement. The roentgenogram at that time revealed an epiphysitis of the upper anterior margin of L_3 (*arrow*). Some vertebral demineralization is shown by the bulging of the intervertebral discs. The symptoms persisted but a roentgenogram at fifteen showed a relatively good bone growth during the previous year. The localized destructive process had become walled off during that interval. At seventeen years the walling off zone had become wider. Considerable growth had taken place anterior to the lesion so that it had moved back from the anterior margin of the vertebra. This confirms the observations of others that the principal growth of a vertebra occurs on the anterior surface of the body of the structure and at its plane surfaces. Observe the lines parallel to the disc surfaces denoting the location of the epiphyses at various times of temporarily delayed growth. The patient was seen from time to time during the following years. The ring epiphysis at the anterior margin of the vertebra had not been destroyed. At thirty-eight years of age the sclerotic zone about the old lesion had become narrower and more sharply defined. The defect had partially filled in with bone. Additional bone growth had left the defect even further from the anterior margin of the vertebra. Many of the horizontal lines were still present but the original biconcave shape of the demineralized vertebral body was no longer observable. (The final examination was supplied by the courtesy of Dr. C. G. Otis of Townshend, Vt.)

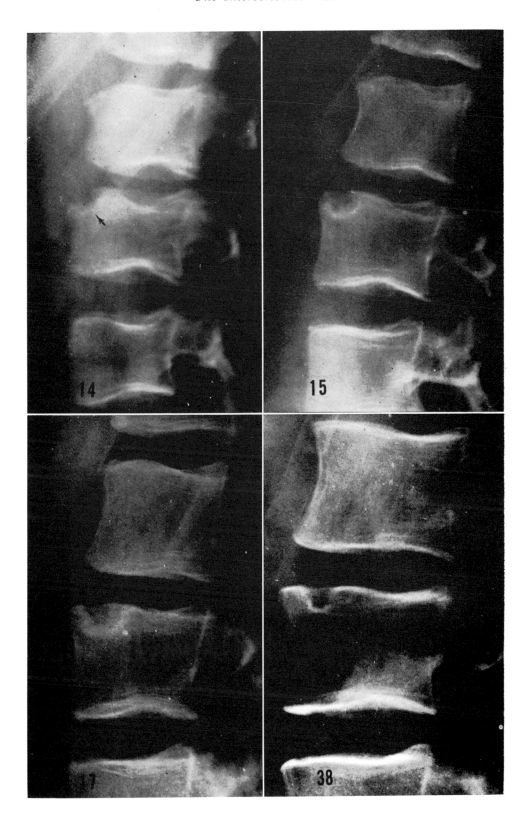

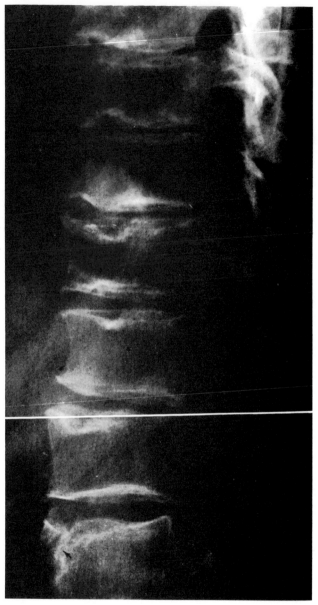

Fig. VIII:21. Forty-seven-year-old farmer with chronic deficiency of the vertebral epiphyses. All epiphyseal plates are wavy and irregular. The tenth thoracic vertebra is flattened and relatively increased in A. P. diameter. The patient was obviously the victim of juvenile epiphysitis. The epiphyseal ring of L_3 became detached and displaced forward by a mass of disc tissue which herniated downward beneath it to appear below on the anterior surface of the vertebra. Calcification of the mass occurred *(arrow)*. The detached epiphyseal ring has been termed a "limbus bone" (Figures XIII:23 and II:17).

Patterson, H. A., *et al:* 1958, *Ann. Surg., 147:* 863–867.

Shapiro, R., *et al:* 1960, *Am. Jor. Roent., 83:* 660–662.

Stephens, H., *et al:* 1954, *Ann. Int. Med., 41:* 823–828.

Pathological Disc Changes

Braisford, J. F.: 1955, *Brit. Jor. Rad., 28:*415–431.

Coventry, M. B., *et al:* 1945, *J. Bone J. Surg., 27:*460–478.

Harris, R. I., *et al:* 1954, *J. Bone J. Surg., 36B:* 304–322.

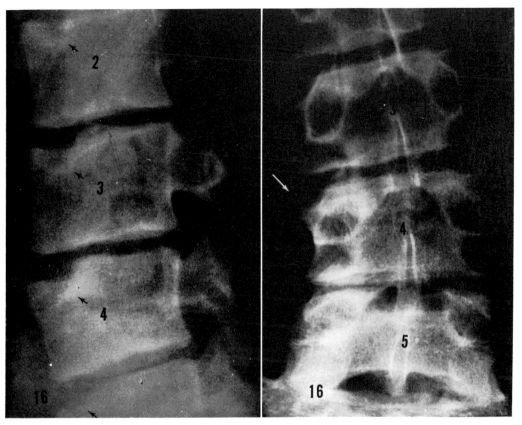

Fig. VIII:22. Epiphysitis in a rapidly growing, well developed youth of sixteen years. This patient was six feet five inches tall, weighing well over 200 pounds and stood with an inclination of his back toward the right side. There was no history of injury but he complained of back pain of increasing severity during the past two years. The pain was not referred but all back movements were limited. Roentgenograms revealed an epiphysitis involving the upper anterior margin of each lumbar vertebra (*black arrows*). There was also a herniation into the under surface of L₃. The upper ring epiphysis of L₄ had become displaced downward, forward and toward the right (*white arrow*). This had allowed the 3rd vertebra and the spine above to become inclined toward the right side. At reexamination nine years later, the patient still complained of lumbar discomfort, all back movements were restricted, and he still remained with a list toward the right side. The roentgenograms revealed the bone deficiencies at the upper anterior corners of the vertebral bodies essentially unchanged. Of some interest is the elevation of bone upon the upper surface of the vertebra immediately posterior to the epiphyseal deficiency. This commonly occurs with vertebral epiphysitis and results in a narrowing of the disc space at that point. These elevations probably indicate an accelerated bone growth stimulated by the epiphysitis.

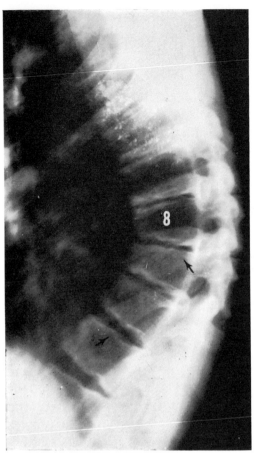

Fig. VIII:23. Kyphosis in an adolescent boy. The lateral projection of this thoracic spine illustrates the typical changes of juvenile kyphosis or Scheuermann's disease. In this type of epiphysitis the entire epiphyseal plate of the vertebra is involved rather than just the epiphyseal ring. The features are: (1) thoraco-lumbar kyphosis beginning during adolesence; (2) wedging or flattening of the vertebrae; (3) irregularity of the epiphyseal plates (*arrows*) and (4) a greater A. P. diameter of the vertebrae at the apex of the

Disc Herniations

Begg, A. C.: 1954, *J. Bone J. Surg., 36B*:180–193.
Lindblom, K., et al: *Jor. Neurosurg., 5*:413.
McRae, D. M.: 1956, *Acta Rad., 46*:9–27.
O'Connell, J. E. A.: 1960, *Brit. J. Surg., 47*:611–616.
Spurling, R. G.: 1940, *Arch. Surg., 40*:375–388.
Staokey, B.: 1940, *Arch. Surg., 40*:417–432.
Webb, J. H.: *J.A.M.A., 154*:1153–1154.

Juvenile Epiphysitis—Scheuermann's

Knutsson, F.: 1948, *Acta. Rad., 30*:97–104.
Knutsson, F.: 1949, *Acta. Rad., 32*:404–406.
Lamb, D. W.: 1954, *J. Bone J. Surg., 36B*:591–600.
Maudsley, R. H.: 1955, *J. Bone J. Surg., 37B*:224–228.
Nathan, L.: 1940, *J. Bone J. Surg., 22*:5–62.
Simon, R. S.: 1942, *J. Bone J. Surg., 24*:681–683.
Wassmann, K.: 1951, *Acta Ortho. Scan., 21*:65–74.

Calcification of Discs

Asadi, A.: 1959, *Am. J. Dis. Child., 97*:282–286.
Peacher, W. G., and Storrs, R. P.: 1956, *Rad., 67*:396–398.
Sandstron, C.: 1951, *Acta Rad., 36*:217–233.
Silverman, F. N.: 1954, *Rad., 62*:801–816.
Walker, C. S.: 1954, *J. Bone J. Surg., 36B*:601–605.
Wallman, I. S.: 1957, *Arch. Dis. Child., 32*:149–150.
Weens, H. S.: 1945, *Jor. Ped., 26*:178–188.

curve than that of those below. The apex of the curve is seen at T_8 in this case. The fundamental pathology is an inadequate production of bone by the deficient epiphyseal plates of the vertebral bodies, a condition aggravated by the kyphosis.

Fig. VIII:24. Specimen showing kyphosis from a male of forty-nine years probably originating in adolescence. A section from T_8 with a magnification X4 shows the deficiency of the epiphyseal plates, a condition which prevented normal bone growth during adolescence. As a result at least five of the mid thoracic vertebrae at the apex of the curve remained flattened and did not grow in height as did their fellows. The roentgenogram also reveals an osteoporosity which has allowed some expansion of the intervertebral discs.

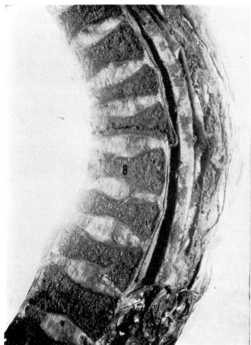
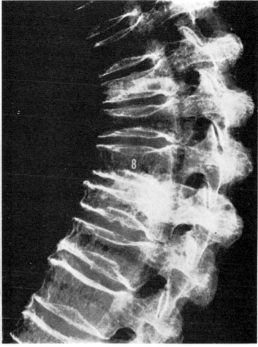

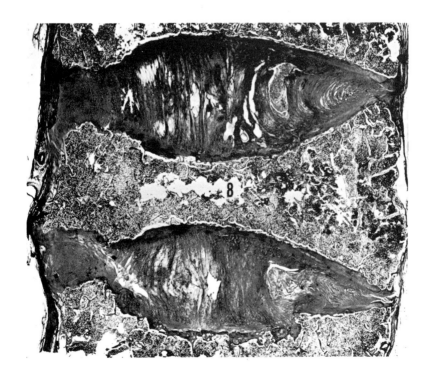

Alkaptonuria-Ochronosis

Black, R. L., *et al:* 1954, *Arch. Int. Med., 93:*75–86.

Cervenansky, J., *et al:* 1959, *J. Bone J. Surg., 41A:*1169–1182.

Eisenberg, H.: 1950, *Arch. Int. Med., 86:*79–86.

Gladstone, M., *et al:* 1952, *Am. Jor. Med., 13:*432–452.

Hertzberg, J.: 1945, *Acta Rad., 26:*484–490.

Martin, W. J., *et al:* 1955, *Ann. Int. Med., 42:*1052.

Pomeranz, M. M.: 1941, *Rad., 37:*294–303.

Sacks, S.: 1951, *J. Bone J. Surg., 33B:*407–414.

Simon, G., *et al:* 1961, *Brit. Jor. Rad., 34:*384–386.

Thompson, M. M.: 1957, *Am. Jor. Roent., 78:*46–53.

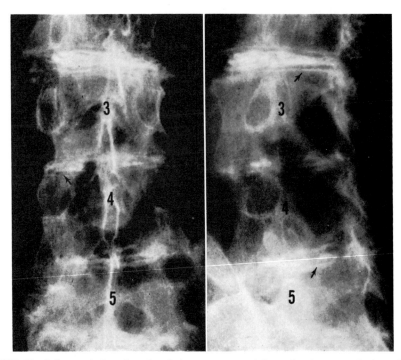

Fig. VIII:25. Ochronosis in a female of sixty-two years. The urine became blackened upon standing and showed alkaptons, justifying a diagnosis of alkaptonuria. There was a history of backache and pain in the joints of ten years duration. Physical examination revealed purple pigmentation of the sclera and the cartilage of the nose and ears. The roentgenograms show increased density, probably calcification of the thoracic discs from the 4th to the 9th inclusive. The lumbar discs, especially L$_2$, were also involved as here visualized. The organic alkapton bodies are normally deposited in the cartilage and produce degenerative changes. The calcium here is deposited in the fibrous tissue of the disc substance while the cartilage plates adjacent to the vertebral bodies remain uncalcified and radiolucent (*arrows*). (Courtesy Syracuse Memorial Hospital.)

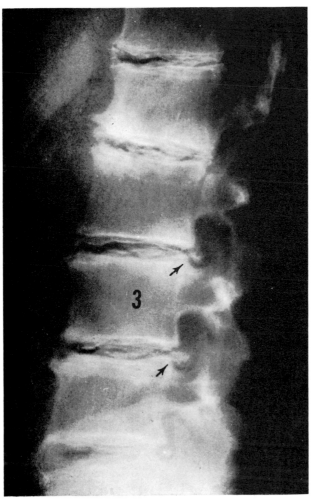

Fig. VIII:26. Ochronosis in a male of sixty-nine years. The degenerated, calcified intervertebral discs show the so-called vacuum phenomenon (see Figure XIV:32). Also note the calcification of the posterior disc herniations *(arrows)*. (Courtesy of the Syracuse University Hospital.)

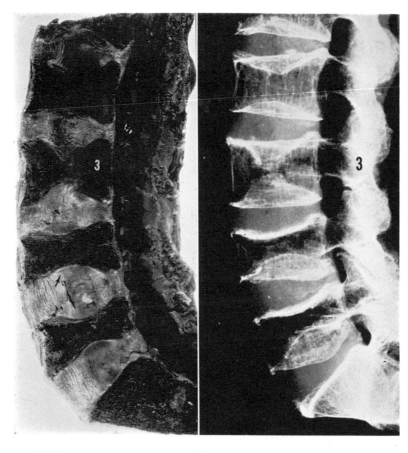

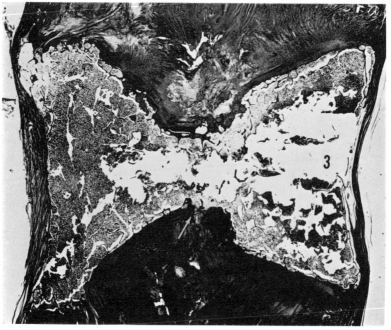

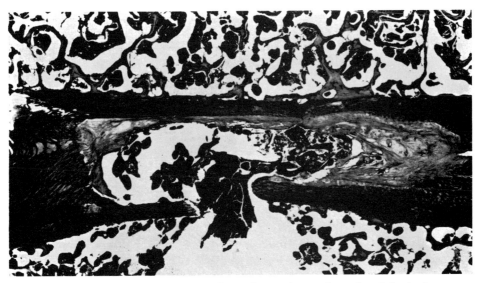

Fig. VIII:28. Metastatic tumor invading the nucleus pulposus thru a break in the lower cartilage plate. This is a section X12 of the 4th thoracic disc from a male of sixty-nine years. The intact disc usually resists metastatic invasion or erosion by a pulsating tumor or aneurism. Once the cartilage plate barrier becomes broken however, invasion is unopposed (see Figure VII:22.)

Fig. VIII:27. Advanced osteoporosis in a female of eighty-one years. The density of the vertebral bodies is actually much less than that of the discs. The inadequate bony structure was unable to counter the imbibition and expansion pressure of the discs, thus producing the so-called fish vertebrae. At some points the cartilage plates of the discs became curved but did not give way (*black arrow*). Elsewhere as at L₃ here seen in section X4 the cartilage plates were unable to resist the pressure and became fractured near the center (*white arrow*).Osteoporosis in the lumbar region usually results in biconcave (fish) vertebrae because of the superimposed weight of the body while the same condition in the thoracic region causes a wedging, since the axis of weight-bearing is in front of the thoracic curve.

Chapter IX

General Conditions

DEGENERATIVE SPONDYLOSIS DEFORMANS

T HIS COMMON condition, popularly miscalled "osteoarthritis of the spine" is largely the result of a wearing out process or attrition of the intervertebral discs as detailed in Chapter VIII. It occurs in later life and is degenerative rather than inflammatory in character. The natural aging changes of dehydration, fragmentation and disintegration of the disc impair the dynamic function of that structure. The degenerative thinning of the disc allows additional movement between the adjacent vertebral bodies with increased bulging of the disc margin. These changes place greater traction stresses upon the attachments of the longitudinal ligaments to the vertebral bodies. Such pulling and shearing stresses are an irritative reaction which promote spur formation. These osteophytes are a stabilizing, compensatory reaction.

As the nucleus pulposus loses its natural turgescence and supporting power, more and more of the weight is carried peripherally by the annulus fibrosus. The annulus ideally resists the centrifugal pressure of a normal weight supporting nucleus pulposus but it is not so well suited to withstand the vertical pressure of the superimposed body weight so that it disintegrates. With advanced degeneration, as the annulus becomes worn out, a direct bony contact of the vertebral plates occurs. Since uncushioned bone does not normally support weight, the vertebrae develop an eburnation of the contacting bony sur-

faces. Direct pressure and friction at the margins of these bony surfaces become a second stimulus to bony spur formation. A somewhat similar process occurs at the covertebral joints of the neck as a result of cervical disc thinning (Figure XIV:1).

Osteophytes projecting into the spinal canal are infrequent since the frail posterior longitudinal ligament attaches only to the discs rather than the vertebral bodies and also because the neural arches carry a major portion of the stress. However since the lumbosacral disc is to some degree wedge shaped, a thinning of that structure may allow pressure and friction between the posterior margins of the fifth vertebra and the sacrum with a resultant eburnation and spur formation at that level (Figures VII:21 and XIV:33). It is noticeable that spurs do not form at those discs in direct contact with the aorta whether that vessel descends on the left side or, as rarely, on the right side of the spine (Figures IX:10 and VIII:11).

In the event of spinal curvature an asymmetrical pressure develops on the concave side of the curve. It is therefore on this side that the osteophytes develop as an additional stabilizing support (Figures VIII:5 and X:14).

Following trauma, a localized spondylosis may result from ligamentous or bony injury at any level of the spine. Spur formation may be evident in four to eight weeks. The timing and character of such spur formation may be of legal importance. Repeat studies are especially valuable. (See Figure IV:18). A post traumatic calcification or spur, developing from haemorrhage or injured soft tissue will first appear blurry and poorly outlined without any cortex. Later it will appear more dense and sharply outlined. Finally after a period of many months the trabeculae and a cortex will give the spur a more mature look (Figure IV:17). A solid bony bridging requires many months or even years to form (Figure IV:25). A generalized spondylosis may be held to be aggravated by an injury if real objective evidence of increased localized spurring is definitely shown roentgenographically within six to twelve months.

Various secondary changes incidental to degenerative spondylosis deformans have been mentioned elsewhere. As the degenerated discs become thinned so that the adjacent vertebral bodies approach each other there is a telescoping or imbrication of the posterior joints. In extreme cases the tips of the articular processes impinge against the pedicle above or the lamina below. Pressure, and to some extent actual weight bearing by the posterior articulations together result in eburnation and even erosion of the underlying bone. The roentgenogram clearly visualizes this evidence of local irritative reaction in structures not primarily designed for weight bearing. The foramina are also encroached upon. The morphological changes of the nerve roots incidental to the foramen constriction are documented in a subsequent chapter (Figures IX:1, IX:2, IX:3, IX:4, IX:5, XIII:16B & D XIII:30 and XIV:40).

Spondylosis, finally, is a more or less universal condition, gradually developing to some degree in practically all spines as a result of the natural aging process. Many of these patients are afflicted with various so-called "rheumatic" symptoms. Even with minimal demonstrable changes the discomfort may at times become quite severe with exacerbations and remissions. On the other hand patients with extensive spondylosis, disc degeneration and massive spur formation may be entirely free of symptoms. The patients may show a decrease in stature and a limitation of motion. Bony demineralization is seen as a result of the aging process, disuse, hormone deficiency or low protein intake and was discussed in Chapter VII. With the lessened resiliency and decreased amplitude of movement the liability to spine trauma is also much greater in these patients.

ANKYLOSING SPONDYLITIS DEFORMANS

Ankylosing spondylitis has been otherwise known as Marie-Strumpell's disease, ankylopoietica, or spondylose rhizomelique. The acute condition is characterized primarily by subcortical bone destruction of the sacroiliacs and other joints followed by ossification in the ligamentous structures of the spine. This disease is probably a spinal manifestation of peripheral rheumatoid arthritis.

The disease occurs first in its active stages as a low grade, chronic, destructive, inflammatory bone condition involving joints of the spine and pelvis. The various connective tissue structures, tendons, fascia, joint capsules and ligaments of the axial skeleton are also involved in this early, painful inflammatory process. Even fascial planes of the muscles may not escape (Figure IX:6).

Healing is characterized by ossifica-

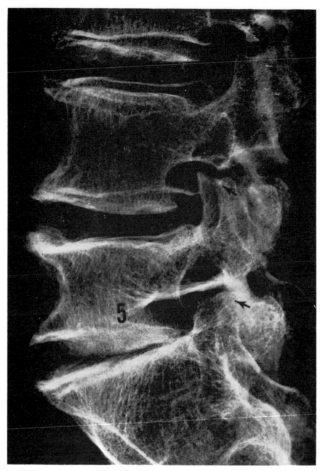

Fig. IX:1. Spondylosis deformans of the lower lumbar spine from a male of eighty years. Degenerative disc thinning has resulted in bony spur formation at the disc margins. The wedge shaped lumbo sacral disc is completely destroyed in back to that the posterior margins of L_5 and S_1 are in direct contact. Note the imbrication of the lower two pairs of posterior articulations. The normally pointed tips of the superior articular processes have become squared off by impingement against the suprajacent pedicles (*arrows*).

tion of connective tissue structures and ankylosis of the joints.

There may be a familial element and infection may play a part. The disease develops in early life, more frequently in young men with a ratio of, males to female, nine to one.

Characteristically the disease first appears as a destructive process involving the sacroiliac joints. These young men complain of low back discomfort grad-ually becoming more painful, with stiffness, pain in the hips and sciatica. The symptoms begin in the lower back but gradually ascend and increase in severity. Respiratory movements may be restricted as the costovertebral articulations become involved (Figure IX:12). The disease is insidious so that a preliminary period, even many years of recurrent symptoms, may intervene before x-ray changes appear.

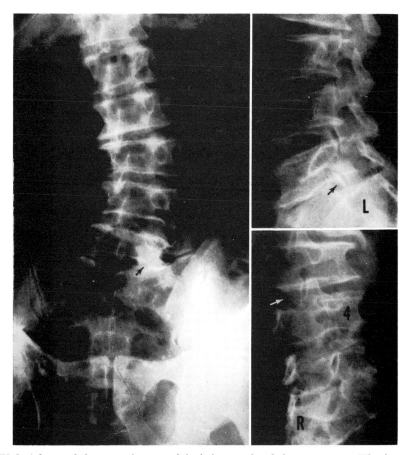

Fig. IX:2. Advanced degenerative spondylosis in a male of sixty-two years. The intervertebral discs are thinned, especially on the right side with some wedging and resultant scoliosis. Spurring is somewhat greater on the side of the concavity. The fifth vertebra is tipped toward the left side with telescoping, impingement and eburnation of its posterior articulation with S_1 (*black arrows*). Since the concavity of the mid lumbar curve is on the right side and with little rotation, the right posterior articulations at that level are telescoped. Telescoping is shown by the manner in which the articular surfaces register opposite to each other (Figure XIV:34). This is seen especially well upon the right oblique study (*white arrow*) as contrasted with the mid lumbar region of the opposite side shown on the film above. The fifth left transverse process also articulates with the ala of the sacrum. This machinist complained of lumbar discomfort, with limited back movements, especially lateral bending toward the left. The patellar reflexes were present but the Achilles reflexes were absent.

In the early stage, because of the subcortical bony destruction, the sacroiliacs appear widened, ragged and blurry (Figure IX:6A). They are bordered by a sclerotic reaction in the adjacent sacrum and iliacs. Later when the joint becomes ankylosed the adjacent sclerosis disappears (Figure IX:6B). Any undestroyed residual cartilage remains entrapped within the ossified capsule (Figure IX:-9).

Reports indicate that about three-fourths of the cases are the gradually developing type characterized by exacer-

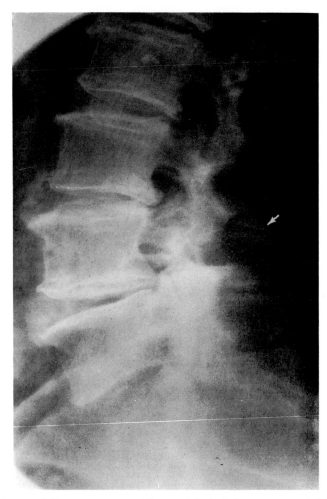

Fig. IX:3. Laborer of sixty-seven years with spondylosis deformans complaining of pain of increasing severity referred down the right leg. There was limitation of motion in all directions. He also complained of paresthesia of lateral surface of the right thigh, the so-called meralgia paresthetica, corresponding to the distribution of the lateral cutaneous nerve to that region. The lateral roentgenogram reveals an extreme lordosis with flocculent calcification and osteophytes involving the degenerated disc margins. There is telescoping of the posterior articulations with foramen encroachment. The lateral cutaneous nerve of the thigh arises from the 3rd and 4th lumbar nerve roots. There is 'kissing" impingement with sclerosis between the dorsal spinous processes (*white arrow*). On the P. A. projection it will be seen that the telescoping 4th and 5th inferior articular processes have eroded notches in the underlying bony surfaces with which they come into contact (*black arrows*). The lordosis plus the telescoping has thrown some weight bearing stress upon these posterior articulations. Note the resultant sclerosis and eburnation of these structures. This patient also has accessory sacroiliac joints one of which has become ankylosed (X). For a discussion of this condition see Chapter XII. (Courtesy of the publisher of *The Journal of Bone and Joint Surgery.*)

bations and remissions which may become spontaneously arrested at any stage. About one-fourth of the patients are victims of the rapid, progressive fulminating type.

Peripheral rheumatoid arthritis complicates the condition in about twenty-five per cent of the patients while in seventy-five per cent of uncomplicated cases the ankylosing spondylitis is held by most American authorities to be a special type of rheumatoid arthritis. Rheumatoid granulomatous nodules have been observed in the vertebral bodies as a destructive lesion simulating, myeloma or metastases.

Rarely a special type of rheumatoid spondylitis may appear as a localized chronic destructive lesion of a vertebral disc and its adjacent vertebral bodies. The involvement is principally anterior. The disc becomes thinned and the involved parts of the vertebrae are sclerotic. The appearance is somewhat that of tuberculosis or pyogenic infection. There is likely to be tenderness to deep pressure over the local area. Ankylosis

develops upon healing of the process (Figure IX:14).

When the inflammatory process has finally subsided ossification of the connective tissue structures takes place. Either as a result of, or a part of, the healing process the fibrous structures gradually turn to bone: The longitudinal ligaments along the vertebral bodies, the capsules of the posterior joints, the inter-spinous ligaments and the ligamentum flavum all become ossified. Healing by osteoblastic activity also occurs at any other area such as: the pubis, ischium, iliac crest, the hips, the costovertebral articulations, the odontoid or even the tempro-mandibular joints if they have been involved. This is a progressive process which may be undergoing different stages at different levels of the spine at the same time (Figures IX:6 to figure IX:11).

The lumbar bodies may appear to have square corners. The lumbar curve becomes straightened but the thoracic region develops a kyphotic curve with the neck thrust forward and fixed in posi-

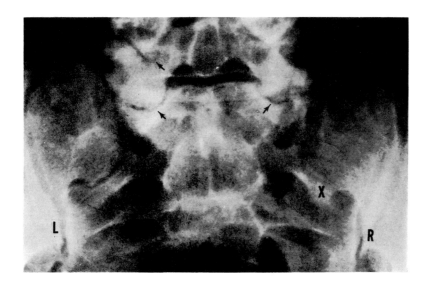

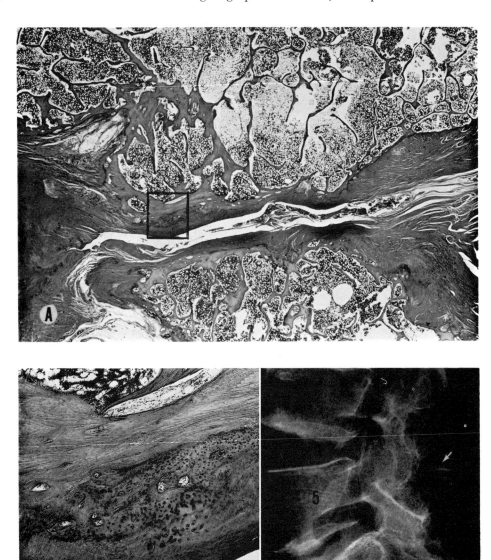

Fig. IX:4. Impingement of the spinous processes in a male of eighty-one years. The photo-micrograph (A) X6 shows the interspinous fissure between the 4th and 5th lumbar spinous processes as indicated by the white arrow upon the roentgenogram. The recurrent pressure has destroyed the continuity of the interspinous ligament. Studies by contrast material have indicated that this structure normally remains intact. A sclerosis of the cortex has been induced by the pressure at the points of contact. Dense ligamentum flavum tissue is visualized at the left. The location of photomicrograph B x40 is indicated by the square on A. It shows that a bumper of fibrocartilage has developed as a result of the intermittent pressure between two bony surfaces which are normally only covered with periosteum. This is an illustration of the so-called "kissing" impingement which may develop between spinous processes. It is painful upon dorsal extension. Note erosion of the vertebral body below pedicle 5 for the artery (see Figures XIV:27 and XIV:28.)

tion. The patient is obliged to turn his body to look behind him. In this late, healed stage of ankylosis the patient has little pain but he has developed a stiff rigid "poker back."

The condition of the intervertebral discs depends upon their state at the time of the ligament ossification. If that process occurred early they may have retained their original thickness, but if later the discs will be thinner. Partially degenerated discs may have bulged before ankylosis and will so finally appear as the so-called "bamboo" spine (Figure IX:10).

In ankylosing spondylitis the ossification is of and in the longitudinal ligaments and is of a more or less homogenious character on the surface of the vertebra (Figure IX:9). While on the other

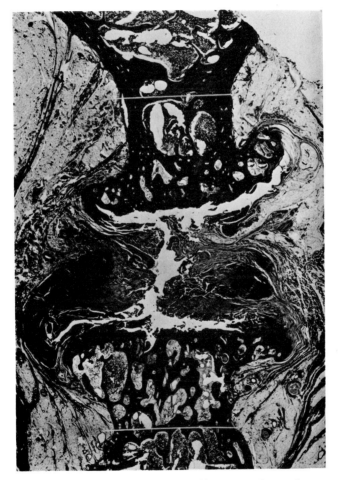

Fig. IX:5. Frontal or coronal section thru two adjacent lumbar spinous processes, X6, male ninety-five years old. Repeated pressure between these structures has destroyed the interspinous ligament. Its fragments are seen each side of the midline. Two mushroom-shaped, dense, bony outgrowths have formed as bumpers upon the adjacent surfaces of the spinous processes. The white lines indicate the orginial cortices of those processes from which the growths first originated. All of the bone therefore between the lines is new growth which has developed as a result of the pressure and other stresses. There has been some fibrocartilage bumper formation (see Figure XIV:37).

hand the spur formation of degenerative spondylosis develops outwards from the surface of the vertebral body (Figure VIII:9). The posterior spinal articulations are not usually ankylosed in degenerative spondylosis. This latter de-generative type of spinal condition appears later in life and is ten times as frequent as the ankylosing spondylitis first seen in the younger individual. Osteoporosis occurs late in both of these conditions. A destructive process in the

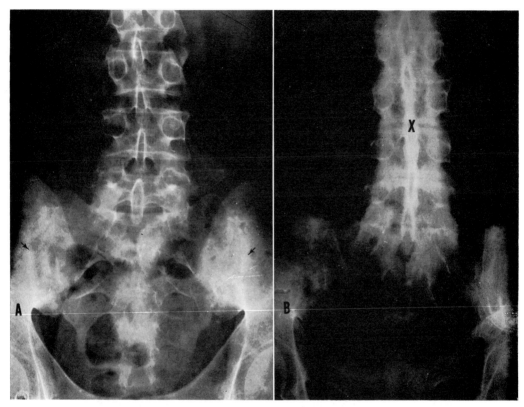

Fig. IX:6. Development of ankylosing rheumatoid spondylitis during a period of fifteen years. Films on the left (A and C) were made at ages of forty-three and thirty-eight respectively. The thoracic spine appeared normal at the earlier examination but the sacroiliacs at forty-three showed the changes of early Marie-Strumpell disease. The widened, blurry, irregular joint shadows with increased density of the surrounding bone indicate the acute inflammatory reaction with subcortical erosion characteristic of the early, active stage of rheumatoid spondylitis (*black arrows*). Those radiographs on the right (B and D) were made at fifty-three years of age. These reveal the late, healed, burned out stage of the disease. Note the ossified lateral longitudinal ligaments of the thoracic spine (*white arrow*) and the ossified interspinous ligament of the lumbar region (X). At fifty-eight years of age this man has developed the ankylosed, "poker back" spine of late Marie Strumpell disease. The films indicate that he has passed the acute painful stage. The sacroiliac joints are now ankylosed with some of the undestroyed articular cartilage entrapped and the surrounding inflammatory reaction has become resorbed during a ten-year interval. Radiographs of this same patient showing destruction of the odontoid which may occur with this disease are shown as Figure IX:7.

$\longrightarrow$

sacroiliac joints and posterior articulations with ankylosis of the latter as well as ossification of the fibrous tissues of the spine, point toward the ankylosing rheumatoid spondylitis.

JUVENILE RHEUMATOID ARTHRITIS

This is a chronic systemic disease of childhood occurring before puberty. The peripheral joints are invariably affected and the spine at some level is involved in about half of the cases. There are visceral lesions with spleno-hepatomegaly, enlarged lymph glands and frequently heart disease. The condition may be related to rheumatic fever. The etiology is unknown altho infection may be a factor.

In the cervical spine the posterior articulations are first destroyed. Then the articular processes and the laminae become fused into a solid bony mass. Since the vertebral bodies can no longer expand in a longitudinal direction and have not the stimulus of movement they remain small and the discs do not enlarge as the child grows. There is less ossification of the paraspinal ligaments than noted in ankylosing spondylitis.

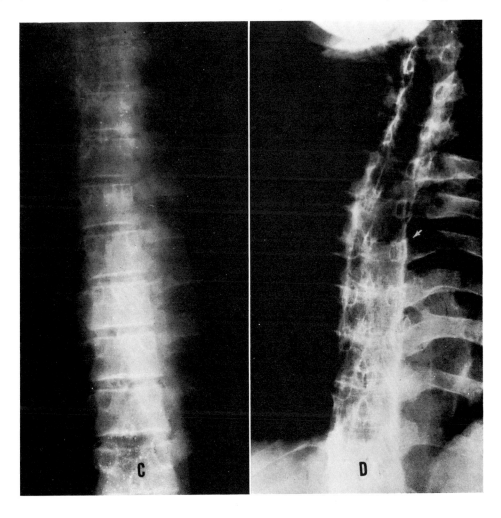

However in both there may be a sub-luxation of the atlanto-axial joint (Figure IX:13).

Contrasting the two diseases; ankylosing spondylitis begins usually at the sacroiliacs in young men after the eighteenth or twentieth year, ascends along the spine and terminates in ossification of all the paraspinal connective tissue structures. Since growth was completed at onset the vertebral bodies and discs preserve their normal size and thickness.

In some cases there is also involvement of the peripheral joints. Juvenile rheumatoid arthritis on the other hand is a systemic disease with involvement of the peripheral joints and visceral structures. It is more common in girls, arises before puberty, and may appear as early as the second or third year. If involved, the cervical spine presents a characteristic appearance with the arches fused into a solid block and the vertebrae of a size noted in childhood (Figures IX:15 and

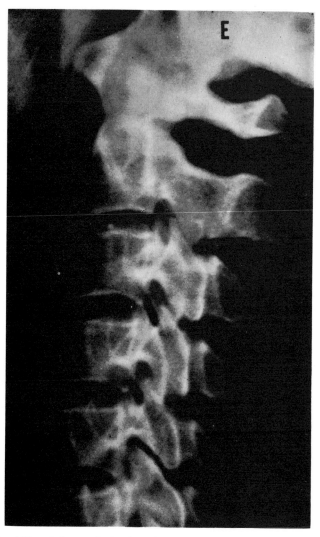

Fig. IX:7. A lateral film of the cervical spine of patient in Figure IX:6 made before the onset of his disease shows the odontoid and other structures apparently normal (E).

IX:16). Compare with Figure III:14 a congenital nonsegmentation of the cervical and thoracic spine, probably not arthritic, wherein the posterior articulations were not destroyed.

PAGET'S DISEASE (OSTEITIS DEFORMANS)

Paget's is a disease of later life and may appear as monostotic or it may involve many bones. Schmorl in a series of 4600 autopsies encountered the condition 138 times, or an incidence of 3 per cent. It was found to be slightly more prevalent in men than in women, a ratio of 7 to 5. The spine is affected in half the cases and the sacrum even slightly more often. In one type the involved bones appear to be made up of coarse thickened trabeculae with loose open spaces or cavities within them. The position and direction of these coarsened

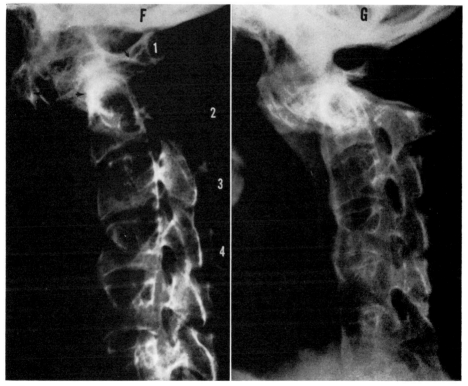

F. The same patient five years later. He has now developed a generalized spondylitis deformans involving the entire spine with partial destruction of the odontoid and extreme spontaneous forward subluxation of the atlas. Arrow-heads indicate the distance between odontoid and the anterior arch of the atlas. Compare the present odontoid with its previous normal appearance (E). There now remains only a narrow space for the spinal cord between the odontoid and the first neural arch (*black arrow*). Laminectomy was performed at once.

G. Seven years post-operative. The patient now has solid bony bridging between the occiput, atlas and the axis as well as between all of the cervical segments. The posterior articulations have disappeared so that the posterior articular processes now form a continuous tubular structure. The odontoid likewise is no longer present. Since the intervertebral discs were not destroyed the intervertebral foramina have preserved their normal size.

trabeculae follow exactly the balancing lines of stress and force. Since the greatest stress in the vertebral body occurs at the cortex and the plane surfaces, these structures necessarily become more dense and the entire vertebra appears on the radiograph as a rectangle with dense margins, the so-called "picture frame" (Figure IX:17). Those coarse trabeculae remaining in the center of the vertebra

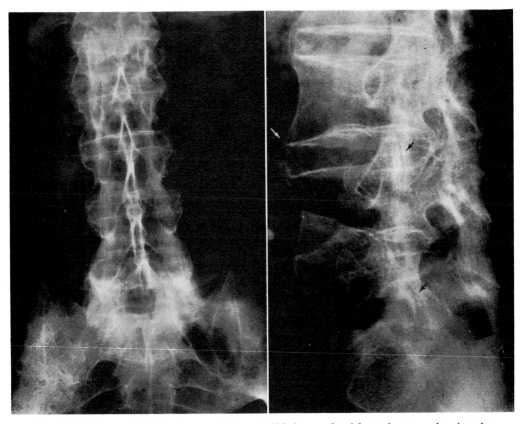

Fig. IX:8. Later ankylosing rheumatoid spondylitis in a male of forty-six years, showing the typical "bamboo" spine, ankylosed sacroiliacs and ossified interspinous ligament. The oblique projection visualizes the "squared" corners of the vertebrae and ossified longitudinal ligaments with their double cortices (*white arrow*). Posteriorly are seen the ankylosed arthritic apophyseal articulations (*black arrows*). At the time of examination the patient was having some chest pain arising in the arthritic costovertebral joints. The intervertebral discs will appear in this disease full thickness or thinned depending upon their condition at the time when they became entrapped by the ankylosing process of ligamentous ossification.

───→

Fig. IX:9. Photograph and roentgenogram showing ankylosing rheumatoid spondylitis in a female of fifty-two years. The longitudinal ligaments and joint capsules are ossified. There is a marked shift in the position of the lines of stress as shown by the rearrangement of the trabeculae. A photomicrograph of the T_{10} posterior articulation X18 shows the cartilage cells entrapped within a completely ankylosed joint. A section thru the sacroiliac joint shows complete ankylosis between the ilium (I) above and the sacrum (S) below. Note the density of the ossified sacroiliac ligament in front (*arrow*).

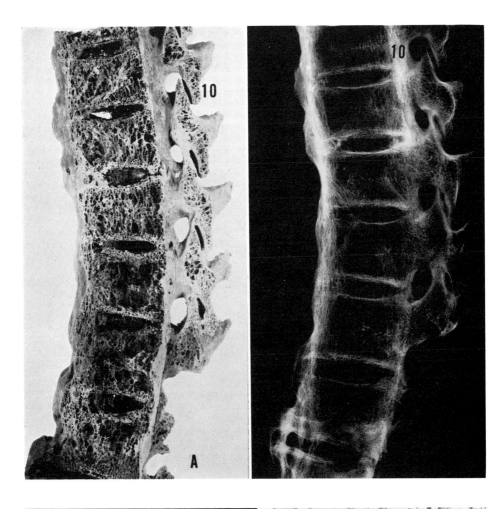

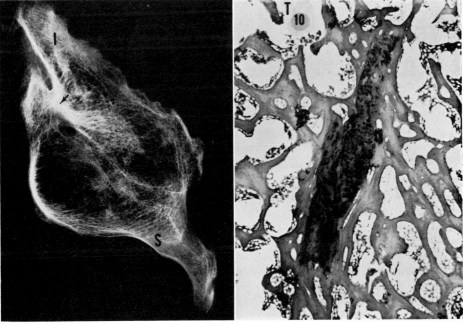

assume a vertical direction, sustaining the pressure stresses between the plates (Figure IX:18).

In a second type of Paget's the trabeculae are closely packed together so that the bone appears to have the density of ivory. Or in other cases, especially late in this disease, the bone takes on a coarsely mottled or "cotton wool" appearance (Figure IX:21).

It is this mottled appearance which is usually seen in the skull when the

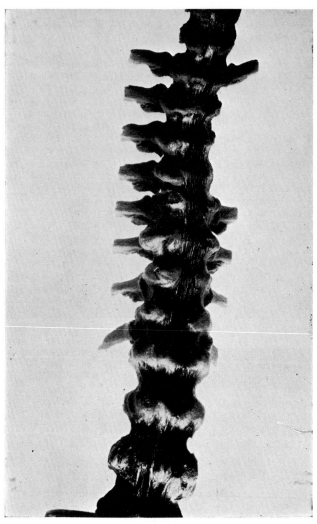

Fig. IX:10. Typical bamboo spine of ankylosing rheumatoid spondylitis with photograph and radiographs showing ossification of the longitudinal ligaments. This bony bridging, developing as ossification of the connective tissue of the longitudinal ligaments, differs somewhat from the degenerative spondylosis spurs which originate in the attachment of those ligaments to the vertebra. Even the frail posterior longitudinal ligament has here become ossified (*white arrows*). The ribs are ankylosed to the spine. Note the absence of spur formation at those points were the aorta is in direct contact with the spine and separate from it only by the anterior longitudinal ligament. That ligament here remains in situ (Figure VIII:11).

calvarium becomes thickened. In spite of its apparent greater density however the bone is really soft. As a result the skull becomes wider and the occiput may become invaginated upward into the cranial cavity producing a basilar impression (Figure III:34). These patients with their proportionally wider head present a somewhat triangular facies. They are said to suffer from hearing deficiency, possibly from lengthing of the auditory nerves.

At times the disease appears first in the calvarium as an osteoporosis circumscripta. This is an area of decreased density, sharply delineated by a definite margin which gradually advances as the area becomes larger. There is some evidence that this may be a vascular disturbance.

The softened bone of Paget's contains less calcium. It has a brittle or chalky character and is subject to fracture. Healing occurs but the disease extends to the callus. At times fissures may appear on the convex surface of the long bones somewhat in the nature of a march fracture (Figure IX:20). Bending of these long bones is a common observation. Weakening of the vertebral body may occur. In the lumbar region with osteoporosis the disc expands but with demineralization in the thoracic area, a wedge vertebra forms and kyphosis results. The bone may become enlarged by periosteal new bone growth (Figure IX:21C). The disease then spreads to this bone the same as it does to the callus. Encroachment of the spinal canal may supervene.

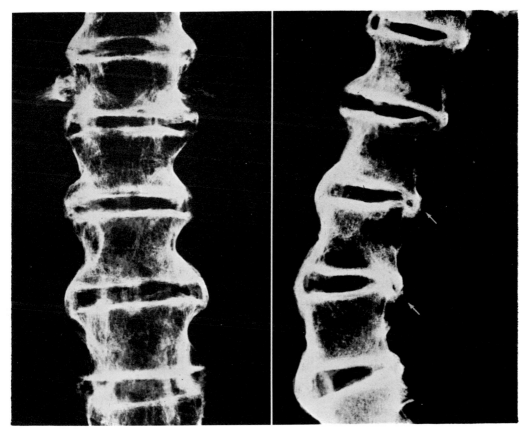

Laboratory studies show the serum calcium and phosphorous normal but the alkaline phosphatase is high. Sometimes this reaches a level as much as twenty times its usual value.

The bone of Paget's disease is at times so soft that it may be cut with a knife. On section the trabeculae are seen to be coarse, thick and irregular, either closely packed together or widely placed with spaces between.

Upon microscopic section the bone of Paget's disease exhibits a characteristic irregular "mosaic" pattern. Irregular segments of lamellar bone are separated by many, short, ragged, wide, dark cement lines. These stain a deep blue with hematoxaline. This produces the characteristic mosaic appearance which is not seen in the adjacent normal bone with its haversian systems about the vessel canals (Figures IX:19 and X:16).

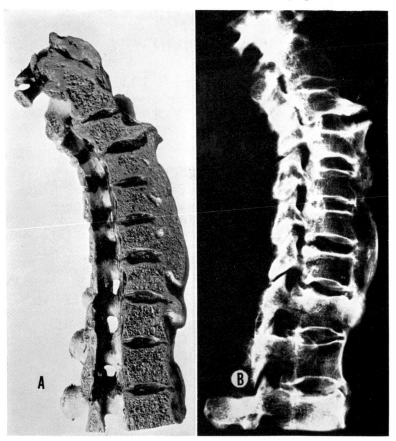

Fig. IX:11. Ankylosing spondylitis in a male of seventy-eight years. There is complete ossification of the atlas and axis into a solid bony block. From C_4 to T_1 the anterior longitudinal ligament has ossified into a solid bony mass with trabeculae and cortex. This is 8 mm. thick at one point. The united cervical vertebrae and discs have preserved their own individual identity. A photomicrograph (C) X5 of the first two cervical segments reveal ossification of the ligamentous structures. The congential disc between the odontoid and the body of C_2 is seen as a persistent rest *(arrow)*. The square indicates the site of the transverse ligament. A photomicrograph (D) X40 shows a portion of the transverse ligament ossified into dense laminated bony tissue. On the right side is a mass of entrapped fibrous tissue which has not as yet undergone this change.

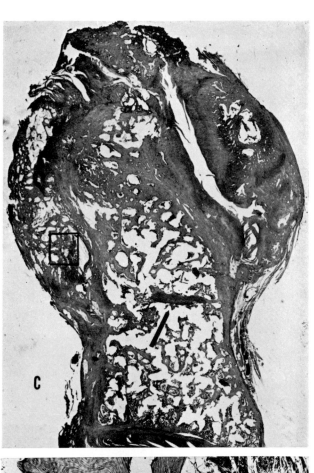

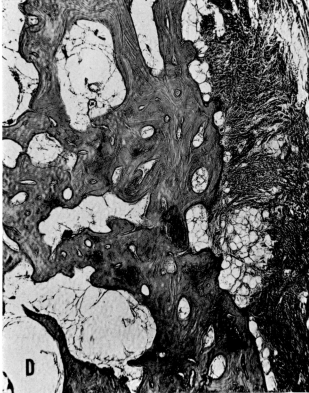

The bone marrow is replaced by fibrous tissue rich in blood vessels.

Osteogenic sarcoma which usually develops in younger individuals is, nevertheless, a not unusual terminal condition to become engrafted upon Paget's disease in these older patients. Cases of involvement at multiple levels have been reported but only bones showing osteitis deformans are involved. The prognosis is grave altho cures have been reported where amputation of an involved extremity was possible.

THE NEUROTROPHIC SPINE

Charcot in 1868 originally described neurotrophic arthropathy in connection with certain chronic nervous disorders. These are characterized by degenerative changes in the posterior columns of the spinal cord. Tabes, syringomyelia or diabetes may be responsible for the demyelization and atrophy of the nerve bundles. Other diseases have been implicated.

The afferent pain impulses are impaired and the proprioceptive stimuli to the cord are diminished while the

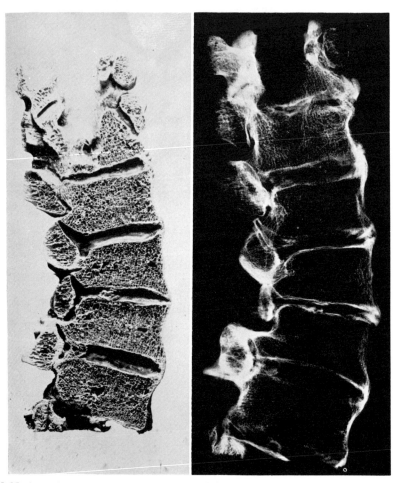

Fig. IX:12. A section from the thoracic spine of the same individual as Figure IX:11 showing ankylosis of the ribs to the vertebral bodies.

motor tract to the joint remains intact. The condition usually occurs in weight bearing joints as a result of trauma, either major or repeated minor injuries. There is weakness and instability. The condition may be asymptomatic or accompanied by root pains and other symptoms of the causal disease.

The roentgenographic manifestations are characterized by a bizarre combination of hyperplastic and destructive bone changes. These may occur in extent out of all proportion to the severity of the pain. Infractions and even spontaneous fractures may occur. Fragmentation with wedging and various types of curvatures may be a feature of the disease. Mushrooming of the vertebra and destruction of the disc were reported by Zucker in his diabetic case. New bone forms in the destroyed area but not in the adjacent bone. Gross thickening of the lamellae and subcortical eburnation results in a dense hypertrophy of the affected bone tissue. Also there may be a massive development of ragged vertebral osteophytes. Figure IX:22 illustrates both destruction and hyperplasia of the spinal structure.

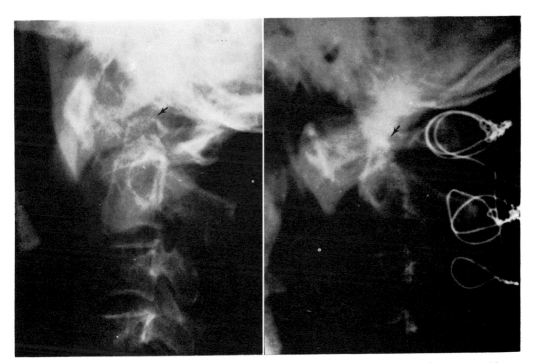

Fig. IX:13. Peripheral type of rheumatoid arthritis with gradual destruction of the odontoid in a young man of twenty-six years (*arrows*). The resultant subluxation of C_1 necessitated operative fixation. There was no other spinal involvement. The sacroiliac joints were destroyed but the apophyseal articulations did not appear to be involved altho the disease had attacked various peripheal articulations. These roentgenograms were made at an interval of fourteen months. One year later the odontoid had completely disappeared. Compare with Figure IX:7 - (Courtesy of the Syracuse V. A. Hospital.)

REFERENCES

Degenerative Changes

Bohatricheck: 1955, *Brit. Jor. Rad., 28:*389–404.

Culver, G. J., *et al:* 1956, *Am. Jor. Roent., 76:* 1157–1160.

Jacobson, H. G., *et al:* 1958, *Am. Jor. Roent., 79:* 677–683.

Kohler, R.: 1959, *Acta Rad., 52:*21–27.

Scott, W. G.: 1942, *Am. Jor. Roent., 48:*491–505.

Smith, C. F., *et al:* 1955, *Am. Jor. Roent., 74:* 1049–1058.

Teng, P.: 1960, *J. Bone J. Surg., 42A:*392–407.

Ankylosing Rheumatoid Spondylitis

Boggenstoss, A. H.: *J. Bone J. Surg., 34A:*601–609.

Boland, E. W., *et al:* 1946, *Rad., 47:*551–561.

Grainger, R. G.: 1959, *Jor. Fac. Rad., 10:*138–150.

Guest, C. M., *et al:* 1951, *Am. Jor. Roent., 65:* 760–768.

Martel, W.: 1961, *Am. Jor. Roent., 86:*223–240.

Middlemiss, J. H.: *Jor. Fac. Rad., 7:*155–166.

Polley, H. F., *et al:* 1947, *Ann. Int. Med., 26:* 240–249.

Rheumatoid Disease Symposium: 1958, *Acta Med. Scand.,* Suppl. 341, *162:*1–261.

Seaman, W. B., *et al:* 1961, *Am. Jor. Roent., 86:* 241–250.

Swezy, R. L., *et al:* 1957, *Ann. Int. Med., 47:*904–921.

Whaley, M. H., *et al:* 1960, *Rad., 74:*54–56.

Juvenile Rheumatoid Arthritis
Still's Disease

Barkin, R. E., *et al:* 1955, *New Eng. J. Med., 253:*1107–1110.

Cass, J. A., *et al:* 1946, *Jor. Ped., 29:*143–156.

Kelley, V. C.: 1960, *Ped. Clin. No. Amer., 7:* 435–456.

Martel, W., *et al:* 1962, *Am. Jor. Roent., 88:*400–423.

Pickard, N. S.: 1947, *Arch. Int. Med., 80:*771–790.

Paget's Disease

Allen, M. L.: 1937, *Am. Jor. Roent., 38:*109–115.

Brailsford, J. F.: 1954, *Brit. Jor. Rad., 27:*435–442.

Kasabach, H. H., *et al:* 1937, *Am. Jor. Roent., 37:*577–602.

Kelley, P. T., *et al:* 1961, *Rad., 77:*368–375.

Poppel, M. H., *et al:* 1953, *Rad., 61:*639–644.

Steinbach, H. L.: *Am. Jor. Roent., 86:*950–964.

Teng, P., *et al:* 1951, *J. Neurosurg., 8:*482–433.

Sarcoma Complicating Paget's Disease

Coley, B. L., *et al:* 1931, *Arch. Surg., 23:*918–936.

Derman, H., *et al:* 1951, *Am. Jor. Roent., 65:* 221–226.

Esposito, W. J., and Berne, Alfred S.: 1960, *Am. Jor. Roent., 83:*698–703.

Goldenberg, R. R.: 1961, *Bull. Hosp. J. Dis., 22:* 1–38.

Jaffe, H. L.: 1933, *Arch. Path., 15:*83–131.

Porretta, C. A., *et al:* 1957, *J. Bone J. Surg., 39A:* 1314–1329.

Schatzki, S. C., *et al:* 1961, *Cancer, 14:*517–523.

Sherman, R. S., *et al:* 1954, *Rad. 63:*48–58.

Summey, T. J., *et al:* 1946, *Ann. Surg., 123:*135–153.

Tabes of Spine
Charcot Arthropathy

Cleveland, M., *et al:* 1959, *J. Bone J. Surg., 41A:* 336–340.

Fig. IX:14. Rheumatoid arthritis in a female of sixty-three years with numerous peripheral joints involved. The patient was complaining of back ache. A destructive process has involved the eleventh intervertebral disc anteriorly with some adjacent bony reaction and kyphosis (A). Displaced disc material is outlined in front by the osteophytes. Paravertebral shadows are visualized on the A. P. projection in this patient (*white arrows*). The fourth lumbar posterior articulation had become destroyed allowing a so-called pseudo spondylolisthesis. Roentgenographically this process may resemble some-what an infection of the disc such as tuberculosis, however the clinical picture should prove helpful in differentiating the two conditions. Reexamination six years later (B) shows limitation of the destructive process and of the surrounding reaction. Paravertebral shadows are no longer visualized.

———————————————▶

Holland, H. W.: 1953, *Proc. Roy. Soc. Med., 46:* 747–752.

Katz, I., *et al:* 1961, *Am. Jor. Roent., 86:*965–974.

Key, J. A.: 1932, *Am. J. Syph., 16:*429–446.

Steindler, A.: 1931, *J.A.M.A., 96:*250–256.

Zucker, G., *et al:* 1952, *Am. J. Med., 12:*118–124.

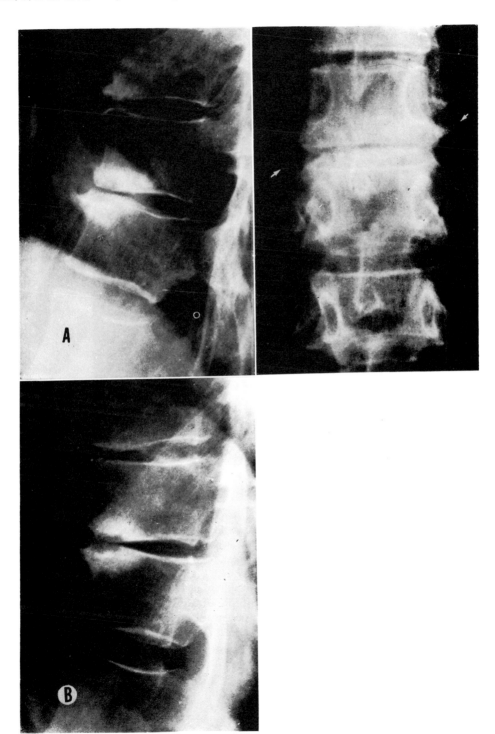

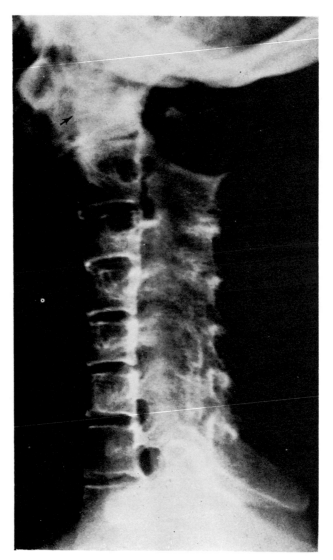

Fig. IX:15. Juvenile rheumatoid arthritis in a male of thirty-four years. There was a history of rheumatic fever for one year beginning at age thirteen with arthritis involving multiple joints. The patient still complained of constant neck pain, occassionally referred down the arms. Note the fused cervical neural arches incidental to the destroyed apophyseal articulations. The vertebral bodies below C_1 are smaller than normal and there is no cervical curve. The atlas however while normal for an adult of thirty-four is relatively larger than the other cervical segments. It will be seen that C_1 is displaced forward so that its anterior arch is well in front of the odontoid, the anterior surface of which is indicated by the arrow point.

(Courtesy of Dr. Thomas J. Rankin.)

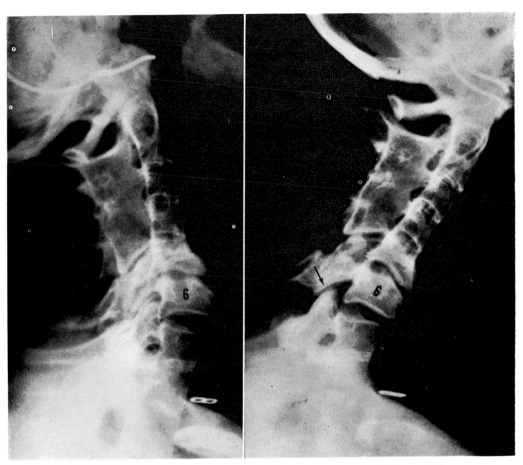

Fig. IX:16. Aged female. Fusion of the second, third, fourth and fifth cervical segments with imprisoned discs but complete disappearance of the posterior articulations, possibly from old juvenile rheumatoid disease or congenital nonsegmentation. Flexion-extension studies show a fusion between the atlas and occiput and very slight, if any, movement between the axis and atlas. The upper cervical spine is practically fused solid. One may note the decreased antero-posterior diameter of the fused segments, both cervical and thoracic. The flatness of the anterior vertebral surface at the C_7 to T_2 disc level somewhat resembles a congenital fusion at that point. These features, as well as the small, round or oval foramina are characteristic of early synostosis. Nearly all movement in this patient's cervical spine occurs at the fifth and sixth discs which are of normal anterior-posterior diameter. Apparently the dynamic function of the part stimulated growth to normal size. The fifth disc has developed advanced degenerative changes. Compare the flexion-extension studies for gliding of the posterior joints (*arrow*) and increased distance between the spinous processes at these two levels as the neck is bent forward. The upper thoracic vertebrae are also fused so that practically all of the upper spine movement occurred at the C_{5-6-7} level with consequent advanced degenerative changes. (See Figure IV:37.)

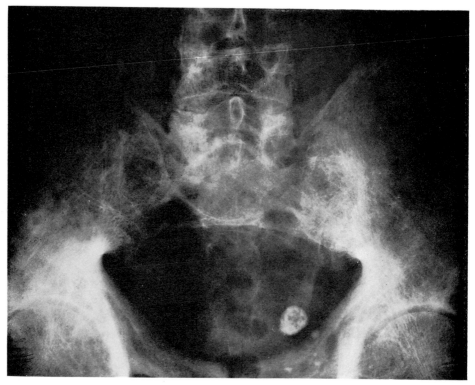

Fig. IX:17. Lower spine and pelvic changes of Paget's disease in a male of seventy-five years. These consist of coarse trabeculations involving the pelvic bones and sclerosis of the vertebral plates. The calvarium was 2 c.m. thick with characteristic cotton wool mottling. He complained of pain in the dorso-lumbar and sacroiliac regions without sciatica but with all movements limited. The Achilles and patellar reflexes were normal.

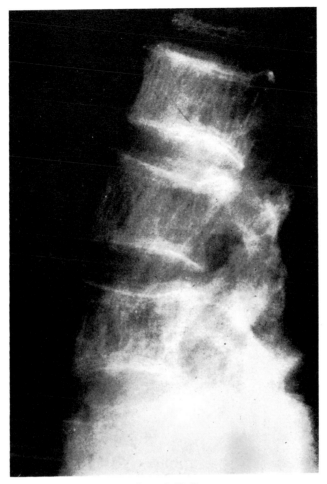

Fig. IX:17 B.

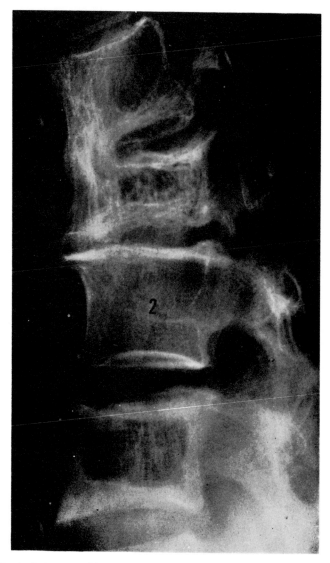

Fig. IX:18. Typical changes of later Paget's in a female of sixty-five years. Softening of the vertebra had previously allowed a compression of L_1. In healing this became fused with the lowermost thoracic segment by coarse trabeculations. The third lumbar vertebra with square corners presents an excellent example of the so-called "picture frame" formation.

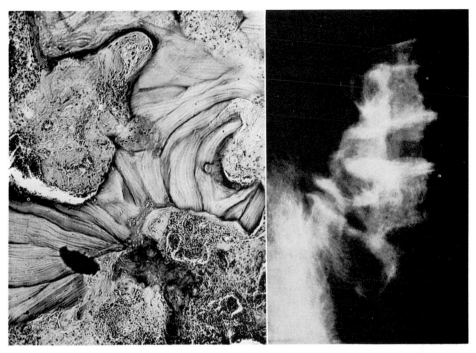

Fig. IX:19. Photomicrograph X 130 from the fifth lumbar vertebra of an individual with Paget's disease showing the typical mosaic pattern in the formation of the trabeculae. The marrow is replaced by fibrous tissue and many blood vessels. The dark oval spot is an artifact (see Figure X:16).

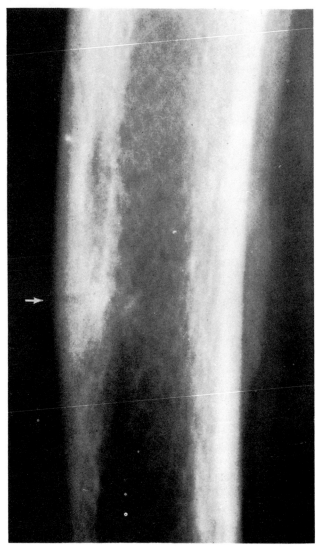

Fig. IX:20. A Milkman-type of pseudo fracture in the lateral cortex of the femur of a seventy-year-old female with Paget's disease *(arrow)*. She continued to suffer from pain in the leg. Six months later upon turning suddenly she sustained a complete spontaneous transverse fracture of this femur. This was followed at once by relief from pain. It healed firmly after insertion of a medullary pin and no longer caused the patient any discomfort.

Fig. IX:21. Generalized advanced Paget's disease of the entire spine in a male of fifty years showing multiple sarcomata at necropsy. A lateral projection of the lumbar region (A) shows the cotton wool type of involvement with bone softening. The 4th and 5th vertebrae have become flattened, widened and biconcave. This is confirmed by the A. P. projection (B) which also shows the pelvic involvement. In the cervical region (C) one notes that as the result of a marked bony hyperplasia the axis has become grossly enlarged and of an ivory-like density. An osteogenic sarcoma developed at the C_4 level displacing backward this

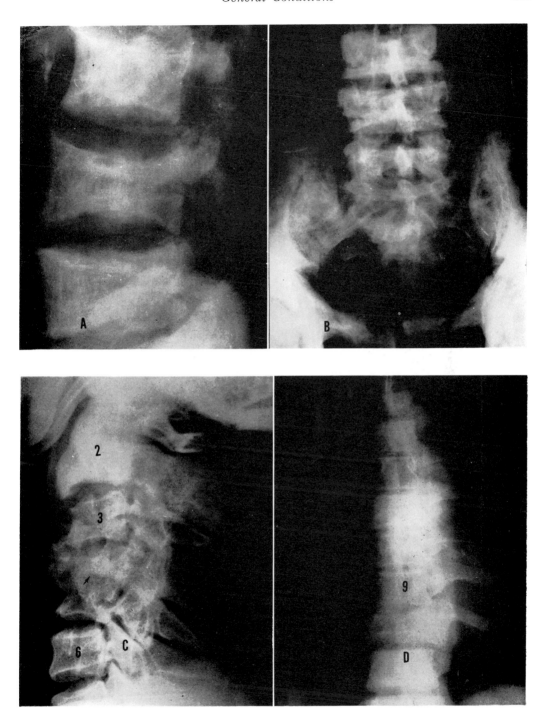

vertebra with its enlarged spinous process (*arrow*). As a result the spinal canal was encroached upon, C_5 was partially destroyed and the tumor bulged forward into the retropharyngeal area. A second sarcoma formed at T_{10} and extended into the paravertebral space on each side (D). There was a history of back ache of increasing severity for four years and paralysis for one year before death.

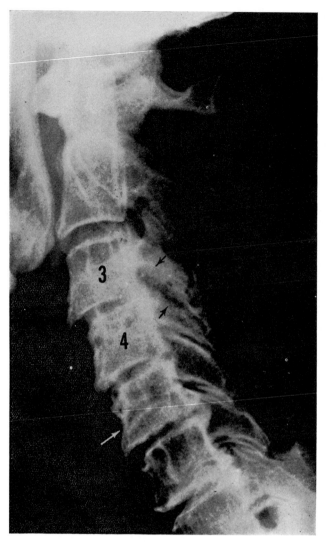

Fig. IX:22. Tabetic spine. This sixty-year-old male with a luetic history complained of pain in the left shoulder with sharp shooting pains in the legs together with a burning sensation. There was tremor and instability of movements. The pupils were sluggish, the Romberg sign was positive and the patellar and Achilles reflexes could not be obtained. A lateral projection of the cervical spine shows eburnation of the 3rd and 4th neural arches with destruction of the articulations between them (*black arrows*). A dark band crossing C_5 (*white arrow*) as well as spur formation of the 5th disc posteriorly indicate arthrotic and hyperplastic changes involving the covertebral articulations. The entire lumbar spine, like the mid cervical, shows advanced eburnation and loss of normal trabecular structure. The left side of L_5 has collapsed allowing a scoliosis toward that side. Disintegration of the lower apophyseal articulations has permitted various subluxations to occur in that region.

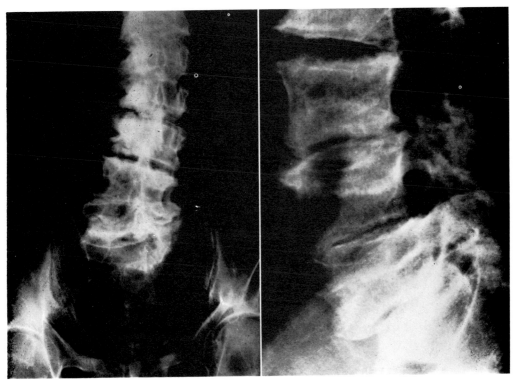

Fig. IX:22 B.

Chapter X

Spinal Curvatures

KYPHOSIS

Of the spinal curvatures the most common is kyphosis (dorsal prominence) of the thoracic region. This produces less actual angulation of the spine than scoliosis or lateral curvature, however for the amount of malalignment the patient's deformity may appear to be even greater.

Kyphosis may result from absent vertebral segments, block vertebrae and other congenital anomalies, wherein the length of the posterior portion of the spine exceeds that of the anterior portion (Figures II:28, II:27, and II:33).

The most common types of postnatal kyphosis are: (1) Juvenile, (2) Senile, (3) Osteoporotic and (4) Infective from tuberculosis. Juvenile kyphosis resulting from an aseptic vertebral epiphysitis was described by the Danish orthopedist Holger Scheuermann. It develops during adolescence if the posterior arch structures of the spine grow more rapidly than the vertebral bodies. The height of the vertebral body increases at the epiphyseal growth zone directly beneath the cartilaginous plate of the disc. Pressure has been shown to inhibit epiphyseal growth. If pressure is uneven on the opposite sides of an epiphysis, that side with the lesser pressure will grow more rapidly. In stoop shouldered asthenic adolescents with inadequate dorsal musculature the thoracic vertebral epiphyses are subjected to greater pressure in front than in back. As a result, the posterior part of the vertebral body grows more rapidly than the anterior and the struc-

ture becomes wedge shaped. The axis of the center of gravity for the head and thorax is well anterior to the thoracic spine. With increased growth this center of gravity is carried further forward at a time when the patient is increasing in height and weight. The resultant additional pressure upon the anterior edges of the epiphyses increases the kyphosis even more. This is accentuated by fatigue and slouching. Aseptic epiphysitis is also a factor.

In addition to the kyphotic deformity, the radiographic picture of dorsal curvature at this age is characterized by the following four features. (1) The wedging or flattening of the vertebral bodies, (2) narrowing of the discs, (3) a ragged, wavy appearance of the disc surfaces caused by irregular ruptures of their cartilage plates and, (4) an increased anterior-posterior diameter of the involved vertebral bodies. This latter is in contrast to the lesser corresponding diameter of the normal vertebral bodies below. Juvenile kyphosis usually involves the thoraco-lumbar region (Figures X:1, VIII:23 and VIII:-24).

A type of senile kyphosis may develop later in stoop-shouldered elderly persons with minimal or no wedging of the vertebral bodies. In this case the pressure upon the anterior margin of the disc destroys the annulus fibrosus producing a wedge shaped disc and allowing the anterior margins of the adjacent vertebral bodies to come into contact. The rims become fused with bony trabeculae replacing the anterior portion of the disc (Figure X:2).

More commonly, senile kyphosis results from osteoporosis, wherein the vertebral body loses its normal strength and succumbs to superimposed pressure or minimal trauma. In this case the mid thoracic vertebrae which may have been entirely normal in middle life gradually become wedge shaped as their anterior margins collapse (Figure X:3 and X:4).

Tuberculosis of the spine or Pott's disease is the most common type of infection to produce a sharp kyphotic gibbus. It usually begins in the vicinity of the disc. The earliest radiographic sign is a thinning or narrowing of that struc-

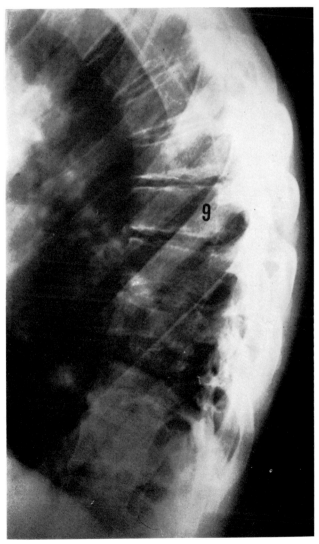

Fig. X:1. Juvenile kyphosis or Scheuermann's disease originating in adolescence but still obvious at midlife. The 9th thoracic vertebra is flattened, its epiphyseal plates are wavy, and the A.P. diameter is increased, even exceeding that of the lumbar bodies. There is also some wedging of the 8th vertebra.

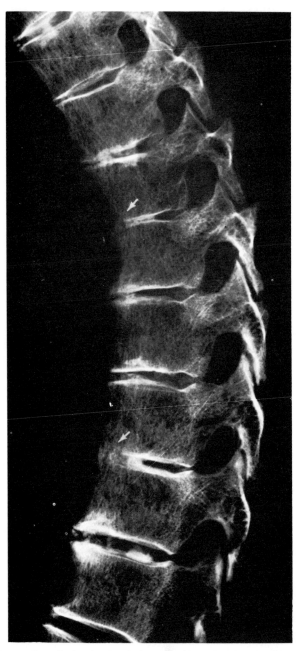

Fig. X:2. Specimen of senile kyphosis of the thoracic spine from a female of seventy-five years. The anterior portion of a disc has become destroyed by pressure and the adjacent vertebral bodies have ankylosed (*white arrows*). The other dics show an earlier stage of the same process. Note there is no wedging of the vertebral bodies, no osteophyte formation and no ossification of the spinal ligaments. These observations rule out: osteoporotic kyphosis, spondylosis deformans and ankylosing rheumatoid spondylitis, respectively. Neither is this the characteristic picture of juvenile kyphosis.

ture. Further destruction of the disc and the adjacent vertebral bodies may be visualized subsequently. The neural arches are likely to be spared. A paravertebral abscess may be seen upon the radiograph of the thoracic region because of its contrast with the lesser density of the lung. Below the diaphram however such an abscess is difficult to visualize unless it contains bony debris or displaces other structures. The infection usually extends beneath the longitudinal ligaments to other vertebrae so that multiple levels become involved. Complete healing may occur with de-

velopment of a solid kyphotic block vertebra. Even with considerable angulation the diameter of the spinal canal appears adequate although cord pressure may result from the pathological process (Figures X:5, XI:10 and XI:8).

Various other conditions which have been mentioned as a cause of kyphosis are spondylitis deformans, compression fracture, Morquio's, gargoylism, or Hurler's disease and achondroplasia (Figures XV:3, XV:5, XV:6 and XV:7). Also wedge vertebrae developing from any destructive process such as Gaucher's or Paget's disease, rickets, malignancy or

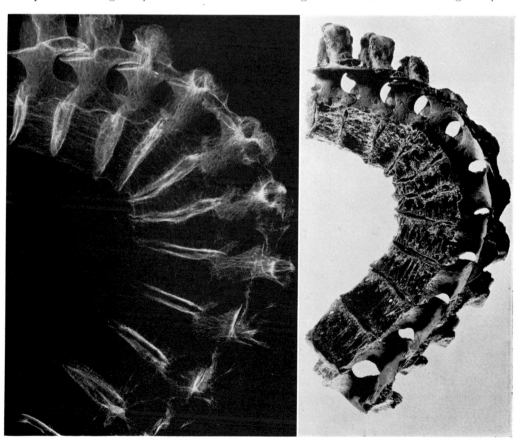

Fig. X:3. Photograph and roentgenogram of a specimen showing advanced osteoporotic kyphosis in an elderly individual. There is generalized resorption of calcium and wedging distortion of the vertebral bodies at the apex of the curve. The few trabeculae still present in the spongiosa are arranged perpendicular to the end plates, thus serving the lines of greatest stress with the minimal amount of bony material.

hyperparathyroidism. Likewise the following conditions may cause either kyphosis or scoliosis: (1) neurofibromatosis, (2) poliomyletis, (3) muscle dystrophy and various other conditions (Figure XVI:10).

Stoop shouldered, kyphotic individuals tend to walk with the head thrust forward and may suffer from emphysema or cardiac disturbance. They develop a compensatory cervical lordosis.

LORDOSIS

Lumbar lordosis, or "swayback" as termed by Jacobson may compensate for dorsal kyphosis or poor posture. It may help to balance the abdomen enlarged by obesity, pregnancy, ascites, or hepatosplenomegaly. Lordosis with the prominent buttocks is characteristic of achondroplasia and certain other dystrophies

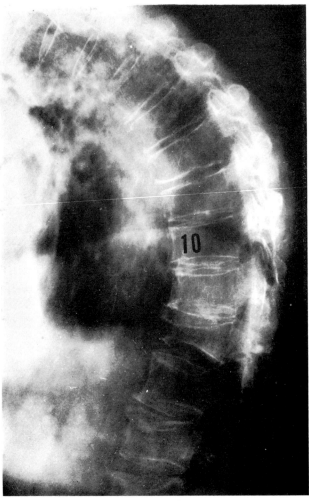

Fig. X:4. Osteoporotic kyphosis in a farmer of eighty-one years. The collapse of T_{12} and L_2 had occurred since a previous examination one year before at which time those vertebrae were osteoporotic but normal in size and shape. Adolescent kyphosis may also have been a factor in this patient's deformity.

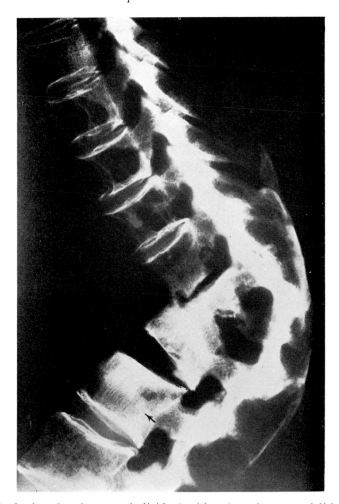

Fig. X:5. Kyphotic spine from an individual with tuberculous spondylitis. A graft of healthy bone inserted many years before united the spinous processes. The ankylosing operation however failed to arrest development of the angulation. Complete destruction of two vertebral bodies at the apex of the gibbus was responsible for the deformity. The infective process, creeping upward beneath the longitudinal ligaments, had involved at least five vertebral bodies above the angulation. At one point the lytic and sclerotic phases of the disease were both present in a single vertebra (*arrow*).

(Figures XV:3 and XV:4). The disturbing feature of lordosis is the resultant shearing stress applied to the lumbo sacral area. Telescoping imbrication of the posterior articulations with joint capsule tension, bony impingement, erosion and eburnation are all potentially painful in these circumstances and have been discussed in Chapter IX. A so-called "kissing" impingement of the spinous processes will cause discomfort upon backward bending. Likewise foramen encroachment may be a clinical factor in the production of sciatica. A substantial number of these patients suffer from low back distress (Figures IX:1, IX:2, IX:3 and IX:4).

SCOLIOSIS

Lateral spinal curvature, frequently combined as a kypho-scoliosis with rotation may be generally classified as: congential, paralytic and idiopathic. We have shown in Chapter II how certain asymmetrical anomalies of the new born such as block vertebrae (nonsegmentation), hemivertebrae or a combination

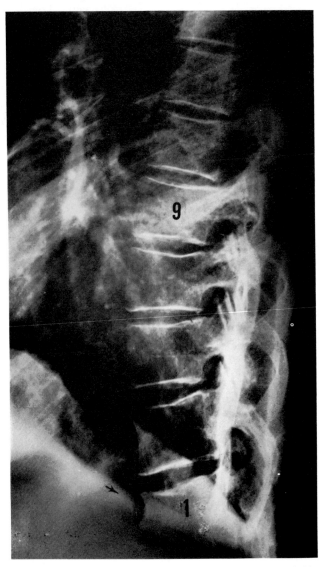

Fig. X:6. Thoracic lordosis in a male of forty-one years. At the age of fifteen this patient had sustained a compression fracture of L_1 (*arrow*). He was treated by traction and dorsal extension on a Bradford frame at a time when the spine was still growing. Here is an example where traction applied to the epiphyseal plates during the growing period together with freedom of weight sustaining pressure resulted in a growth acceleration of the vertebral bodies. The fractured lumbar vertebra remained wedge-shaped. (Its outline is here retouched.) The A.P. diameter of the mid thorax decreased but this was compensated somewhat by a forward bulging of the anterior chest wall laterally.

of these may be responsible for the development of a congenital scoliosis, which increases as the child grows (Figures II:30, II:31, II:32, II:34, II:35, II:36, and X:7).

Paralytic scoliosis, on the other hand, results from a disturbed muscle balance, the contraction of the stronger unparalyzed muscles tending to throw the spine out of alignment. Paralytic scoliosis resulting from poliomyelitis may appear at any age irrespective of the stage of skeletal development. Unilateral paralysis of the intercostals allows the ribs to drop down and the individual develops a convexity on the weak side. Alignment of the pelvis is important (Figures X:8, X:9 and X:10). The scoliosis may be a

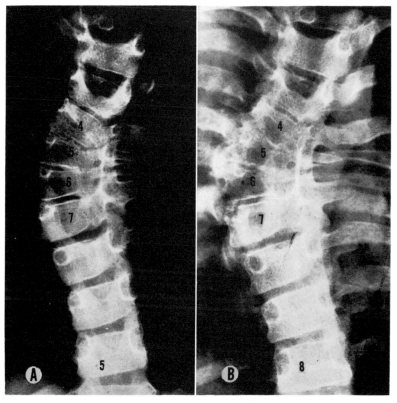

Fig. X:7. Scoliosis in this girl developed as the result of a congenital asymmetrical nonsegmentation. When first seen at five years of age (A) there was a complete unilateral synostosis of the 4th, 5th, 6th, and 7th thoracic vertebrae on the left side with a scoliotic convexity toward the right. Upon reexamination at eight years (B and C) it is seen that the curvature had increased. Growth of the fused segments occurred on the right side but was impeded on the left. It will be noted that the lower spine was relatively straight at eight years and that no rotation had yet occurred. At fourteen years (D) the thoracic scoliosis had increased and she had developed a compensating, rotary, thoraco-lumbar curvature to the left. The discs and the vertebrae at the convexity had become wedge shaped. The primary thoracic curvature did not become rotated because the 4th, 5th, 6th and 7th neural arches had fused into a solid mass on the left side. The cortex of this mass is outlined by white curvilinear lines (*arrow*). The secondary scoliosis continued to increase, the discs became increasingly distorted and a fusion was necessary. The post operative condition is seen at sixteen years (E) by courtesy of Dr. Dwight Needham, Syracuse, N. Y.

serious complication depending upon the particular muscle group which is paralyzed as well as the degree of weakness. In some cases it is rapidly progressive. Paralytic scoliosis may also result from muscular atrophy or thoracoplasty. In the latter the convexity of the curve is toward the resected ribs. Splinting from an empyema may likewise result in a scoliosis, concave on the affected side (**Figure X:11**).

IDIOPATHIC SCOLIOSIS

The so-called idiopathic scoliosis which appears in growing children more commonly toward the right side is the real curvature problem. This, like all scoliosis, is characterized by rotation toward the convexity of the curve, lateral flexion and hyperextension of the spine. It is increased by asymmetrical growth of the epiphyses, gravity and by unbalanced muscle action. As in the kyphotic, that side of the epiphysis on the convexity of the curve grows more rapidly than that portion of the epiphysis subjected to the greater pressure on the concave side.

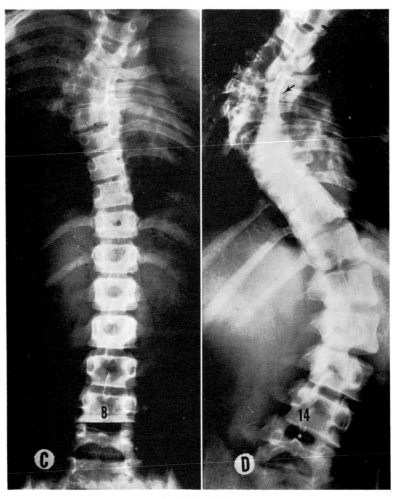

Fig. X:7 C & D.

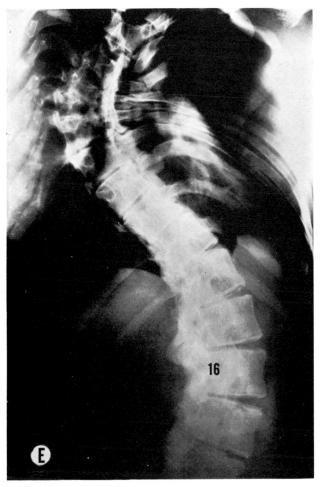

Fig. X:7 E.

This increases the wedging of the vertebral body and the resultant curvature is aggravated. The curve is more prominent when the patient is standing.

There is a type of idiopathic infantile scoliosis appearing in very young children as a single curve which usually resolves by five years of age without treatment. Rarely however, as reported by Scott, it may become progressive and reach a severe degree of deformity. Idiopathic scoliosis develops and increases during the rapid growth period at and immediately preceding puberty. When growth ceases the deformity remains stationary. There is little change in the idiopathic type after the sixteenth or seventeenth year when the spinal epiphyses have become united. Progress of the curve may cease spontaneously at any time. For some unknown reason, girls are the principal victims, various figures giving the frequency of four to nine times that of boys (Figures X:12 and X:15).

Many theories have been proposed to explain the origin of idiopathic scoliosis, such as a weakness of the muscles on the convex side or a displacement of the ring epiphysis like a slipped epiphysis of the hip (Figure VIII:22). In scoliosis the

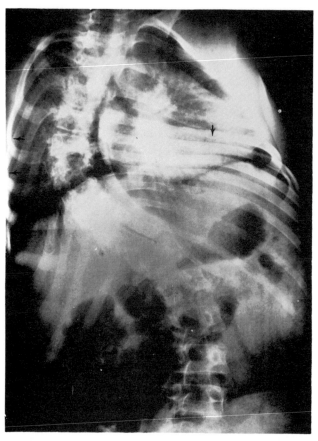

Fig. X:8. Paralytic scoliosis in a boy of 12 years. At fifteen months of age this patient was the victim of poliomyelitis involving the intercostal muscles. The weakened right inter-costals were overbalanced by those on the left side so that he developed a primary thoracic curve convex toward the weakest or right side. The arrows indicate the approximate plane of the mid axilla on each side. The ribs are much more widely separated at the convexity. The secondary curves above and below could be straightened by bending toward the left. (Courtesy of Dr. Horton Murray and Memorial Hospital.)

posterior part of the spine (the neural arches and their ligaments) is shorter than the column of the vertebral bodies because of its slower growth. The growth of these elements comprising the spinal canal is governed by the growth of the spinal cord which they protect. This author believes that the possibility of a neurological factor in the etiology of idiopathic scoliosis is worthy of exploration. Other theories proposed are a possible endocrine disorder with hor-

mone imbalance or a disturbed growth factor affecting the development of the epiphyses.

Since the posterior structures are tight and shorter than the column, they act as a bow string to increase the curvature and rotation. During anterior flexion this bowstring arrangement forces the spine to rotate even more toward the convex side. This causes the increased bulge of the posterior chest wall when the child bends forward. The posterior articular processes are deformed by the excessive asymmetrical stresses to which they are subjected. Those on the convex side are somewhat larger as a result of the pulling strain. Since the chest wall bulges backward on the convex side it becomes necessary to use special care in positioning the patient for supine radiography. During growth the ribs offer some resistance but gradually accommodate themselves to the changed stresses of the rotation. The vertebral bodies and the discs become distorted in shape and foramen encroachment results (Figure X:13).

The spine can be straightened passively at first but soon the structural changes appear. Later after the process has become arrested compensatory features develop. Ligamentous structures and muscles on the convex side undergo extensive hyperplasia while spur formation and bony bridging develop at the disc margins on the concave side of the curve. In this manner some measure of stability is restored. Eventually complete ankylosis may occur (Figure X:14). Examination of the intervertebral discs at a curvature invariably reveals a degeneration of these structures on the concave

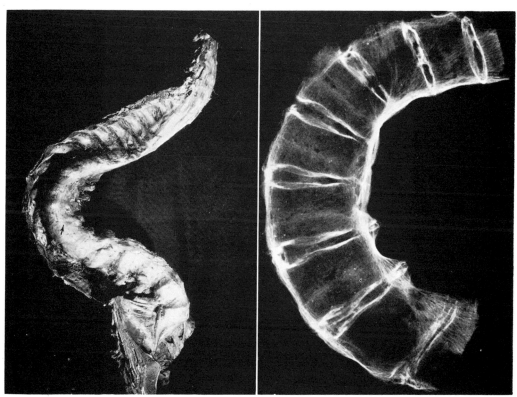

Fig. X:9. Paralytic kyphoscoliosis in a male of sixty-nine years. Pressure by the aorta had eroded a concavity within the hollow of the curvature (*arrow*). The radiograph made from a section at the apex of the curve shows the vertebral bodies almost devoid of trabeculae except at the concavity where they fan out compatible with the lines of stress. The extreme degree of rotation had resulted in gross deformity of the chest cavity. Posteriorly on the convexity of the chest the strap-like levator costae muscles extending from the transverse processes to the ribs had become markedly hypertrophied. The paralysis had involved the intercostals and paraspinal muscles on the right side.

side of the curve (Figures VIII:5 and VIII:6).

The primary structural curve produced by the deforming factor may develop at any level of the spine, lumbar, thoracic or even lower cervical. A secondary compensating curve develops in the opposite direction to balance the body weight. This can be straightened by lateral flexion toward the concave side and increased by flexion toward the convexity. In lateral bending the flexion of the spine is somewhat restricted on the side of the convexity but less or not at all on the side of the concavity (Figure X:-15).

Observation of the patient presents not only a backward rotation of the chest

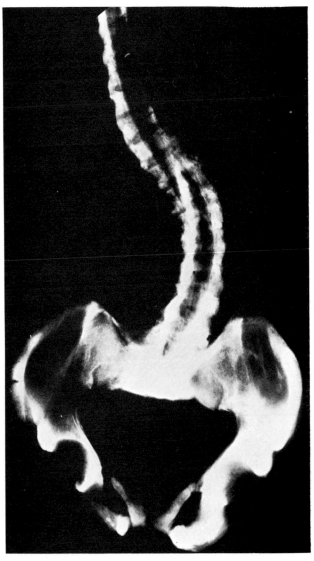

Fig. X:10. Paralytic scoliosis in a female of seventy-seven years. The left ilium is definitely smaller than the right and the distorted pelvic cavity is smaller on the left side. There was obviously inadequate lower left extremity musculature and probably involvement of certain lower left paraspinal muscles as well.

on the convex side but usually a contralateral depression of the shoulder and prominence of the hip.

Idiopathic scoliosis in most cases, progresses slowly and becomes arrested spontaneously. Less commonly the progess may be rapid and reach a severe grade of deformity before spontaneous arrest at the end of the growth period.

The prognosis depends somewhat upon the length of the curve, the degree of rotation, age of onset, rapidity of deterioration and the site of the primary angulation. Those cases developing early, in the thoracic region and with rapid deterioration, have the poorest prognosis.

The deformity tends to reduce the patient's vital capacity and the cardiovas-

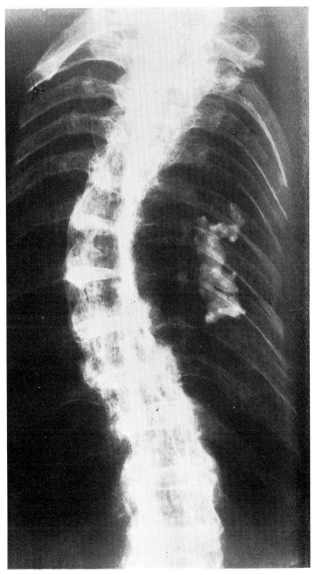

Fig. X:11. Specimen showing scoliosis with old empyema in a female of eighty-six years. The calcification is visualized adjacent to the left posterior chest wall. Note the fanning out of the bone trabeculae to follow the lines of stress within the thoracic spine.

cular function may be impaired. The growth rate is likely to be reduced and the patient remains underdeveloped. There is little pain at first but later as arthritic changes occur in the distorted posterior joints (Figure X:13) discomfort may prove to be a troublesome problem. Further deterioration with disc degeneration produces encroachment of the intervertebral foramen (Figure VIII:6C). Rarely the spinal cord may be involved with resultant paraplegia.

Spinal curvatures, notably scoliosis, have been caused by various other conditions. A softening of the vertebra as by Paget's may result in scoliosis (Figure X:16). Intensive radiation therapy exposing one side of the spine in a young child has produced deformity by locally restricting enchondral bone growth. Children with osteogenesis imperfecta may develop spinal curvatures because of their inherent deficient bone-forming powers. A substantial percentage of pa-

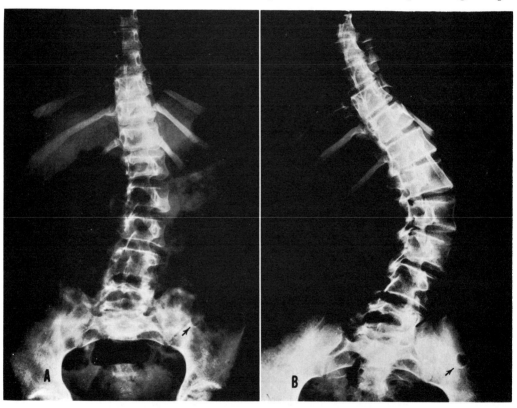

Fig. X:12. Idiopathic scoliosis in an adolescent girl of thirteen years (A). The condition was progressive and three years later at the age of sixteen had reached the state shown in B. Note wedging of the discs. The curvature increased under conservative treatment so that a fusion of the spine was done at eighteen years. The patient was reexamined fifteen years later or twenty years from the first examination (C and D). She now had a solid graft extending from the sacrum to the thoracic area incorporating the neural arches. The space posterior to the lordotic lumbar spine was well filled in with bony tissue (X). At the age of thirty-three she was suffering no discomfort and was well able to discharge all the duties of a housewife with three children. The small round area of decreased density originally noted in the ilium at the first examination was still present unchanged twenty years later

(*arrows*).   ⟶

tients with neurofibromatosis develope spinal curvatures. These result from the destructive process involving the bone. This destruction may be caused by direct tumor pressure or by transmitted pulsation (Figure XVI:10).

REFERENCES

Kyphosis

Bingold, A. C.: 1953, *J. Bone J. Surg., 35B*:579–583, Congenital.

Gulledge, W. H., *et al:* 1950, *J. Bone J. Surg., 32A*:900–903.

Roaf, R.: 1960, *J. Bone J. Surg., 42B*:40–59.

Lordosis

Jacobson, H. G., *et al:* 1958, *Am. Jor. Roent., 79*:677–683.

Scoliosis

Arkin, A. M.: 1952, *J. Bone J. Surg., 34A*:47–54.

Cobb, J. R.: 1958, *J. Bone J. Surg., 40A*:507–510, Editorial.

Farkas, A.: 1954, *J. Bone J. Surg., 36A*:617–654.

Ponseti, I. V., *et al:* 1950, *J. Bone J. Surg., 32A*: 381–395.

Hunt, J. C., and Pugh, D. G.: 1961, *Rad., 76*:1–20, Neurofibromatosis.

James, J. I. P.: 1954, *J. Bone J. Surg., 36B*:36–49.

James, J. I. P.: 1954, *Brit. Jor. Rad., 27*:511–523.

Johnston, A. D., *et al:* 1961, *J. Bone J. Surg., 43A*:865–875.

McCarroll, H. K.: 1960, *J. Bone J. Surg., 42A*: 965–978, Biopsy.

Salter, R. B.: 1960, *J. Bone J. Surg., 42A*:31–49, Compression.

Scott, J. C., *et al:* 1955, *J. Bone J. Surg., 37B*: 400–413, Infantile.

Smith, A. D. F.: 1958, *J. Bone J. Surg., 40A*:505–507, Historical.

Somerville, E. W.: 1952, *J. Bone J. Surg., 34B*: 421–427.

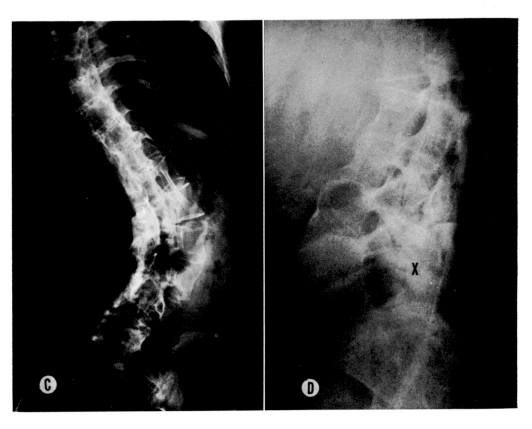

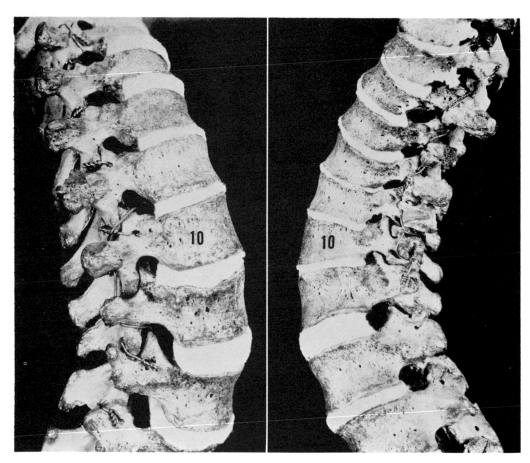

Fig. X:13. Photographs of the right and left sides of a mounted specimen of thoracic scoliosis convex to the right in a male of fifty-nine years. The 8th, 9th and 10th vertebral bodies are wedge shaped, smaller on the left. On the concave side the neural arches have short pedicles, the posterior joints are telescoped and distorted and the intervertebral foramina are encroached upon. By contrast, on the convex side the pedicles are longer, the posterior articulations are not imbricated and the foramina are adequate. The separate photo shows the under surface of T_{10} with massive hyperplasia about the posterior articulation and asymmetry of the vertebral body.

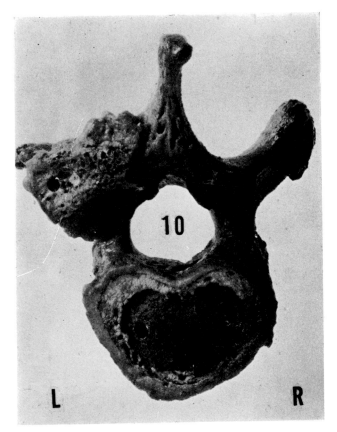

Fig. X:13 C.

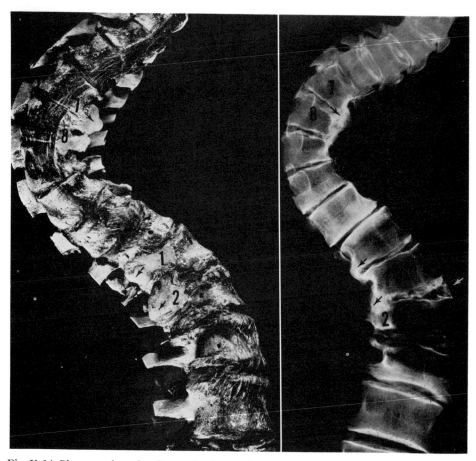

Fig. X:14. Photograph and radiograph of a specimen of scoliosis probably of the idiopathic type. The condition is obviously of long duration. Solid bony bridging on the concave side has developed at the thoracic and the thoraco-lumbar curves (*black arrows*). T_7-T_8 and T_9 are united, also T_{12}-L_1-L_2 and L_3. Bone formation has developed within the convex side of the disc at the L_1-L_2 level (*white arrow*). By these means and also by a strong hypertrophy of the ligamentous structures on the convexity of the scoliotic curves a balance of the axial skeleton is maintained.

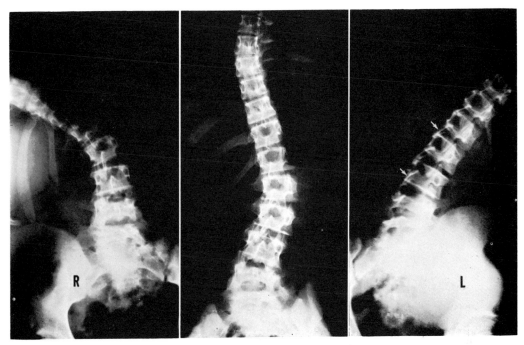

Fig. X:15. Dynamic studies in a fourteen-year-old girl with iodiopathic scoliosis, lumbar convex to the left. These movement studies with the patient standing show excellent flexion toward the right side with straightening of the secondary curves. Bending toward the left or convex side however is definitely restricted. Normally upon lateral bending to the left there is a rotation of the lumbar spine toward the right side. In this individual the structural change in the scoliotic lumbar curve precludes this usual rotation so that bending toward the side of her convexity is resisted.

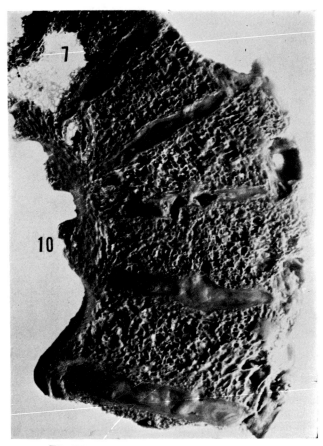

Fig. X:16. Scoliosis in a male of sixty-nine years. This specimen from the mid and lower thoracic region is suggestive of Scheuermann's disease with widened, wedge shaped vertebral bodies. The roentgenogram and the photomicrograph however are characteristic of Paget's disease. The section (S) taken from the 4th or uppermost vertebra of the film shows the typical mosaic pattern of that condition and the photo shows the characteristic bone architecture of that disease. See figure IX:19.

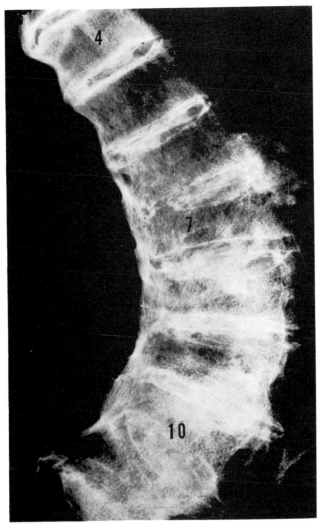

Fig. X: 16 B.

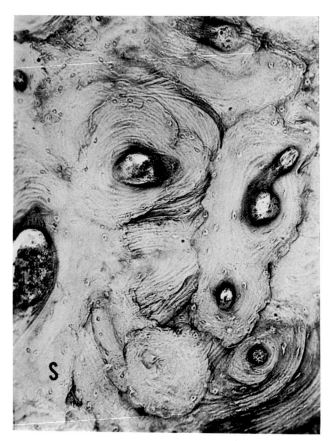

Fig. X:16 C.

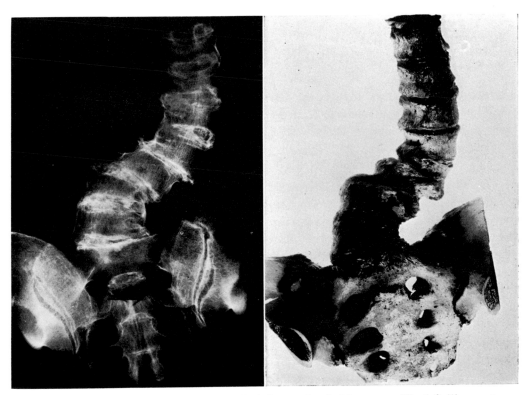

Fig. X:17. Extreme degree of lumbar scoliosis in a male of eighty years. The left iliac crest had become rounded off and had developed a busa where it was impinged upon by the tenth rib. The vertebral bodies are not only rotated but the second and third lumbar segments have subluxated toward the left side. Also the fourth and fifth are wedge shaped, being partially collapsed on the left side and with the left side of the pelvis elevated. There was a fusion of the third, fourth and fifth posterior articulations on the left.

Of some interest were the various adaptations of the soft tissue structures which had arisen to stabilize this, the principal weight supporting portion of the spine. On the left side, in front, the psoas muscle had developed a Y-shaped origin attaching to both the upper and lower lumbar areas separately. Posteriorly on the left a heavy sacro-spinalis muscle extended upward over the convexity and a strong aponurosis of dense fibrous tissue fanned out above the left posterior superior iliac spine. This was supplemented on the left by deep strong ligamentous structures arising from the ilium and attaching to the transverse and articular processes of the convexity from L_3 upward. Adaptations on the right side were entirely different. Anteriorly a fibromuscular band extended from the iliac crest to the twelfth rib and the L_1 transverse process. Also ligamentous structures extended from the right ilium to the fourth and fifth transverse processes. Posteriorly on the right, the support-ing aponurosis extended upward only to L_4 - a much lower level than it did on the left. From an observation of the specimen one might conclude that the condition probably occurred early and that the individual had lived an active life thereafter.

Chapter XI

Infective Spondylitis

INFECTIVE PROCESSES involving the spine may usually be classified as caused by pyogenic organisms or tuberculosis. Other miscellaneous organisms of lesser importance will be mentioned later.

PYOGENIC SPONDYLITIS

Osteomyelitis of the spine is usually a hematogenous infection by the staphlococcus or streptococcus originating from the skin or subcutaneous tissues elsewhere. It may result however from lumbar puncture or some other diagnostic or therapeutic procedure to the spine. One group of cases has followed infection within the pelvic cavity, supposedly by venous extension. This supposition is based on the work of Batson demonstrating the direct continuity between the pelvic and the vertebral venous systems.

The clinical picture is that of sudden, excruciating, back pain unrelieved by medication. The muscles are spastic with the back held rigid and bending only at the hips. There is a pyrexia, leukocytosis and other evidence of toxemia. There may be tenderness to pressure and pain upon percussion directly over the affected segments.

The roentgenogram of the vertebra appears normal in the beginning. However, since the destructive process first develops about the terminal arterioles in the vertebral body beneath the cartilage plate, the infection is soon able to penetrate into the disc. This structure, once it is invaded, seems to have very little defensive power and the nucleus pulposus is quickly liquified. The first change to be visualized by the x-ray is a thinning of the disc.

In childhood especially, the disc is more frequently involved. At this age it may be infected primarily since the vascularity of the disc persists until adolescence (Figure I:17). At times only the ring epiphysis is involved (Figures VIII:20 and VIII:21).

After three or four weeks the trabeculae contiguous to the thinned disc are destroyed, giving to that area a fuzzy roentgenographic appearance. This is soon followed by an osteoporosis of the

---

Fig. XI:1. Early bacteremic osteomyelitis of L_2 and L_3 in a male of fifty years. At the first examination (A) there was a history of low back pain of two months duration. The blood culture was positive for staphlococcus aureus and there was lumbar muscle spasm with severe pain upon motion. The undersurface of L_2 presented an irregular moth-eaten appearance where the vertebral plate had been destroyed (*arrow*). There was some thinning of the intervertebral disc and spur formation. The roentgenograms B and C were made three and one-half months later. During that interval there had been additional thinning of the L_2 disc with development of minimal kyphosis. The vertebral bodies had then reached the sclerotic, healing stage. Note the increased bone density in L_2 and L_3 adjacent to the partially destroyed disc. The final examination visualized a typical healing pyogenic spondylitis. (Courtesy of the University Hospital.)

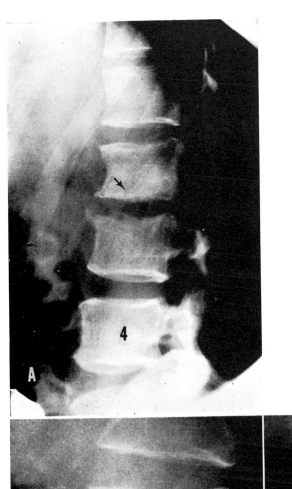

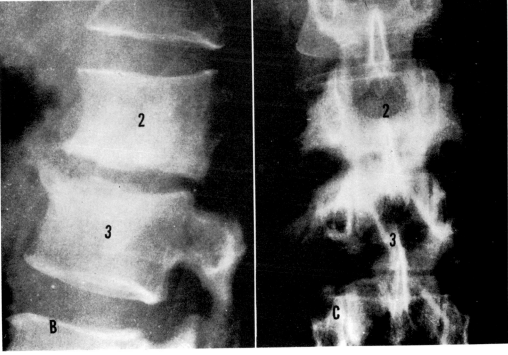

entire vertebra as the trabeculae of the structure become destroyed. In the more virulent pyogenic type of infection this may occur within four to six weeks of infection. A somewhat milder, insidious type of spinal osteomyelitis may develope more slowly with subacute symptoms,

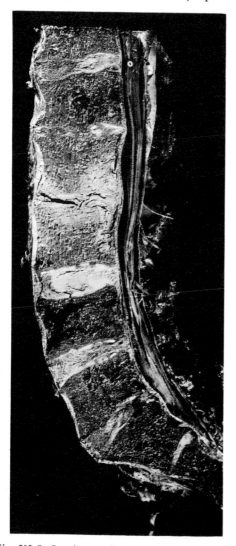

Fig. XI:2. Specimen of pyogenic spondylitis involving L_2 and L_3 with the disc between them. There is some bulging of the posterior longitudinal ligament. The fracture of L_4 occurred postmortem. There was a history of old osteomyelitis of the left femur and hip reactivated with "vague pain in the back" three years before death.

boring back pain, loss of weight, etc. Although this is usually the picture of early tuberculosis rather than pyogenic spinal disease, it may occur with organisms of lower virulence.

Pyogenic spondylitis heals by bone production, the osteoporotic vertebra being replaced by dense sclerotic bone after two or three months (Figures XI:1, XI:2 and XI:3). This process continues with further thinning of the disc and increasing density. Osteophytes develope and fusion of adjacent vertebral bodies into a single block vertebra may have occurred by the end of a year. This process may become arrested at any point but there is no restitution of the structures to their original normal state.

During the active stage the infection may be confined by and spread beneath the anterior and lateral longitudinal ligaments (Figures XI:4 and X:5). The posterior longitudinal ligament is not attached to the vertebral body at all (Figures VIII:6 and I:7). Thus unopposed extension to the spinal canal or the neural arches may result in epidural abscess, cord damage or a meningeal syndrome.

Abscess formation elsewhere may develop either with a pyogenic or with a tuberculous infection. Involvement of the psoas muscle, particularly in the child, may cause the thigh to be held in a flexed position, with a complaint of pain in the hip. Involvement of the joint may be ruled out by: (1) no pain to deep pressure behind the joint, (2) trocarteric percussion not painful, (3) backward extension the only painful movement. Tenderness to pressure and pain upon percussion over the lumbar region would indicate the true origin of the psoas muscle spasm.

Spondylitis of the discs may occur, especially in children, following injury.

It is thought that trauma to the blood vessels with a resulting endarteritis and thrombosis predisposes to the infective process.

Spondylitis secondary to pelvic infection appears in a somewhat older age group. It may follow childbirth or operation upon the genitourinary organs. The venous plexus within the spinal canal and the paraspinal veins are without valves. They constitute a drainage system originating within the pelvis. Batson has shown that they may be filled by strong retrograde pressure and has postulated that they are a route for the passage of carcinoma or infective metastases originating within the pelvis (Figures XI:5 and XI:6).

TUBERCULOUS SPONDYLITIS

Tuberculosis of the spine is merely the localized mainifestation of a generalized systemic disease. It develops at the terminal arterioles of the adult vertebral body as a result of hematogenous dissemination. As in the pyogenic type, the earliest roentgenographic evidence of tuberculous spondylitis is a thinning of the intervertebral disc. The progress of the tuberculous disease is much slower than that of the pyogenic. The lytic stage, characterized by osteo-porosis and tubercules within the normal hematopoietic bone marrow may persist for six months or a year. Later the bone marrow of the involved vertebra is replaced by fibrous tissue with a proliferation of dense sclerotic trabeculae, removal of sequestra and organization of the abscesses (Figures XI:7 and XI:8). Further healing results in additional sclerosis and fusion of adjacent segments. Complete healing may require two or three years. The disc is replaced by fibrous scarring

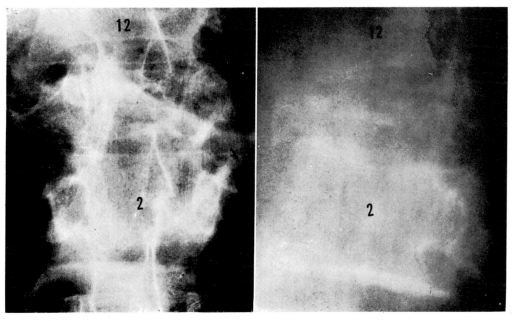

Fig. XI:3. Osteomyelitis from staphlococcus aureus septicemia in a male patient of seventy-two years. Compression of the first lumbar vertebra, paravertebral abscess and cord bladder, complicated the systemic condition. The vertebral body is almost completely destroyed but the discs appear to have escaped. (Courtesy of the University Hospital.)

and there is late calcification or ossification of the paraspinal exudate. Both lytic and sclerotic areas may appear in a single vertebra at the same time (see L:4 and Figures XI:9c and X:5). It is difficult to visualize these changes on the roentgenogram of the patient.

Increased density like that noted in aseptic necrosis has been attributed by Cleveland et al to an interrupted blood supply to some area of the bone. The arterial supply enters the vertebral body by many small vessels penetrating the entire circumference of the structure (Figure I:19). There are additional longitudinal arteries on each side within the spinal

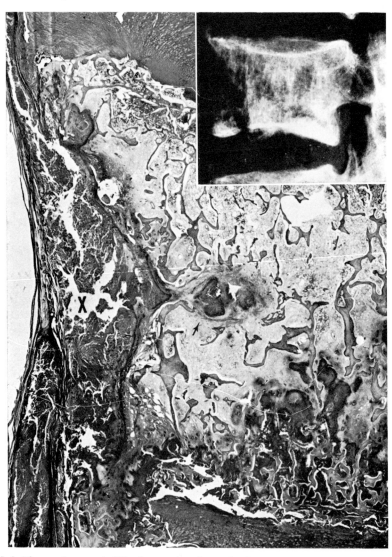

Fig. XI:4. Photomicrograph X5 of a section from the lumbar vertebra (*inset*) of a male of sixty-seven years. Osteomyelitis at the lytic stage has largely destroyed the bone but has left the discs intact. At the left is a large collection of purulent material (X) underlying the anterior longitudinal ligament. At the center is a small abscess in direct continuity with a nutrient foramen on the anterior surface of the vertebra (*arrow*). Another extensive area of marrow involvement is noted just above the lowermost disc.

canal which give off branches that enter the nutrient foramina beneath the posterior longitudinal ligament. Within the vertebral body are venous spaces which finally exit thru the posterior nutrient foramina into the loose valveless plexus of the spinal canal.

So-called "cold" burrowing abscesses may develope, especially beneath the longitudinal ligaments or the psoas muscle (Figures X:5 and XI:4). If a secondary, mixed infection, developes it is likely to stimulate a sclerotic reaction of the bone with increased density and sequestrum formation (Figure XI:10).

A miscellaneous group of diseases endemic in certain countries has been reported as causing spondylitis. Of these may be mentioned: Actinomycosis, Blastomycosis, Coccidiomycosis, Toxoplasmosis, Samonella, Typhoid, Paratyphoid and Syphilis as well as Undulant Fever from Brucella Mellitensis. Both lytic and productive lesions occur. There are no characteristic roentgenographic findings so that the diagnosis depends upon the clinical picture of the local disease.

REFERENCES

Pyogenic Spondylitis

Batson, O. V.: 1940, *Ann. Surg., 112*:138–149, Anatomy.

Campbell, J. A., *et al*: 1954, *Am. Jor. Roent., 72*: 229–246, Neurological.

DeFeo, E.: 1954, *Rad., 62*:396–401, Pelvic.

Doyle, J. R.: 1960, *J. Bone J. Surg., 42A*:1191–1200, Children.

Henson, S., *et al*: *Surg. Gyn. Obst., 102*:207–214, Pelvic.

Jamison, R. C., *et al*: 1961, *Rad., 77*:355–367, Children.

Lame, E. L.: 1956, *Am. Jor. Roent., 75*:938–952, Pelvic.

Leigh, T. F.: 1955, *Rad., 65*:334–342, Pelvic.

Pritchard, A. E., *et al*: 1960, *J. Bone J. Surg., 42B*:86–89, Children.

Saenger, E. L.: 1950, *Am. Jor. Roent., 64*:20–31, Children.

Scherbel, A. L., *et al*: 1960, *J.A.M.A., 174*:370–374, Pyogenic.

Wiley, A. M., *et al*: 1959, *J. Bone J. Surg., 41B*: 796–809, Anatomy.

Tuberculosus

Auerbach, O., *et al*: 1944, *Am. Jor. Roent., 52*: 57–63, Pathology Tbc.

Cleveland, M., *et al*: 1942, *J. Bone J. Surg., 24*: 527–546, Tbc.

Finder, J. G.: 1936, *Surg. Gyn. Obst., 62*:665–676, Pathology Tbc.

Guri, J. P.: 1946, *J. Bone J. Surg., 28*:29–39, Pyogenic vs. Tbc.

Hollock, H., *et al*: 1954, *J. Bone J. Surg., 36A*: 219–240, Tbc.

Poppel, M. H., *et al*: 1953, *Am. Jor. Roent., 70*: 936–963, Tbc.

Miscellaneous

Aguilar, J. A., *et al*: 1961, *Jor. Neurosurg., 18*: 27–33, Brucella.

Baylin, G. J., *et al*: 1953, *Am. Jor. Roent., 69*: 395–398, Fungus.

Greenspan, R. H., *et al*: 1957, *Rad., 68*:860–862, Samonella.

Reeves, R. T.: 1954, *Rad., 62*:55–60, Fungus.

Sgalitzer, M.: 1960, *Abst. Am. Jor. Roent., 85*: 789, Syphilis.

Stenström, R.: 1958, *Acta Rad., 49*:355–360, Samonella.

Zammit, F.: 1958, *Brit. Jor. Rad., 31*:683–690, Brucella.

Fig. XI:5. Female, thirty-seven years of age. Possible embolism and infarction of C_4. Within a few hours following a difficult thirty-six hour labor the patient complained of a stiff neck. The pain became rapidly worse so that she could not elevate the head without help. Pain radiated to the shoulders and down the arms. Tests for tuberculosis, syphilis and brucellosis were negative.

A. Film made one month after onset shows some destruction of the fourth and fifth cervical bodies and the interposed disc.

B. Twenty months later there is some evidence of healing but with angulation, and wide separation of the corresponding spinous processes. The lower anterior corner of C_4 has become split off allowing the remainder of the vertebra to become displaced backward. It has tipped forward on a transverse axis producing the angulation with separation of the posterior joint surfaces as well as the spinous processes.

C. Seven years after onset there is complete healing with ankylosis and relief of symptoms. The partial loss of C_4 exaggerates the separation of the spinous and articular processes. Batson has shown that increased intra-abdominal pressure by straining, forces blood from the utero-vaginal veins into the vertebral venous system. The latter is without valves and extends the length of the spinal canal. It is possible that this patient may have sustained a post-partum embolus passing by way of the intravertebral plexus and lodging in the fourth cervical body.

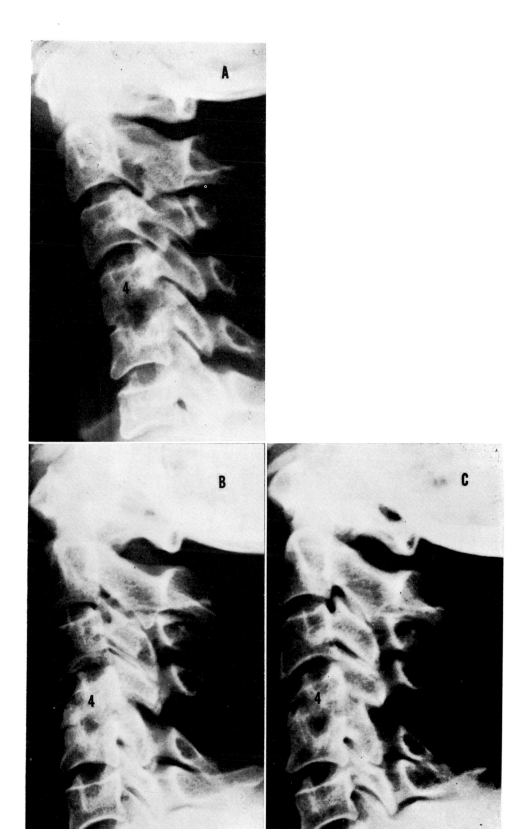

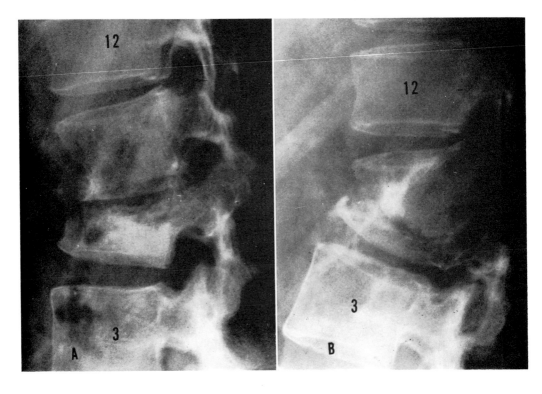

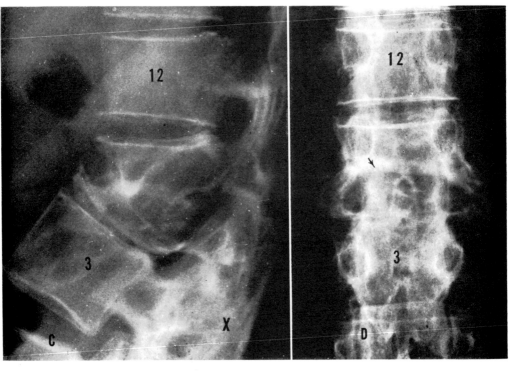

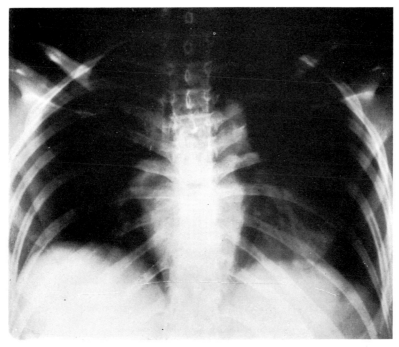

Fig. XI:7. Tuberculosis of the mid thoracic spine with paravertebral abscess in a young woman of twenty-one years. Kyphosis is indicated even on the P. A. projection by the radiating arrangement of the ribs.

Fig. XI:6. Female thirty-four. Destructive process involving L_1 and L_2 with operative fusion and complete healing thirteen years later. The destructive process began in L_2. There was kyphosis, local pain and spasm aggravated by attempted movement. The patient had been operated for tubal disease six months before. The Wasserman was negative. The chest films were repeatedly normal and gastric contents examined for tuberculosis failed to reveal any organisms, however her condition was diagnosed as tuberculous of the spine. She was treated for one year by fixation in plaster without relief and with increase of kyphosis. (A and B were made one year apart.) The patient was then fused with material from a bone bank and remained in fixation by cast for one year. The A.P. and lateral films C and D were made twelve years later. The patient was entirely asymptomatic at that time. The continuous bone graft (X) extended from T_{12} to L_3. The first and second lumbar vertebrae had developed a solid bone block with the underlying second disc bulging upward into it (*arrow*). The adjacent intervertebral foramina were encroached upon and the kyphosis had increased fifteen degrees in twelve years. One cannot be certain whether this infective spondylitis was tuberculosis or resulted from the pelvic inflammatory disease.

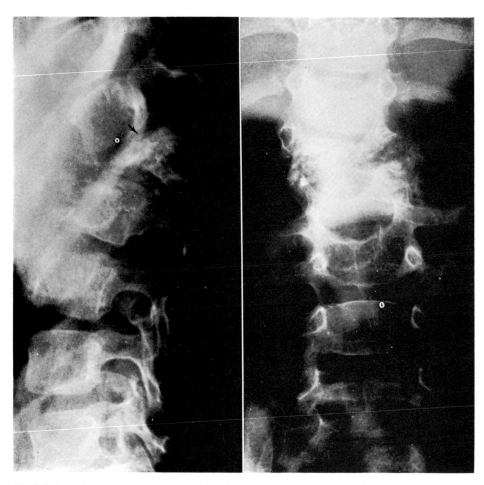

Fig. XI:8. Active tuberculosis of the spine in a boy of two years. Debris from the completely destroyed two uppermost lumbar vertebrae has become displaced paravertebrally and backward into the spinal canal (*arrow*). The next two vertebrae are already involved and the typical angular gibbus is well established. Extension occurs beneath the longitudinal ligaments (see Figure X:5) so that involvement is usually more extensive than it appears on the roentgenogram.

Fig. XI:9. Photograph and radiographs showing Specimen 2333 from a female of sixty-nine years. Extensive destruction of the lower spine by tuberculosis involving T_{12}, L_1-L_2-L_3 and L_4. T_{12} and L_2 have collapsed and L_1 shows cavitation. There is an encroachment of the spinal canal and development of paravertebral abscess formation with generalized demineralization. The upper posterior portion of L_4 is increased in density while the remainder of the vertebra is osteoporotic.

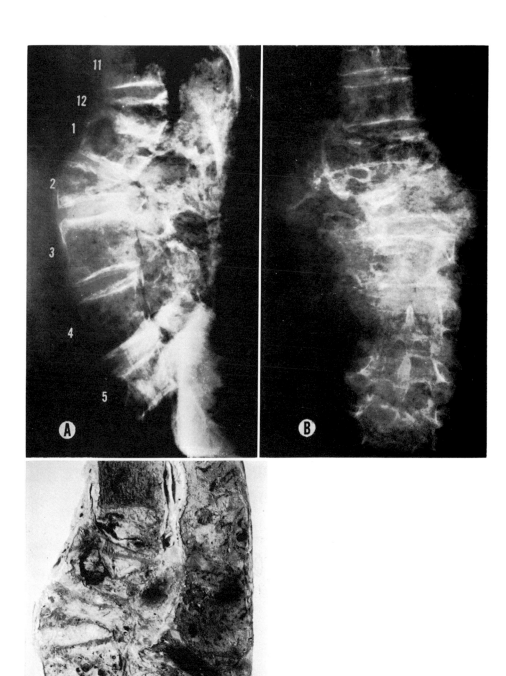

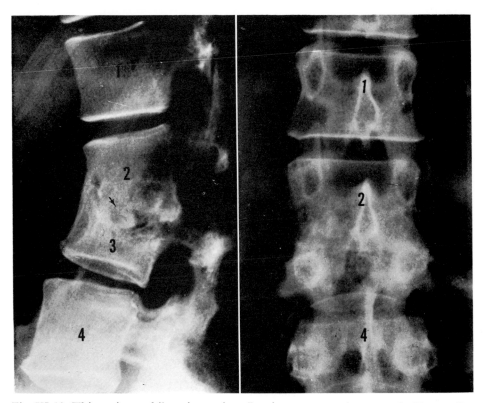

Fig. XI:10. This patient, while prisoner in a Russian concentration camp in Eastern Po-
land, had developed tuberculosis of the chest and spine at twenty-eight years of age. She was
treated in a plaster jacket at that time. These radiographs made eight years later show a
fusion of L_2 and L_3 with a kyphosis at that level. Recent pain and the presence of an increased central density (*arrow*) indicate the probability of sequestrum development.

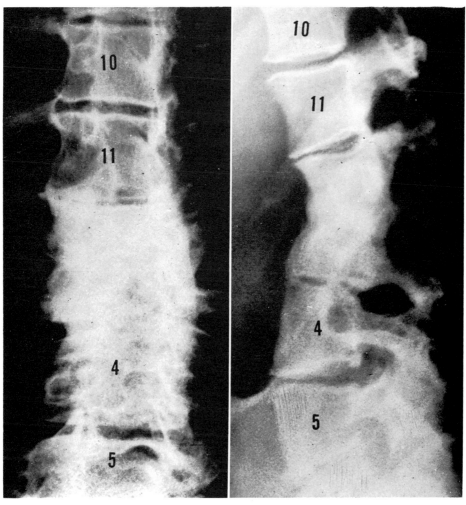

Fig. XI:11. Healed tuberculosis of the spine in a male of forty-one years with development of a kyphotic block vertebra comprising the T_{12}, L_1, L_2 and L_3 vertebrae. (Courtesy of the Syracuse Memoral Hospital.)

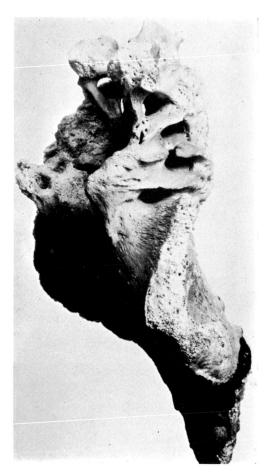

Fig. XI:12. Specimen from an individual with an old healed tuberculosis showing fusion of the L_2-L_3-L_4-L_5 and S_1 arches into a single kyphotic block. The vertebral bodies are entirely lacking with their place occupied by a cavity.

Chapter XII

Observations at the Lumbo Sacral Level

THE DYNAMIC function of the lumbo-pelvic skeletal mechanism is not only to afford a movable support to the torso but also to supply stability and maintain the erect position. This is accomplished at a point where the downward thrust of body weight meets the counter-upward thrust of the lower extremities.

The two innominate bones may be considered as forming an inverted arch with its apex at the pubis. The upward thrust of the femurs is applied to the convex sides of this arch at the hip joints. This force is conveyed upward along the true pelvic brim and presses the ilia against the sides of the sacrum (Figure XII:1).

The bony surfaces of the auricular-shaped sacroiliac joints are covered with hyaline cartilage and are somewhat irregular in contour. They correspond to the first and second segments of the sacrum (Figure XII:13). The successful and efficient function of the sacroiliac joint depends upon the integrity of the sacroiliac ligaments holding the joint surfaces in contact.

IMPORTANCE OF THE LIGAMENTOUS STRUCTURES

At the lumbo sacral level the ligaments not only hold the sacroiliac joints in firm contact but also by the downward thrust they draw the bony surfaces more firmly together. In fact these ligaments actually support a substantial portion of the superimposed body weight.

The sacrum, seen from in front and below, has somewhat the shape of a keystone but it does not serve as such in the usual sense. Upon cross-section it is seen to be wider in front than behind, so that with the sacrum in its normally inclined position with the anterior surface downward the narrow side of the keystone is above, rather than below. This places the weight-carrying burden almost entirely upon the sacroiliac ligaments, especially the strong ones in back. These short ligaments suspend the sacrum between the ilia, supporting it almost entirely except for the irregularities of the sacroiliac joints (Figure XII:2). The contiguous surfaces of these joints being nearly vertical do not offer bone-to-bone support like the knee, hip or the intervertebral discs (Figure XII:14).

The sacrum may be considered somewhat as a rigid inclined platform with a transverse slightly movable axis of support at about the level of the second sacral segment. The downward thrust of the superimposed body weight, exerted at the promontory, tends to tip the upper anterior end of the sacrum downward and forward. This tilting movement is countered posteriorly by the sacrosciatic ligaments joining the lower end of the sacrum with the ischium (Figure XII:3).

Of some possible concern is the relaxation of the pelvic ligaments which occurs in the female pelvis during parturition.

The fifth lumbar vertebra, resting

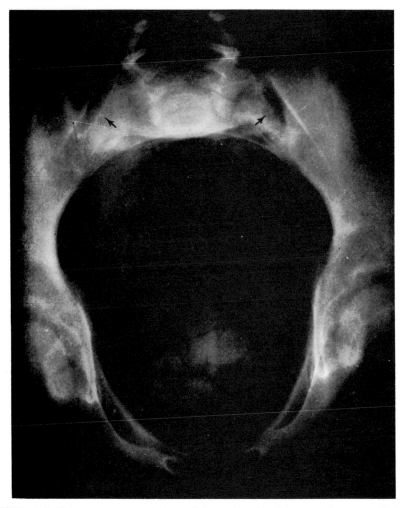

Fig. XII:1. A.P. Roentgenogram of the pelvis made with the central ray parallel to the anterior surface of the sacrum. The iliac bones form an inverted arch with its apex at the pubis. The upward and inward thrust of the femurs is applied to the sides of this arch at the hip joints. Thence the pressure is carried upward by the iliac bones to be directed against the sides of the sacrum. Note that the planes of the sacroiliac joints (*arrows*) are separated more widely in front and below than they are in back.

$\longrightarrow$

Fig. XII:2. Radiograph and photograph (*from below*) of a section of the pelvis made at the level of the true pelvic brim. The specimen is from a male seventy-five years old. The sacrum is wider in front and below. It is suspended by the strong posterior sacroiliac ligaments (*whitened on the photograph*). The sacrum is not a true keystone structure. The inverted innominate arch clearly shows the stress lines of weightbearing extending upward from the acetabula. There are only slight bony irregularities in the contour of the sacroiliac joints (*white arrows*).

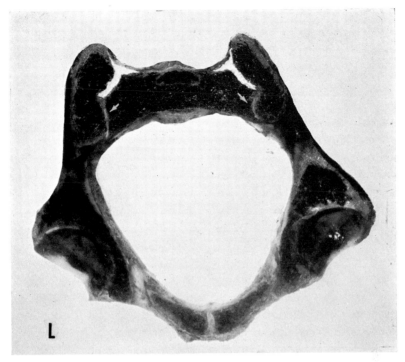

Fig. XII:2 B.

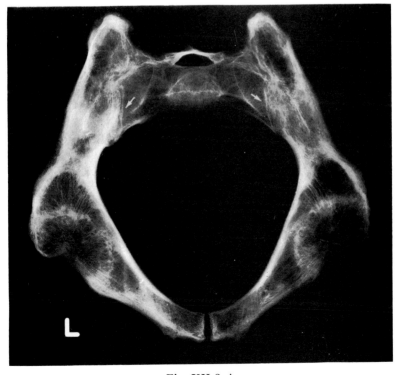

Fig. XII:2 A.

upon the inclined plane of the sacrum, is also partially suspended as in a hammock by the very strong ilio-lumbar ligaments. These structures extend from the fifth transverse processes upward and backward to become inserted in the iliac crests. As a result the fifth lumbar vertebra with the superimposed body weight is supported, not only on the sacrum, but also by these sturdy ileo-lumbar ligaments. Their attachment to the iliac crest is frequently the site of pain and tenderness to pressure following low back trauma.

From these considerations it is apparent that, except for the abdominal weight carried by the iliac wings and those slight bony irregularities of the sacroiliac joints, the body weight above the pelvis is largely supported by the ligamentous structures of the lumbo-pelvic region. This fact together with the shearing stresses of the lordotic lumbo-sacral curve are undoubtedly responsible for many of the low back symptoms incidental to the upright position of homo sapiens (Figures XII:4, XII:5 and XII:6).

In about one half of the cadaver specimens examined I was able to identify a lateral lumbo sacral ligament extending backward and laterally from the disc, the fifth vertebral body and the transverse process, to the ala of the sacrum. This bridges the fifth lumbar nerve root immediately below the intervertebral foramen, forming a tunnel for that structure beneath the psoas muscle (Figure XII:7). This ligament is variable. It may be quite strong and firm, thin and ferestrated or even absent entirely. In case of lumbo-sacral disc degeneration it contributes to the lateral spur formation producing a bony canal for the fifth nerve root. Rarely such a spur may actually impinge upon and compress the nerve at the promontory (Figure XII:8).

LUMBO-SACRAL NERVES

The fourth lumbar root contributes to the innervation of both the anterior thigh, via the femoral nerve, and the sciatic distribution thru the lumbo-sacral plexus. Its lower branch descends in front of the fifth transverse process to join the fifth lumbar root. Together these dip over the brim of the pelvis at the sacroiliac joint changing their direction about 60°. On one specimen studied, a forward bulging of the sacroiliac joint produced an obvious displacement of the nerve toward the pelvic cavity.

Fig. XII:3. Lateral projection of the spine and pelvis from a preadolescent female. The axis of weightbearing drawn through the femoral head transects the lumbo sacral joint and passes through the lower lumbar bodies. It lies entirely anterior to all of the thoracic vertebrae. The upward thrust from the hips is carried by the ilium toward the second sacral segment (*arrows*). This is the point of support for the sacrum. The white dotted lines indicate the position of the sacrosciatic ligaments. These structures fan out and upward from the ischial spine on each side to balance the downward thrust of the body weight applied at the promontory.

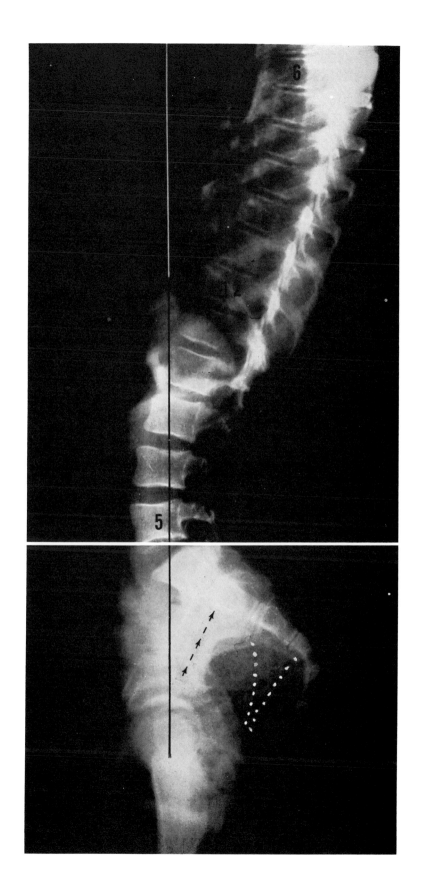

LUMBO SACRAL MOVEMENT

In the mobile cervical spine, as shown in Chapter IV, the A. P. movement results from a to and fro gliding of the vertebral bodies upon each other. In the lower lumbar region however, where stability is more important than mobility, the flexion-extension motion is achieved by a rocking movement of the vertebral bodies upon each other. As this occurs the discs assume a wedge shape with the wider edge toward the convexity of the curve. There is also a telescoping of the posterior joints and a consequent change in the sizes of the intervertebral foramina (Figure XII:9). In cases of instability from loss of disc substance or neural arch deficiency the comparative flexion-extension studies reveal a forward-backward gliding movement at the lumbo-sacral level with the flat surfaces of the disc parallel. This is similar to the movement seen normally in the mid cervical region. Various Scandanavian workers have shown that an unstable vertebra may even move backwards upon anterior flexion. Dynamic studies of this type may indicate early evidence of low back instability which is not apparent upon the plain roentgenograms. The method also helps to estimate the degree of any such in-stability which is apparent radiographically (Figures XIII:36 and XIII:37).

Again, dynamic flexion-extension studies at the lumbo sacral level as in the cervical region help to evaluate any diminished amplitude of spinal movement. Such decreased motion occurs as a normal change in the soft tissues incidental to senescence. However, lessened mobility resulting from traumatic disturbance of the articulations, ligaments or other soft tissues may be visualized by such dynamic studies.

The lumbar spine is capable of anterior flexion, retroflexion, lateral bending, circumduction and rotation. At the lumbo sacral level movement is almost entirely in the A.P. direction. Lateral movement occurs principally above L_5. The widest side of the wedge shaped disc normally occurs on the convexity of the curve. In certain cases of disc or soft tissue disturbance however the dynamic studies may reveal the disc wedge to be wider on the concave side (Figure XIV:25).

Mention is frequently made of the lumbo sacral "angle" as applied to the anterior surfaces of L_5 and the sacrum at the promontory. Of greater clinical significance is the lumbo sacral "curve"

————————————————————————→

Fig. XII:4. Large spur on the fifth disc producing a bony canal for the fifth left nerve root (N). The photograph also shows the attachment of the iliolumbar ligament to the crest of the ilium at X. This corresponds to a point of tenderness to deep pressure frequently complained of by patients with low back pain. In certain cases this attachment becomes ossified. After photographing the specimen a coronal section one-half inch thick was then removed for this roentgenographic study. The film (*reversed*) reveals increasing degrees of disc degeneration from above downward. The lumbo sacral disc is completely destroyed. Sections of the spurs indicate that these outgrowths arise in the attachments of the longitudinal ligaments at the sides of the vertebral bodies. The possible relationship of lumbo sacral disc spurring to fifth root encroachment is obvious.

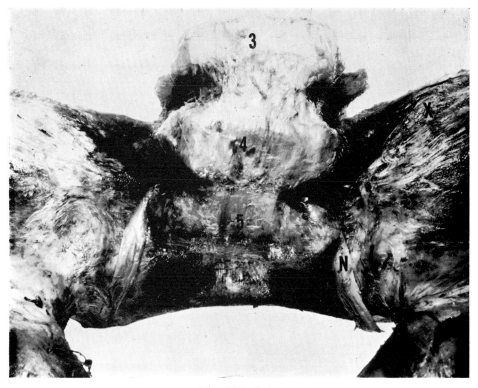

Fig. XII: 4 A.

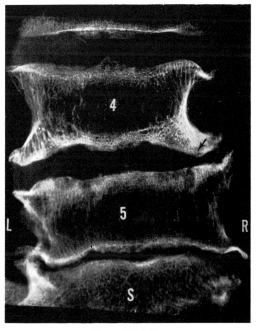

Fig. XII:4 B.

which is that arcuate line corresponding to the posterior surfaces of the vertebral bodies or the anterior wall of the spinal canal. Its proximity to the cauda equina and the posterior arch structures renders this an area of crucial importance.

ACCESSORY SACROILIAC ARTICULATIONS

Accessory sacroiliac articulations occur in about one third of the older patients and of these, in turn, about one third show evidence of arthritic changes. One or two such joints may appear on either or both sides between the ilium and the posterior surface of the sacrum.

The sacrum is normally formed by the fused elements of five primary vertebral segments. The alae, in front, originate from the costal elements. Posteriorly, the transverse processes join to form the crests which are lateral to the posterior sacral foramina (Figures I:14 and I:-

20). The ear-shaped, cartilage-covered, articular surfaces arise from the anterior portions of the first two segments corresponding to the alae of the sacrum. There is a sacral tuberosity above and behind the articular surface on either side (Figure XII:13).

The antero-inferior portions of the adjacent surfaces of the sacrum and the innominate bone form the true ear-shaped sacro-iliac joint. Only about one half of these adjacent surfaces is actually in contact at this joint. The remaining portions, separated by a deep cleft one-eighth to one-quarter of an inch wide, are connected by the strong posterior sacro-iliac ligaments. However, articular facets may develop a bridge across this space and thus form accessory sacro-iliac joints. These are above, behind, and entirely separate from the true sacroiliac joints. They are movable, diarthrodial articulations, with joint space, capsule, and articular surfaces. In their normal condition they should be considered asymptomatic (Figure XII:10). Two types of accessory sacroiliac articulations may be identified. The more common superficial accessory sacroiliac joint is seen between the posterior superior iliac spine and the lateral crest of the sacrum, opposite the second posterior sacral foramen. Prominent facets surmounted by articular cartilage develop at these points. The superficial joint is very close to the body surface and, if arthritic, it may be tender to deep pressure. It is separated from the true sacro-iliac joint by a foramen through which pass branches of the superior gluteal nerve

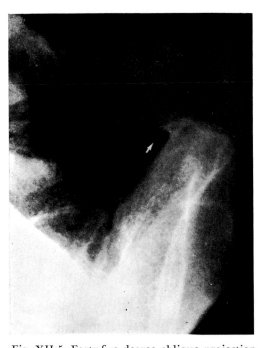

Fig. XII:5. Forty-five degree oblique projection to show a spur on the right ilium at the attachment of the ilio-lumbar ligament (*white arrow*). The condition was unilateral. This fifty-nine-year-old man complained of pain in the right iliolumbar angle and tenderness to deep pressure directly over this point.

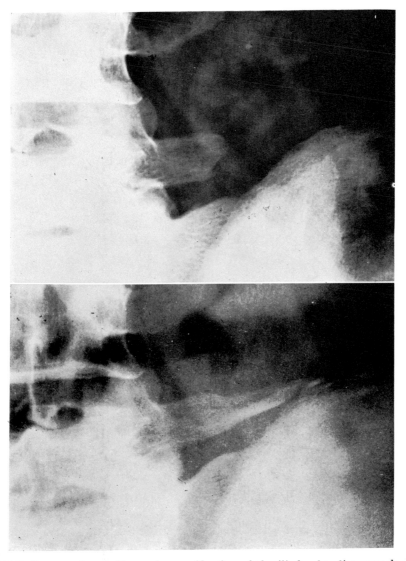

Fig. XII:6. Comparative studies to show ossification of the ilio-lumbar ligament during a period of eighteen years. Roentgenogram above was made at forty years of age. Below is a reexamination of the same patient at fifty-eight years. Back pain was present although it was probably caused by various degenerative changes.

and artery. This foramen constitutes a useful landmark for identifying the superficial accessory sacroiliac articulation. It lies between that vicarious joint and the true sacroiliac joint (Figure XII:11).

The deep articulation, less frequently found, develops between the large roughened tuberosity of the ilium and the smaller sacral tuberosity. It is found opposite the first posterior sacral foramen (Figure XII:12).

The deep and superficial types may occur together in the same individual. Occasionally, the two types become fused to form a large accessory sacroiliac, en-

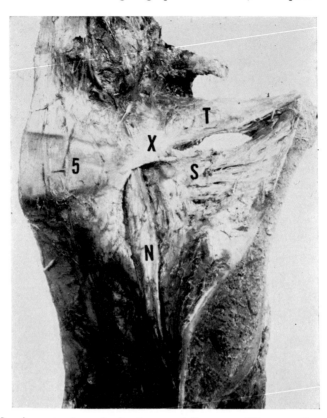

Fig. XII:7. Specimen to show the lumbo sacral ligament (X) extending from the fifth disc, the vertebra, and the transverse process (T) to insert on the ala of the sacrum (S). This ligamentous bridge separates the fifth nerve root (N) from the psoas muscle. The dissection also illustrates how the fifth lumbar vertebra is partially supported as in a hammock by the strong ilio-lumbar ligament extending from the fifth transverse process to the crest of the ilium.

tirely separate from the true joint. This may encompass the sacral tuberosity and the crest of the sacrum down to the second posterior foramen. Articulation for an enlarged fifth transverse process occasionally simulates the appearance of a third articulation, such as that reported by Giraudi.

The planes of the normal and the accessory articulations may form an angle amounting to as much as 60 degrees. In other words, two bones articulate at two separate movable surfaces the planes of which are at a considerable angle. The resultant sheering stress constitutes a mechanical hindrance to any customary movements between the ilium and the sacrum. This may contribute in part to the arthritic changes so frequently noted (Figure XII:14). Complete bony ankylosis has also been observed (Figure IX:3). Patients with accessory articulations frequently complain of low back pain, sciatica, muscle spasm limitation of motion, or tenderness to deep pressure over the accessory joint.

Peterson, in 1905, and Derry, in 1911, reported on the incidence of accessory articulations in sixty-three and 192 specimens respectively. The incidence in

Peterson's series was 16 per cent; in Derry's 10.4 per cent. Trotter, in a study of 958 anatomical specimens, found an incidence of 36 per cent. Her findings "supported the belief that the . . . articular facets are covered by hyaline cartilage and separated by an articular cavity and that the joint is surrounded by a capsule." She also stated that "the incidence of accessory articular facets was found to increase with increase in age." Our study of 185 specimens of half sacra revealed accessory sacroiliac joints in 18 per cent. Of the 163 ilia examined, 16 per cent revealed accessory articular facets.

No figures are available for asymptomatic individuals. However in a review of 200 consecutive roentgenographic examinations of private patients, most of whom complained of low back pain with or without sciatica, 33.5 per cent of patients were found to have accessory sacroiliac joints. In 42 per cent of these patients the condition was bilateral. The superficial type occurred about four times as frequently as the deep type. Of the total number of such vicarious joints, 64 per cent showed no arthritic changes, 36 per cent were 'obviously arthritic and six per cent were ankylosed. Roentgenographic changes considered as indicative of an arthritic process were thinning and irregularity of the joint space, bony exostoses of joint margins, and

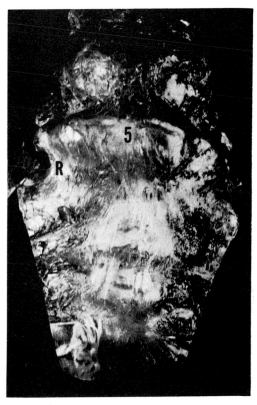

Fig. XII:8. Anterior view of the lumbo sacral articulation from an individual of seventy-seven years. On the left side of the fifth disc a spur compressed and flattened the nerve root and was adherent to that structure (*arrow*). A spur on the right side (R) produced a tunnel for the nerve but compression and perineural fibrosis had not yet developed as they had on the left.

eburnation of the subjacent bone. (Figures XII:15, XII:16, XII:17, and XII:-18).

SACRALIZATION

Sacralization of the lowermost or first presacral lumbar vertebra is congenital and develops early. I have observed a unilateral sacralization in the sections of a ten weeks' fetus still in the chondrogenous stage. It is frequently encountered and easily identified during infancy. The bilaterally symmetrical type is seldom responsible for symptoms but the asymmetrical, unilaterally sacralized lower segment may be responsible for symptoms in various ways (Figures XII:-19 and XII:20).

The structural asymmetry produces an imbalance in the stresses at the lumbosacral support level. There is

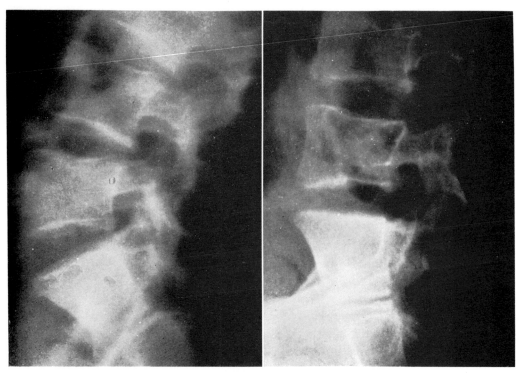

Fig. XII:9. Lateral projection of the lumbo sacral articulation at the full limits of movement. Note the wedge shaped discs, widest on the convex side, the telescoping posterior articulations and the alteration in size of the intervertebral foramina.

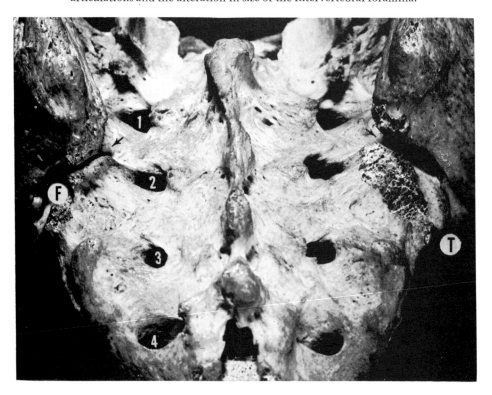

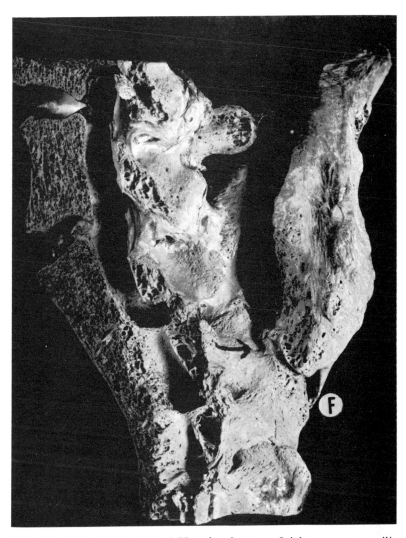

Fig. XII:11. Specimen from male, aged fifty, showing superficial accessory sacroiliac joint (*arrow*) with arthritic spur formation. The nutrient foramen shadow (F) foreshortened, is seen to the right of and below the accessory joint. (Courtesy of the publisher of *The Journal of Bone and Joint Surgery*).

←

Fig. XII:10. Articulated specimen, showing bilateral superficial accessory sacroiliac articulations (*arrows*). Facets on the posterior superior iliac spines articulate with corresponding facets on the sacrum. These are of the superficial type and are opposite the second posterior sacral foramina. The posterior surface on the right side has been removed, revealing the edge of the articular surface. The foramen for branches of the superior gluteal nerve and artery is clearly shown on the left side between the accessory and true sacro-iliac joints (F). The true sacroiliac joint is seen above T on the right side. (Courtesy of *Radiology* and *The Journal of Bone and Joint Surgery*.)

usually an asymmetry in the planes of the posterior articulations and the enlarged transverse process may also articulate with the ilium. These patients in the beginning experience low back pain only during periods of fatigue. Subsequently, arthritic changes develop as a result of pressure and movement at the vicarious joint between the enlarged lowermost transverse process and the ala of the sacrum. Incidental to these painful arthritic changes bony spur formation occurs along the margins of the joint. Late bony ankylosis may finally immobilize this abnormal articulation to bring a welcome relief of symptoms (Figures XII:21, XII:22 and XII:23).

The bony spur formation, projecting

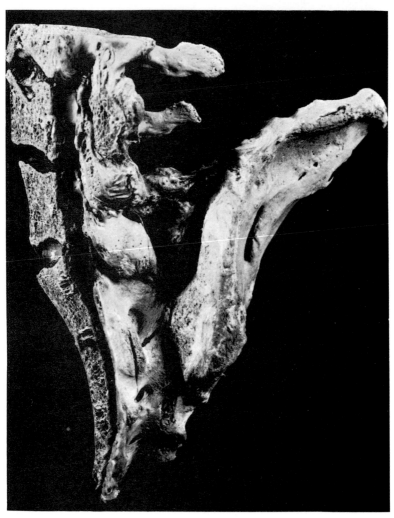

Fig. XII:12. Specimen from a male, seventy-five years old. Deep type of accessory sacroiliac articulation is seen opposite the first posterior sacral foramen. The usual cleft between the ilium and posterior surface of the sacrum is bridged by this vicarious articulation (*arrow*). The articulation is separated from the true sacroiliac by a passage for the nerve and blood vessels. There is no connection between this joint and the old fractures of the third and fourth vertebral bodies and of the right ilium, which occurred twenty-five years before death. (Courtesy of publisher of *The Journal of Bone and Joint Surgery.*)

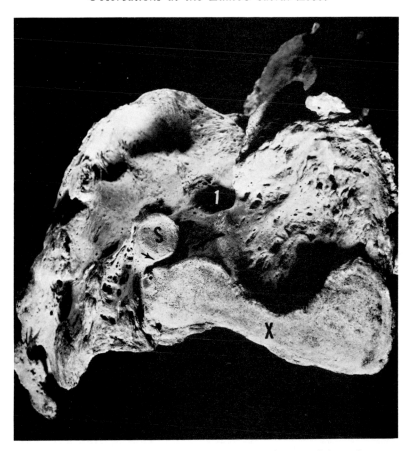

Fig. XII:13. A sacrum viewed from the right side. Note the round facet for an accessory sacroiliac articulation (S) above and behind the true, so-called auricular, sacroiliac articulation (X). Note also the space between these articular surfaces for passage of the nerve and blood vessels (*arrow*). In all of the cases studied, the accessory and the true sacroiliac joints were found to be separate. The second posterior sacral foramen lies behind the round facet. The first posterior foramen (I) lies just above the ridge of the sacral tuberosity. The first segment of the coccyx is fused to the sacrum. (Courtesy of the publisher of *The Journal of Bone and Joint Surgery*.)

forward from the arthritic joint, underlies the fourth lumbar nerve root as it passes downward to join the lumbosacral plexus. Symptoms indicating root pressure have been observed in certain of these patients. The first was a young woman of thirty-one years who developed weakness in the left leg with paralysis of the peroneal muscles during pregnancy. Postpartum, she also complained of pain in the back. Radiographic study showed a bilateral sacralization but with an arthritic process and projecting spur formation particularly marked on the left side. One might postulate that a counterpressure by the baby's head could have been responsible for her referred nerve symptoms during the pregnancy. She made a complete recovery and when reexamined twenty-three years later, backache was no longer present. Radiographs at that time revealed a complete ankylosis of the sacralized articulations. The case shown as

Figure XII:21 altho the same age is not the patient above reported.

The spur formation is best visualized with the patient supine and then rotated about 45 degrees toward the affected side.

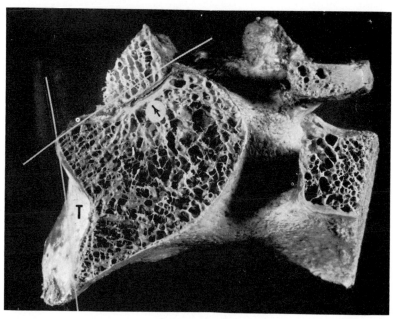

Fig. XII:14. Transverse section through the left half of a sacrum at its first foramen. The plane of the true sacroiliac articulation (T) forms an angle of 60 degrees with the plane of the accessory joint (*arrow*). This would seem to constitute a mechanical disadvantage to any normal movements of the true sacroiliac joint. Note the cartilaginous articular surfaces, the joint space, and the capsule of this vicarious articulation (*arrow*).

OSTEITIS CONDENSANS ILII

Osteitis condensans ilii is a circumscribed condensation of the ilium adjacent to the sacroiliac joint.

It is encountered much more frequently in women, many of whom complain of recurrent back pain. However, its clinical significance is debatable and its presence may be purely incidental. The etiology is unknown, pregnancy, lordosis and obesity having been considered in this connection. The condition is not an arthritis, there is no evidence of an inflammatory process and the usual tests for sacroiliac involvement are lacking. Neither the sacrum nor the sacroiliac joint appear to be involved.

As seen on the oblique projection the area of increased density appears to extend from the articular surface of the ilium outward into the substance of the bone (Figure XII:25A). The involvement may be small or large and either unilateral or bilateral. The margin may be somewhat lobulated but is usually sharply demarcated. When biopsied the condensed sclerotic bone is found to be made up of thickened irregular trabeculae with smaller lacunar spaces (Figures XII:25C and D).

In a study of some biopsy material Rendich and Shapiro report: "no osteolytic or osteoclastic changes . . . no evi-

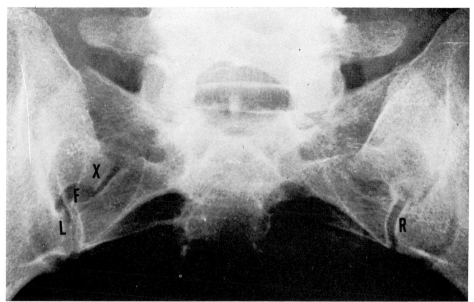

Fig. XII:15. Female, thirty-eight years old, with tenderness to deep pressure over the left posterior superior iliac spine (X). There was no tenderness on the right side. The accessory sacroiliac is well outlined by the narrow zone of eburnation on each side of the joint space. Slightly below and laterally lies the foramen for branches of the superior gluteal nerve and artery (F). This foramen separates the accessory joint from the true sacroiliac immediately below it (L). This is probably an example of early arthritic process while the corresponding accessory sacroiliac on the right side does not show evidence of such reaction. The R and L of each figure indicate the posterior limit of the true sacroiliac.

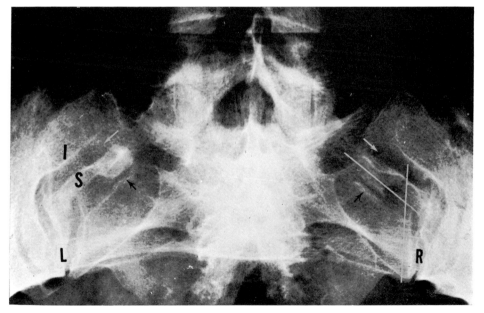

Fig. XII:16. Female, twenty-seven years old, complained of recurrent low back pain worse on the left side. The superficial accessory sacroiliacs show some early arthritic change (*black arrows*). White arrows indicate the space between the tuberosity of the ilium (I) and the sacral tuberosity (S). Actual contact of these with deep joint formation is not present in this instance. The white lines on the radiograph indicate as in Figure XII:12 the angle between the true and the accessory sacroiliac articulations.

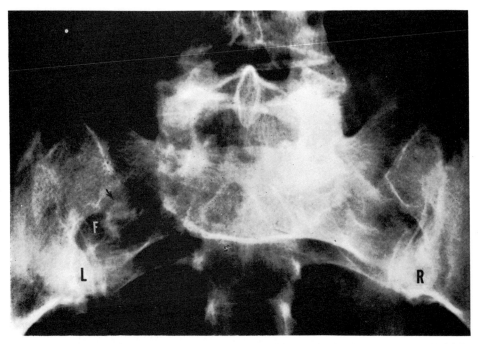

Fig. XII:17. X-ray of female, sixty years old, who had had pains in the low back and thighs for three months past. The film reveals a superficial accessory sacroiliac on the left side with an arthritic spur projecting laterally into the adjacent nutrient foramen (*arrow*). Compare with specimen shown in Figure XII:9 in which, however, the spur is on the medial side of the joint. The foramen (F) lies between the accessory and the true sacroiliac (L). The patient complained of tenderness to deep pressure over the posterior superior iliac spine on the left side. There is also an accessory joint on the right side which shows little evidence of arthritic change. When interviewed seven and one-half years after the original examination she had some low back pain, but only after heavy lifting. (Courtesy of the publisher of *The Journal of Bone and Joint Surgery*).

dence of overactivity of osteoblasts or osteoclasts . . . these cells conspicuous by their absence." There was no evidence of an inflammatory process discovered.

Rarely the condition may appear in a somewhat cystic form (Figure XII:27).

Subsequent examinations have shown the condition still present. Differential diagnosis must include a consideration of Paget's disease, metastases, Marie Strumpell's or sclerosing osteomyelitis.

SACRAL CYSTS

Perineurial sacral cysts are not uncommon, seven examples of the condition having been encountered by this author in a recent series of approximately 150 cadavers, an incidence of nearly five per cent (Figures XII:28, XII:29, XII:30 and XII:31). They may or may not produce symptoms referrable to the sciatic nerve or the caudal nerve roots. They are non-neoplastic, originate in the sacral canal outside the arachnoid and usually develope from the covering of the dorsal nerve root near its ganglion. These cysts may be multiple or single and occur most frequently on the second or third sacral root. If they communicate with the subarachnoid space they may be visualized by myelography (Figures XII:32 and XII:33). However such a communication is not the usual rule, in which case myelography is valueless.

The nerve fibers usually lie in the wall of the sac and as the cyst enlarges they become stretched over its periphery.

Other more distant sacral nerves become displaced by the cyst or pressed against the wall of the canal. This fixation or the pressure upon the nerve roots is probably responsible for the clinical picture. Some of these patients complain of pain or tenderness upon deep pressure directly over the sacral canal. The etiologic role played by these structures in sciatic and sacro-coccygeal syndromes seems to be well established. Paresthesia and urinary disturbance with sensory changes over the buttocks and perineal area may be encountered. Low back pain or sciatica with other sensory or motor deficits of sacral root distribution indicate a consideration of sacral cysts as the possible causal factor.

Since these cysts enlarge slowly the cortical shell of the surrounding adjacent bone appears on the radiograph as a white curvilinear line. The increasing pressure within the sac produces a gradual expansion which elevates the

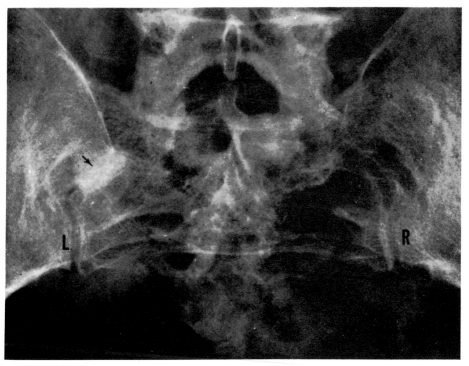

Fig. XII:18. Roentgenogram of a female, sixty-six years old, who complained of low back pain and sciatica on the left side. The patient has a left superficial accessory sacroiliac showing arthritic changes with eburnation of the underlying bone (*arrow*). Note the foramen between this joint and the true sacroiliac. The patient complained bitterly of pain upon deep pressure over this abnormal articulation. The plane of this joint forms an angle of nearly 60 degrees with that of the true sacroiliac. (Courtesy of *Radiology* and *The Journal of Bone and Joint Surgery*.)

dorsum of the sacral canal and/or erodes forward into the substance of the sacral body. Because of the white curvilinear line surrounding the cyst the condition may be visualized upon the radiograph without the aid of myelography (Figures XII:34, XII:35, and XII:36). Cysts are frequently encountered radiographically especially on the lateral projection of the sacrum. This is particularly true if there is a bulging backward of the dorsal wall of the sacral canal. They are visualized less clearly upon the P. A. projection.

Good stereoscopic studies are essential to avoid misinterpretation of other curvilinear shadows such as:

1. The cortices of various normal sacral contours; the pedicles, foramina and intersegmental junctions.

2. Incomplete closure of the neural arches.

3. Tumor formation.

4. Air in the bowel. Figures XII:37 and XII:38.

Laminograms or good stereoscopic studies will obviate these confusions.

REFERENCES

Lumbo Sacral Region

Cornwell, W. S., and Ramsey, G. H.: 1957, *Rad.,* *69*:70–73, Anatomy.

Ghormley, R. K.: 1958, *Rad., 70*:649–653, Anatomy.

Hertzmark, M.: 1960, *Bull. Hosp. Joint. Dis., 21*:50–64, Anatomy.

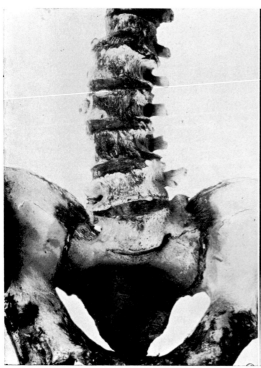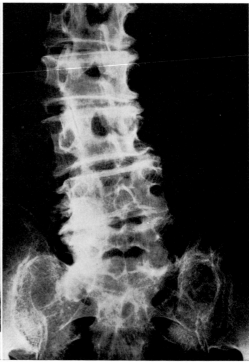

Fig. XII:19. Asymmetrical sacralization of the first presacral segment with an enlarged transverse process on the left side. The right side of this segment has become ankylosed to the ala of the sacrum and there is minimal resultant scoliosis. In this individual there were the normal five sacral segments and five lumbar segments. Unilateral sacralization results in various unbalanced stresses and secondary compensatory developments at the point of weightbearing.

Hosner, E., *et al:* 1952, *Acta Rad., 37*:141–149, Movement.

Hosner, E., *et al:* 1953, *Acta Rad., 39*:225–230.

Jirout, J.: 1956, *Acta Rad., 46*:55–60, Movement.

Jirout, J.: 1957, *Acta Rad., 47*:345–348, Movement.

Jirout, J.: 1958, *Acta Rad., 48*:361–365.

Knutsson, F.: 1944, *Acta Rad., 25*:593–609, Movement.

Mensor, M. C., *et al:* 1959, *J. Bone J. Surg., 41A*: 1047–1054.

Meschan, I., *et al:* 1958, *Rad., 70*:637–648, Anatomy.

Soloren, K. A.: 1955, *Acta Ortho. Scand., 27*:1–127.

Sutro, C. J., *et al:* 1960, *Bull. Hosp. Joint Dis., 21*:42–49, Anatomy.

Tang, S. S.: 1953, *Am. Jor. Roent., 69*:399–412, Motion.

Wilson, J. C.: 1959, *J.A.M.A., 169*:1437–1442, Anatomy.

Accessory Sacroiliacs

Derry, D. E.: 1911, *J. Anat. & Physiol., 45*:202–210.

Giraudi, G.: 1936, *Radiol. Med., 23*:987–994.

Peterson: 1905, O.V.C.E., *Anat. Anzeig., 26*:521–524.

Seligmann, S. B.: 1935, *Anat. Anzeig., 79*:225–241.

Trotter, Mildred: 1937, *Am. Jor. Phys. Anthrop., 22*:247–261.

Trotter, Mildred: 1940, *J. Bone J. Surg., 22*:293–299.

Osteitis Condensans Ilii

Gillespie, H. W., and Loyd, Roberts: 1953, *Brit. Jor. Rad., 26*:16–21.

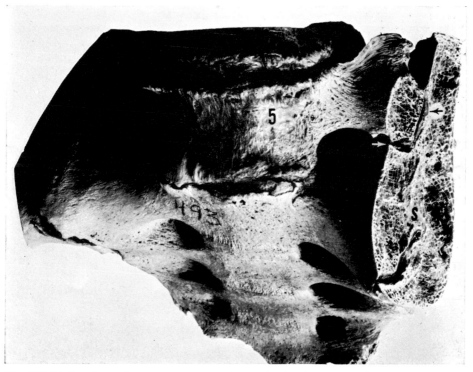

Fig. XII:20. Specimen showing asymmetrical sacralization in a male of seventy-nine years. The articulation between the enlarged L_5 transverse process and the ilium is indicated by the black arrow. The white arrow indicates the vicarious joint between the enlarged transverse process and the ala of the sacrum. Both of these articulations are lined by hyaline cartilage. Normally the sacroiliac joint is lined by this tissue but in this individual ankylosis of the sacroiliac had occurred at the point S. The disc space between S_1 and the sacralized presacral segment is always thinner than normal and in this case it contained two small intercalary ossicles.

Hare, H. F., and Haggart, G. E.: 1945, *J.A.M.A.,* *128*:723–727.

Hertzmark, M.: 1960, *Bull. Hosp. Joint Dis., 21:* 50–64.

Knutsson, F.: 1950, *Acta Rad., 33:*557–569.

Rendich, R. A., and Shapiro, A. V.: 1936, *J. Bone J. Surg., 18:*899–908.

Rojko, A.: 1960, *Acta Ortho. Scan., 29:*108–120.

Schipp, F. L., and Haggart, G. E.: 1950, *J. Bone J. Surg., 32A:*841–847.

Segal, G., *et al:* 1954, *Am. Jor. Roent., 71:*643–649.

Ude, W. H.: 1952, *Minnesota Med., 35:*541–543.

Wells, J.: 1956, *Am. Jor. Roent., 76:*1141–1143.

Sacral Perineurial Cysts

Abbott, K. H., *et al:* 1957, *J. Neurosurg., 14:*5–21.

Archer, V. W., *et al:* 1948, *Rad., 51:*691–695.

Baker, G. S., *et al:* 1952, *Proc. Staff. Meet., Mayo Clin., 27:*231–234.

Hadley, L. A.: 1960, *Am. Jor. Roent., 84:*119–124.

Hyndman, O. R., *et al:* 1946, *J. Neurosurg., 3:* 474–486.

Jacobs, L. G., *et al:* 1954, *Rad., 62:*215–221.

Rexed, B. A., *et al:* 1959, *J. Neurosurg., 16:*73–84.

Schreiber, F., *et al:* 1951, *J. Neurosurg., 8:*504–509.

Schurr, P. H.: 1955, *J. Bone J. Surg., 37B:*601–605.

Seaman, W. B., *et al:* 1956, *J. Neurosurg., 13:*88–94.

Strully, K. J.: 1956, *J.A.M.A., 161:*1147–1152.

Strully, K. J., *et al:* 1954, *Rad., 62:*544–549.

Taheri, Z. E., Riemenschneider, P. A., and Ecker, A.: 1952, *J. Neurosurg., 9:*93–95.

Tarlov, I. M.: 1953, *Sacral Nerve-Root Cysts,* Charles C Thomas, Springfield, Ill.

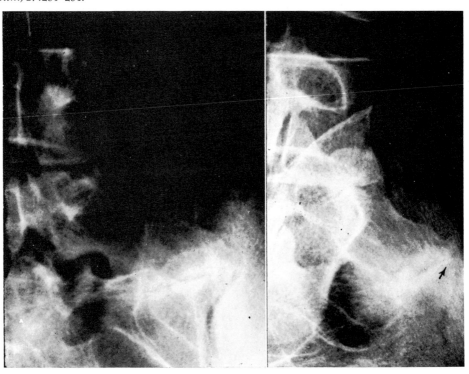

Fig. XII:21. Female, thirty-one years old, struck low back in automobile accident eight months before examination with subsequent attacks of left sciatic pain. Patellar reflexes normal, left Achilles reflex absent. Radiographs reveal unilateral sacralization of a sixth lumbar segment on the left side. This vicarious joint shows advanced arthritic changes. Examination in the 45 degree oblique projection reveals spur formation projecting forward into the pelvic cavity *(arrow)*. It is probably to some degree responsible for the sciatica and reflex changes.

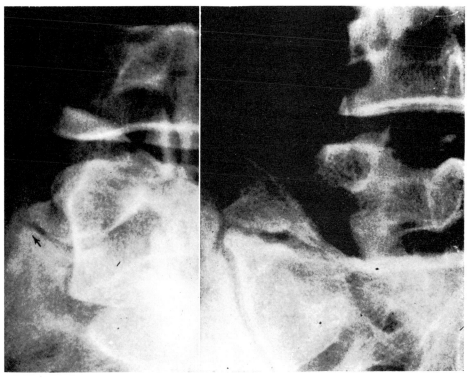

Fig. XII:22. Mechanic, thirty-four years old, complained of increasing localized pain following injury. No radiation or disturbed reflexes. Radiographs reveal an asymmetrical sixth lumbar segment sacralized on the right side. In this oblique projection this vicarious joint shows evidence of arthritic change and spur formation *(arrow)*. Here is an example of a previously asymptomatic anomaly in a sturdy, well developed male who developed symptoms only following trauma.

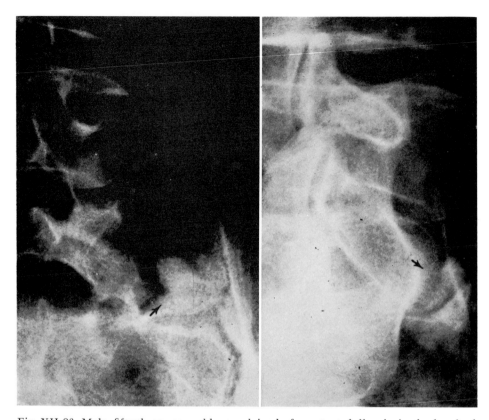

Fig. XII:23. Male, fifty-three years old, complained of constant dull pain in the low back and left gluteal region following a sprain two months before. He stood with his weight carried on the right foot. There was spasm of the lower lumbar muscles and some limitation of movement. The patellar and Achilles reflexes were normal. The radiographs show a massive bony spur formation (*arrows*) projecting upward and forward from the left arthritic vicarious joint. One cannot ascribe the recent symptoms to the pre-existent condition, however it may have been a predisposing factor to be aggravated by the trauma in this older patient.

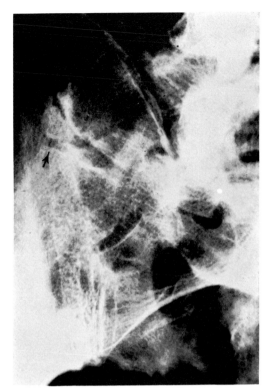

Fig. XII:24. Male of sixty-four years, with unilateral arthritic sacralization on the right side.
There are two secondary ossification centers entrapped within the vicarious joint (*arrow*).

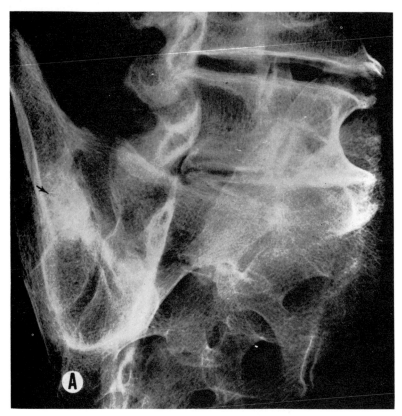

Fig. XII:25. Roentgenogram (A) showing osteitis condensans ilii from a male cadaver of seventy-five years. The specimen (B) was sawed thru to show the dense, circumscribed, somewhat lobulated area of ivory-like bone, adjacent to the sacroiliac joint (*arrows*). There is no involvement of the sacrum. The removed fragment has been rotated outward to show the texture of the bony structure. The photomicrograph C (X8) shows the difference in the trabeculae. Those on the right from the sacrum are slender with large lacunar spaces between them. The sacroiliac joint space is in the center. On the left are the short thick trabeculae with small lacunar spaces from the sclerotic area of the ilium. The photomicrograph D (X40) shows the laminated morphology of the sclerotic trabeculae.

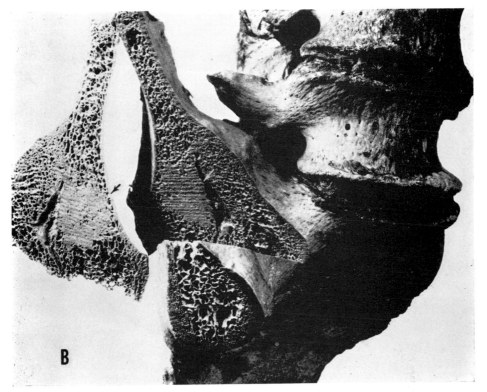

Fig. XII:25 B.

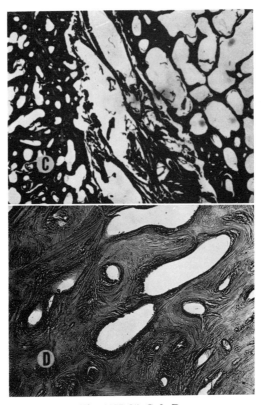

Fig. XII:25 C & D.

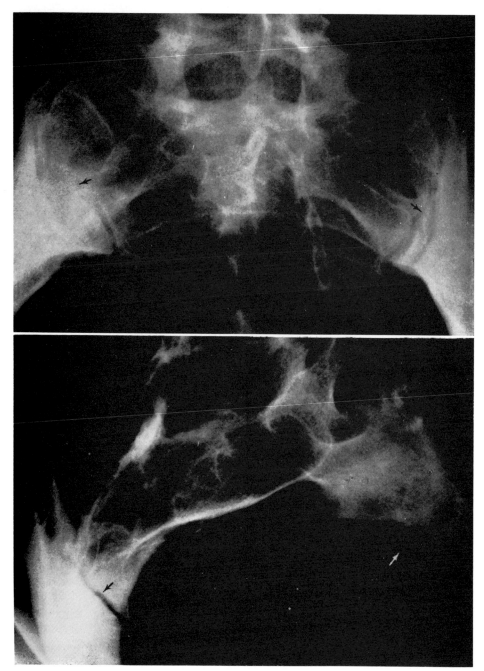

Fig. XII:26.Osteitis condensans ilii in a woman of fifty-nine years. This housewife is the victim of rheumatoid arthritis. Coincidental with each of four pregnancies she has developed low back pain aggravated by sitting but not referred down the legs. The A.P. and oblique studies show the typical areas of sclerosis of the ilium (*arrows*). The patient has a spina bifida occulta below the first sacral arch.

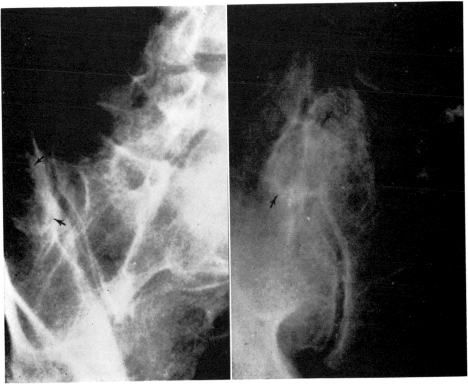

Fig. XII:27. A cystic type of osteitis ilii in a male of sixty years, possibly in the nature of a chondroma. This arises at the surface of the sacroiliac joint and extends into the substance of the ilium (*arrows*).

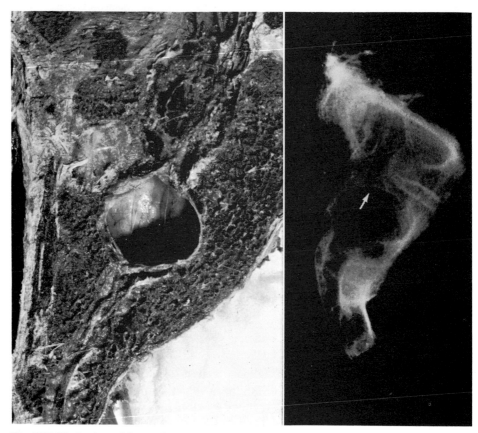

Fig. XII:28. Perineurial sacral cyst involving the left third sacral root of a seventy-seven year old female. The nerves were incorporated into the sac wall and had become displaced laterally. The arrow indicates the white curvilinear line limiting the cyst proximally.

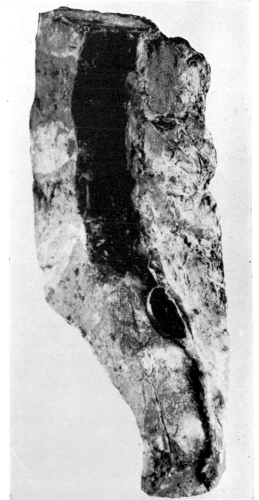

Fig. XII:29. Photograph and roentgenograms showing the right side of the sacrum from a male of eighty-nine years. The erosion is noted to the left of the midline. The cyst had developed on the third sacral root displacing that structure together with the other more distal roots. Note the white curvilinear line (*arrow*) indicating the limit of bony erosion forward into the second sacral segment.

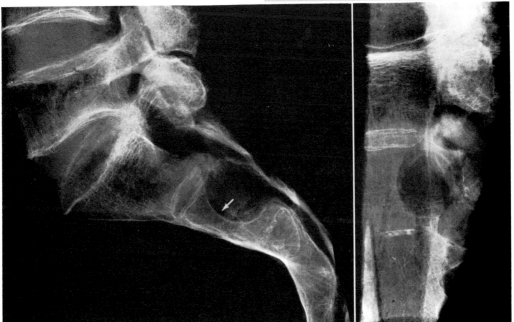

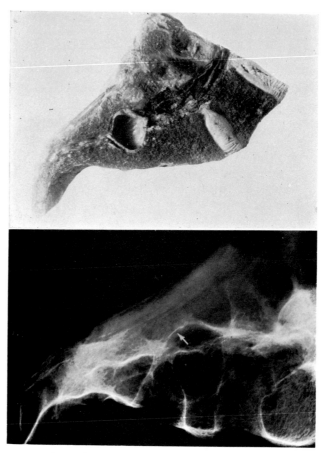

Fig. XII:30. In this specimen the cyst, arising on the left third sacral root, not only eroded forward into the substance of the second sacral segment but also expanded backward into the spinal canal elevating its dorsal wall (*white arrow*).

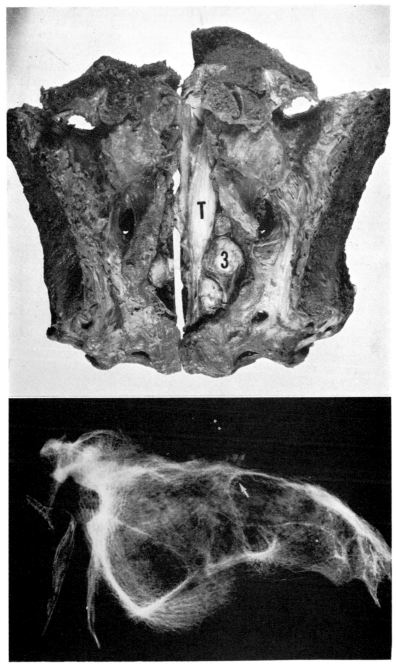

Fig. XII:31. Cadaver specimen showing multiple perineurial sacral cysts; all are outside the theca (T). The third left root is cystic and there are cysts on the second, third and fourth roots on the right side. The roentgenogram visualizes erosion of the spinal canal (*arrow*). Multiple cysts are less common than the solitary type. (Courtesy *American Journal of Roentgenology.*)

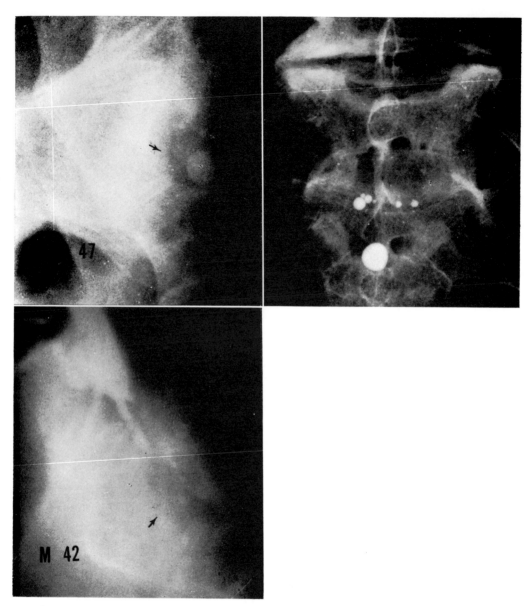

Fig. XII:32. A man of forty-seven years complained of recurrent, incapaciting pain radiating down the left leg with paresthesia. At times there was spasm of the calf muscles on each side. Note the bony erosion at the distal portion of the second sacral segment (*arrow*). The large droplet of oil below the tip of the theca remains in the cyst from a myelogram done five years before.

Radiograph M, made at the time of the original myelography, showed the erosion of the cyst already present (*arrow*). A small droplet of contrast medium had entered the structure during the procedure. Nearly all of the oil was later removed from the canal but a small amount remained and subsequently collected within the cyst. The condition, although present at the earlier examination, remained unrecognized at that time. It would seem that if oil does enter a sacral cyst its evacuation from that structure is unlikely.

→

Fig. XII:34. Incidental finding indicating an asymptomatic sacral cyst in a male of thirty-seven years who sprained his back while at work. Note erosion of the dorsal surface of S_2 (*arrow*) and the backward bulging of the spinal canal.

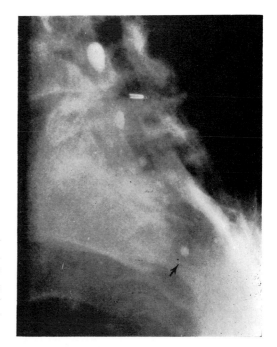

Fig. XII:33. Male fifty-three years of age complaining of low back pain, limitation of motion and tenderness to deep pressure over the midline of the sacrum. The sacral cyst (*arrow*) eroding S$_2$ and containing opaque medium was neither recognized at the operation nor at the myelographic examination.

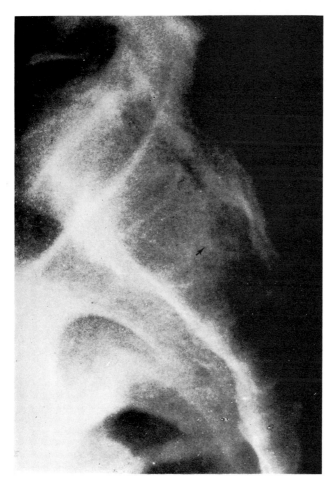

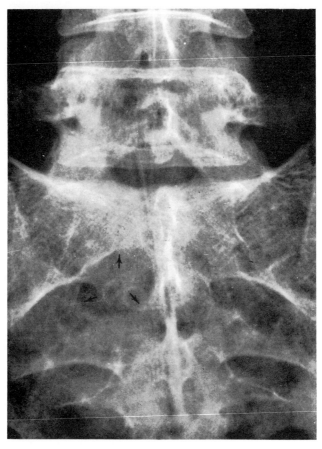

Fig. XII:35. Female patient, age fifty-six years, with oval deficiency in the dorsal wall of the spinal canal on the left side at the S_2 level *(arrow)*. Stereoscopic studies were essential in this examination.

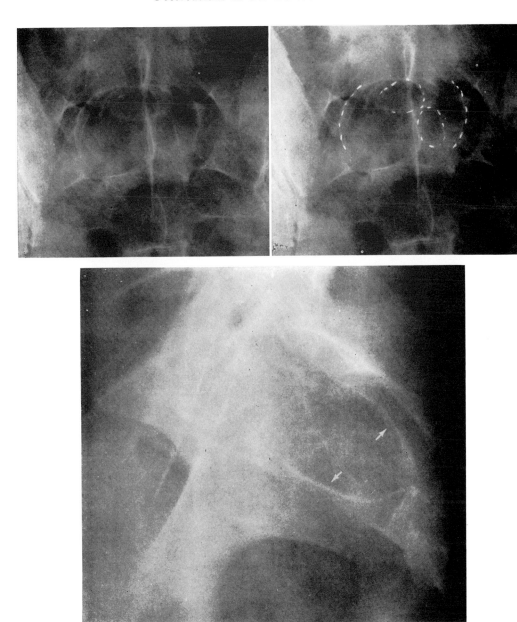

Fig. XII:36. Male, fifty-nine years, with multiple sacral cysts. Observation over a period of ten years has shown some enlargement in a dorsal direction. He complains of increasing pain over the sacrum aggravated by deep pressure at this point. There is backache and pain referred to the calves of both legs but not aggravated by increased intra-abdominal pressure. The Achilles and patellar reflexes are active and there is no perineal paresthesia. Stereoscopy clearly differentiates one large and two small cavaties involving principally the second sacral segment and its spinal canal. These are indicated by white dots in the P. A. projection and white arrows in the lateral view. The symptoms have continued but the patient refuses operation. (Courtesy of *American Journal of Roentgenology.*)

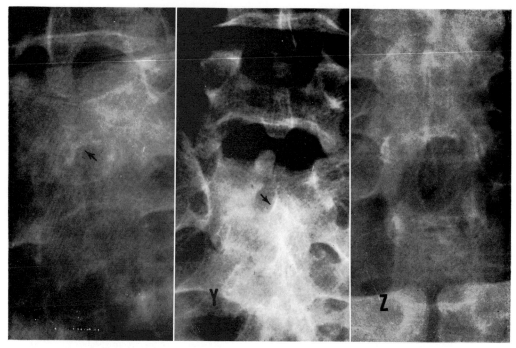

Fig. XII:37. A group of three roentgenograms showing negative shadows bounded by curvilinear white lines and overlying the sacrum which might be mistaken for perineurial sacral cysts (*arrows*). X, a female of sixty-four years with a circular area of calcification within the S_1-S_2 junction. Y, a female of forty-nine years with a neural arch incompletely closed. Z, a white curvilinear line limiting a small collection of bowel gas. Good stereoscopic studies should resolve such confusing possibilities.

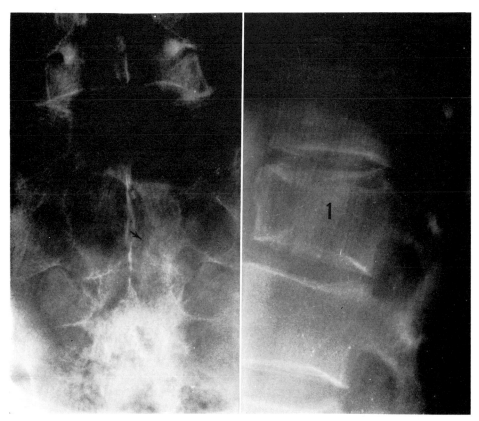

Fig. XII:38. Myeloma of the sacrum in a male of fifty-eight years (*arrows*) offered some confusion until a destructive lesion with bone collapse was discovered in the first lumbar vertebra.

Chapter XIII

Spondylolysis and Spondylolisthesis

DEFICIENCY IN THE NEURAL ARCH

Since one of the principal functions of the neural arch is to stabilize the spine (others being cord protection and muscle attachment), the integrity of that structure in the lower lumbar region is especially important. At the lumbosacral level the 5th lumbar vertebra supports the superimposed weight of the body upon the inclined plane of the sacrum. The necessity for bony continuity of the 5th lumbar pedicle and inferior articular process articulating with the posterior surface of the sacral articulation is obvious. A deficiency in the neural arch or spondylolysis may or may not be complicated by a displacement of the vertebral body or spondylolisthesis. Anatomical studies illustrate some of the changes which occur in the neural arch incidental to this type of bone deficiency (Figures XIII:1, XIII:2 and XIII:3).

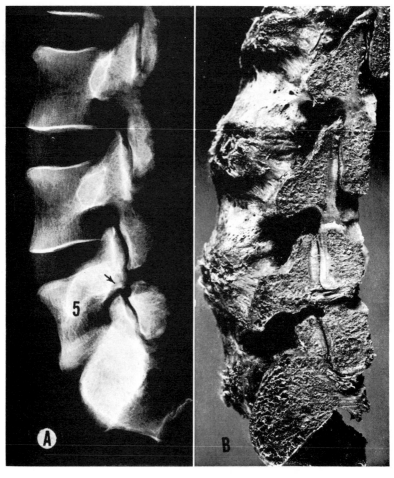

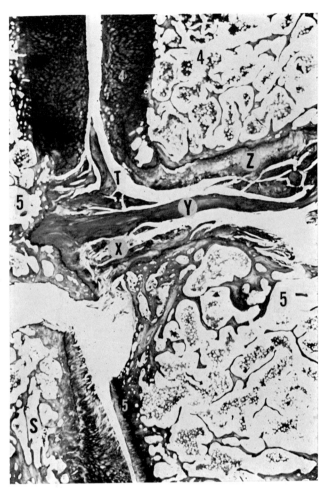

Fig. XIII:1. Photograph, radiograph and section from a male eighty-nine, showing that the ability of the 5th arch to stabilize the lumbar body upon the inclined plane of the sacrum has been completely lost because of a break in the continuity of the 5th neural arch (*arrow*). The useless detached 5th inferior articular process has been bypassed and some attempt at stabilization has occurred as the articular process of the sacrum has developed contact with the undersurface of the 5th pedicle. The defect in the arch (X on the section) between the two fragments of the 5th inferior articular process has become filled in with fibrous tissue. A fibro-cartilage bumper (Z) entirely different in character from normal hyaline articular cartilage has developed at the tip of the 4th inferior articular process to articulate with the detached portion of the 5th neural arch below. The hyaline articular cartilage of the 4th and 5th joints is visualized above and below, respectively. One may note some thinning and early degenerative fibrillation of the 5th joint cartilage but the cartilage of the upper joint appears normal. Compare the 4th and 5th joints in the photograph (B). There is a tab of synovia (T) projecting upward between the joint surfaces above. The lower margin of the fibrous capsule of the 4th joint (Y) has remained continuous but it has become thinned and stretched out.

OBLIQUE STUDIES

Stereoscopic oblique studies made partially supine but with the sagittal plane approximately 45 degrees to the horizontal have accorded the best visualization of the arch defect. The perpendicular central ray is centered slightly below the level of the anterior superior iliac spine. A shadow simulating a break

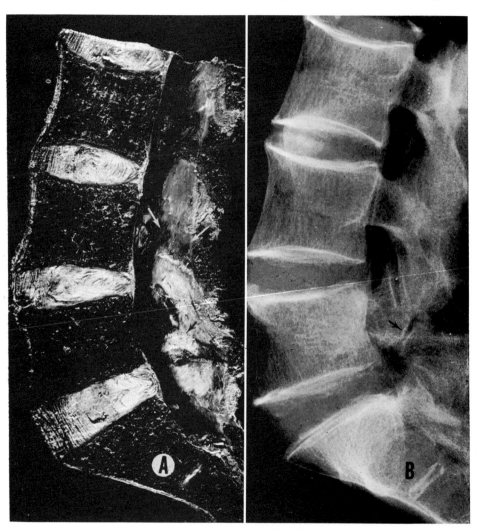

Fig. XIII:2. Female, ninety-three, with a break in the 5th neural arch, spondylolysis but without any spondylolyisthesis or slipping. Photograph taken from the medial side shows a continuation downward of the 4th joint capsule to cover this break in the arch (*black arrow*). Note on the arch above that the bone is entirely continuous between the white arrows from the 4th pedicle to the spinous process. The radiograph and the section reveal a bony cortex on each side of the dehiscence. The photomicrograph X5.5 shows the band of fibrous tissue crossing the bony defect of the 5th arch (X). There is a narrow darker zone of fibrocartilage adjacent to the bony tissue on each side but there is no true hyaline cartilage or joint space. Fibrous elements of the 4th and 5th joint capsules are visible above and below (4 and 5).

in the neural arch may occur on the 45 degree oblique film if the roentgen tube is centered too far cephalad.

On the oblique film of the normal lumbosacral area the 5th posterior articulation is shown beneath or anterior to the 4th. In cases of lordosis or spondylolisthesis, the 5th articulation is seen posterior to the plane of the 4th joint (Figure XIII:35). An occult spondylolisthesis may be suspected even without roentgen confirmation of forward slipping in patients with bilateral 5th arch defect wherein the plane of the 5th posterior articulation lies well posterior to that of the 4th. In this case a lateral roentgenogram made with the patient standing may resolve this uncertainty.

As seen in the oblique film the deficiency in the isthmus of the 5th neural arch usually lies between the tip of the sacral articular process and that of the inferior articular process of the 4th vertebra. These two structures may even approximate each other and appear with the fragments of the 5th neural arch flanking them on each side. This dehiscence or deficiency of bone between the articular processes of L_4 and S_1 is the characteristic feature of a break in the 5th neural arch (Figure XIII:4).

A defect in the isthmus of the neural arch of the 5th lumbar vertebra is present in about five per cent of all adult spines. Since the unconfirmed reports of Rambaud and Renault in 1864, this condition has been considered to be of congenital origin. There is some evidence (Figures XIII:22, XIII:23 and XIII:24, as well as the studies of Roche and Rowe) that an atypical cleavage line across the arch may occur congenitally in the upper lumbar region. However there is little evidence to substantiate a congenital break in the 5th neural arch as the usual cause of spondylolysis. Rowe and Roche

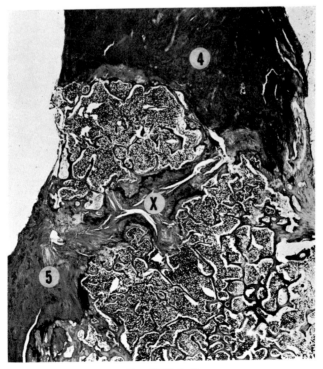

Fig. XIII:2 C.

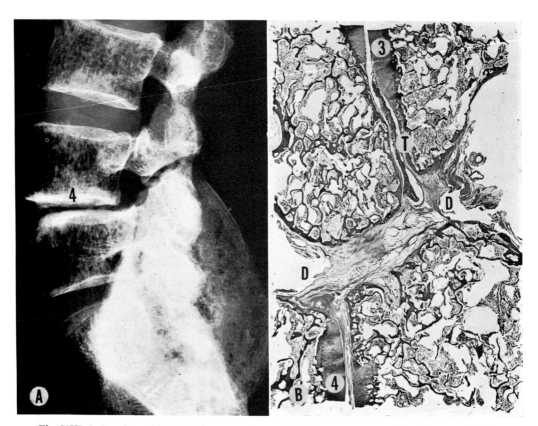

Fig. XIII:3. Specimen No. 5210 from a male aged 78. Roentgenogram showing spondylolisthesis from a break in the 4th neural arch and degeneration of the 4th disc. Section B was made through the break in the 4th neural arch. This defect is seen passing diagonally across the mid-portion of the field (D-D). It contains only fibrous tissue. There is no true joint surface or cartilage between the two parts of the 4th arch but in both the roentgenogram and the section one may identify a distinct cortex on each side of the deficiency. Within the fibrous tissue are a few small open spaces lined with a single layer of cells but no true joint spaces. At the edge of the section above and below are cartilages of the 3rd and 4th posterior joints (3 and 4). A long tab of synovia (T) projects into the former. Pinching of these common synovia tabs between the articular surfaces is a possible cause of the sudden acute pain which at times may follow stooping. (Courtesy of the *American Journal of Roentgenology*.)

———————————————————————————————————
                                                          ——————————→

Fig. XIII:4. Lateral and oblique studies of a specimen showing first degree spondylolisthesis from a break in the 5th neural arch. The photograph A shows that the break in the 5th arch is bridged by the dark ligamentous tissue at 5. Compare with the 4th arch above. A part of the lamina of the 5th vertebra, flattened in front, remained attached to the pedicle and was carried forward with that structure (*arrows*). This constitutes an encroachment upon the passage for the sacral nerve roots. Note the wide break in the continuity between the two fragments of the 5th neural arch as visualized on photograph C. The tip of the articular process of the sacrum is thrust upward into this space nearly to the 4th inferior articulation and articulates with the 5th pedicle. The alignment of the 4th and 5th posterior joints together with the transverse space between them not infrequently takes the form of a cross, as seen in this photograph. (Courtesy of the publisher of *The Journal of Bone and Joint Surgery*.)

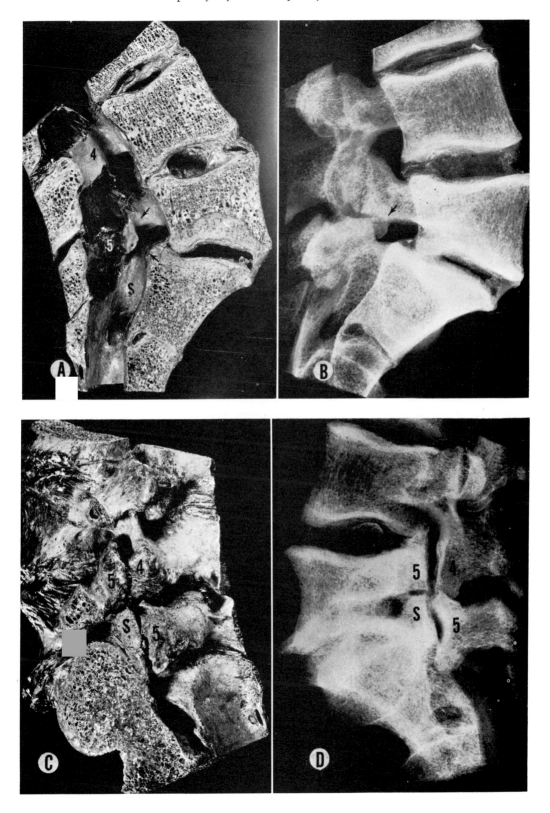

in reviewing the studies of 509 fetal spines, including their own series of fifty-three stillborn infants, were unable to find any evidence of a congenital defect in the isthmus of the neural arch of the 5th lumbar vertebra. Also, in the sixty-nine spines of fetal and newborn subjects studied by this author in the Anatomy Department of the New York State Medical College at Syracuse, not a single specimen showed any evidence of a defect in the isthmus of the 5th neural arch. Various congenital anomalies are encountered in this region and it is conceivable that such a congenital defect may occur rarely but certainly not in five per cent of all individuals. One must conclude, therefore, that the condition usually develops after birth.

In this connection, a glance at the neural arch of the newborn shows the isthmus and the inferior articular process on each side as a sturdy, spatula-shaped structure designed at this period to cover over the spinal canal (Figure XIII:5). The two sides unite across the midline at the end of the first year. At birth the spine is nearly straight and the various curves, cervical, thoracic and lumbar, develop only after the child begins to

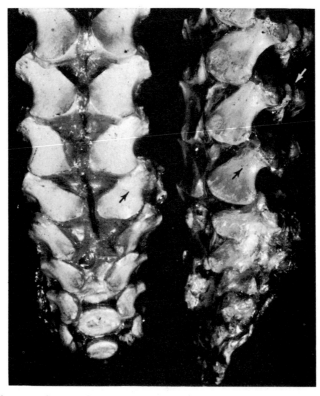

Fig. XIII:5. Photographs X2 of newborn lumbar spines showing the posterior and lateral surfaces. The black arrows indicate the wide sturdy structure of the isthmus or pars interarticularis of the neural arch as it appears at this time. The separate spatula shaped elements of the neural arches cover over the spinal canal. These become united at about one year of age. The white arrow indicates the neuro-central junction where the pedicle fuses with the centrum at about four or five years of age. The lumbo sacral curve has not yet developed at this time. There is only one ossification center for each side of the neural arch and the isthmus is really its strongest part.

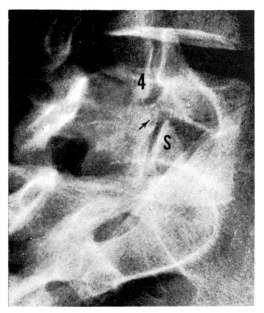

Fig. XIII:6. Female, fifty years old, fell on slippery steps three weeks before, striking on buttocks. Maximum pain in right iliolumbar angle. The roentgenogram reveals an unusually slender right 5th isthmus lying above the sharp tip of the sacral articular process (S). Probable double fracture line crosses the narrowest portion of the arch at this point *(arrow)*. The film illustrates how the slender pars interarticularis in a patient of asthenic habitus may possibly be subjected to the "cutting pinchers" type of trauma. This possibility is not accepted by all observers.

trauma or gradually over a period of time (Figure XIII:6).

Few cases of a break in the 5th neural arch have been reported in young children. Kleinberg discovered this condition in a little one of seventeen months who had only been walking a few weeks. Hitchcock mentioned a female of four years with a spondylolysis or defect in the neural arch. When reexamined at twelve years after a severe fall on the buttocks she had developed spondylolisthesis. Other authors have reported the condition in children but it seems to be rare

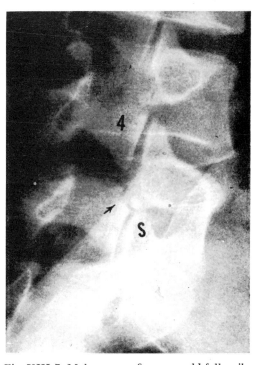

Fig. XIII:7. Male, twenty-five years old fell striking the sacrum three days before examination. All movements were guarded. He indicated the right iliolumbar angle as the site of maximum pain and there was local fingerpoint tenderness and palpable crepitation at that point. The right oblique radiograph shows a fracture of the 5th neural arch *(arrow)* corresponding to the point of crepitation. The trauma obviously resulted from the impact transmitted to the isthmus by the superior articular process of the sacrum (S).

assume the upright position. As the lower lumbar curve develops, with its resultant shearing stresses, two significant anatomical changes occur. The interarticular isthmus of the arch becomes relatively longer and more slender and at the same time comes to lie between the tip of the superior articular process of the sacrum and the tip of the inferior articular process of the 4th lumbar segment. Opposing pressure upon a slender isthmus of the 5th arch between these points may conceivably sever that structure by attrition or as by a pair of cutting pliers. This action is favored by increasing degrees of lordosis and might occur by a single

in early infancy. The condition usually develops by the 20th year and the incidence remains about the same thereafter. Once developed there is seldom additional displacement although the disc may become thinned. A substantial number of patients is entirely free of symptoms.

Taillard, in his excellent monograph, has recorded the trophostatic dysplasia theory of spondylolysis formation as developed by Meyer-Burgdorff and other German writers. The condition is termed by these authors a "creeping fracture." A "strain deossification" with gradual fragmentation is said to occur

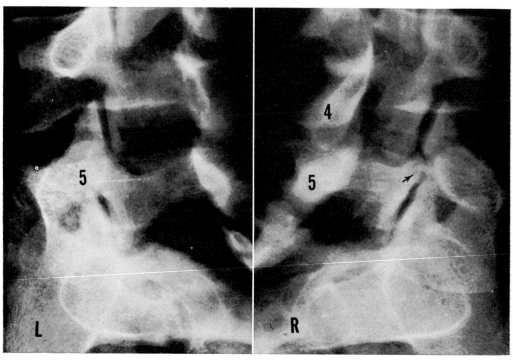

Fig. XIII:8. After a tackle during a football game, this eighteen year old patient emerged from a pile of players with a severe localized pain in the back. He had never previously suffered back pain. When examined eleven months later he complained of "grating" and pain in the right iliolumbar area which sometimes radiated down the right lower extremity. This was aggravated by dorsal extension. There was finger-point tenderness over the right side of the neural arch of the 5th lumbar vertebra and palpable crepitation over this area upon movement of the back. The right oblique roentgenogram (R) made eleven months after injury showed a unilateral break in the neural arch of the 5th lumbar vertebra (*arrow*) with evidence of fragmentation of bony tissue at this point. When seen two years after injury the patient still complained of right-sided back pain and "grating" upon dorsal extension. This author was no longer able to palpate the crepitation at the time of the second examination. The left side of the 5th neural arch (L) is intact. Re-examination five and one half years after injury showed resorption of the fragmented bony tissues. The appearance was that of a clean-cut ununited fracture. The patient did not develop a spondylolisthesis. A comparison of the 4th and 5th neural arches reveals the compensatory increase of density which has developed in the 5th arch as a result of the unilateral break.- Incidental to this unbalanced support a part of the forward and downward stress from the pedicle of the intact left side is carried across to the inferior articular process on the right. (Courtesy of *The Journal of Bone and Joint Surgery*.)

as a result of the chronic overload trauma upon the isthmus, especially in the presence of lordosis. This dissolution is considered as somewhat analogus to the Looser's "Umbauzonen" or transformation zones such as seen in the march fracture. Probably no single etiology is responsible for all cases of break in the continuity of the neural arch.

While history of an adequate producing injury is seldom obtainable from patients with spondylolysis there is evidence that the 5th neural arch like any other bone in the body may succumb when subjected to excessive strain (Figures XIII:7, XIII:8, XIII:9 and XIII:10). In these patients apparently no attempt at bony union occurred. In fact, because of the shearing stress and the difficulty of immobilization a solid bony union is not to be expected. However, the following observations would seem to indicate that healing with bony callus formation may actually occur upon occasion.

BONY MASSES PROJECTING INTO THE SPINAL CANAL

In a certain number of cases with a defect at the pars interarticularis, we have been able to visualize a smooth, rounded, bony callus formation projecting from the defect medially and forward into the spinal canal. Considerable encroachment upon the passage may result at this level. Some of these patients give a history of severe injury, others do not. Where present, such callus would seem to be evidence of fracture healing. The condition is visualized upon the posterior-anterior roentgenograms as a dense shadow bulging medially into the lumen from the lateral wall of the spinal canal.

On the 45 degree supine oblique studies, the posterior articulations of the lowermost side, joined by the isthmus or pars interarticularis, appear overlying the vertebral bodies. If the patient, for instance, is turned partly up onto the right side to show the right posterior joints, the cortex of the right pedicle enface will be seen overlying the vertebral body and immediately anterior to the right isthmus. The tear-shaped profiles of the laminae of the neural arches of the left or uppermost side are seen posteriorly behind the spinal canal. If a callus-like bony mass is present it will be seen on the oblique view posteriorly, as a dense sharply delineated, rounded shadow projecting from the lamina forward into the canal (Figures XIII:11 and XIII:12).

In certain cases a section of the lamina may remain attached to the pedicle and be carried forward with that structure (Figure XIII:4). The profile of this fragment, as seen in the oblique study, is usually flattened anteriorly. It may become incorporated with the bony mass and reunited with the detached fragment of the arch (Figure XIII:15).

Bone formation may also result from a rubbing of the bony surfaces together as shown by specimen No. 278 from the Terry Anatomical collection at Washington University. In this specimen there was a bilateral break in the neural arch of the 5th lumbar vertebra with a substantial mass of bone projecting medially from the left pedicle into the canal adjacent to the defect. The roentgenogram of one of our anatomical specimens showed a bony mass at the neural arch defect. This proved to be an ossicle 7 x 12 mm in size (Figure XIII:16). Gill, Pheasant and other surgeons have repeatedly removed bony masses of this character which were producing pressure upon the 5th nerve root opposite a break in

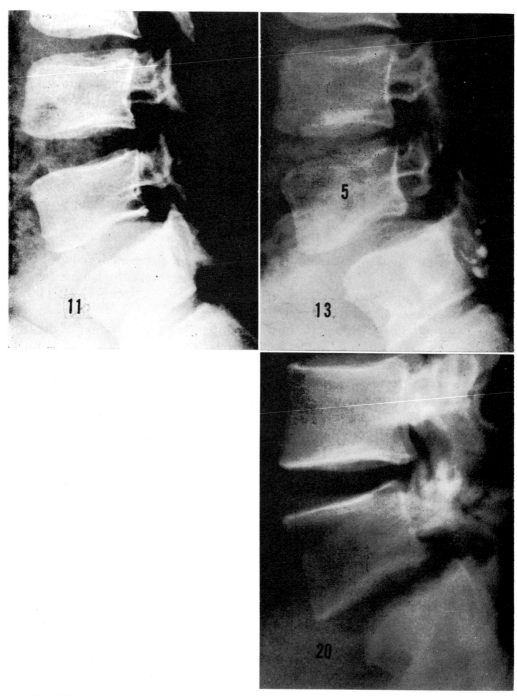

Fig. XIII:9. Spondylolisthesis developing after trauma. Boy eleven years old, injured in football pile-up, suffered severe back pain for a period of time, but made an uneventful recovery. Oblique radiographs at that time showed the slightest suggestion of a dehiscence of the 5th isthmus but no spondylolisthesis (*black arrow*). Three months later after bending over he developed acute pain in the back, referred to the right leg, with muscle spasm and lost patellar reflex. Radiographs at that time showed definite bilateral spondylilisthesis. He was immobilized in plaster five months. Later radiographs at thirteen years showed

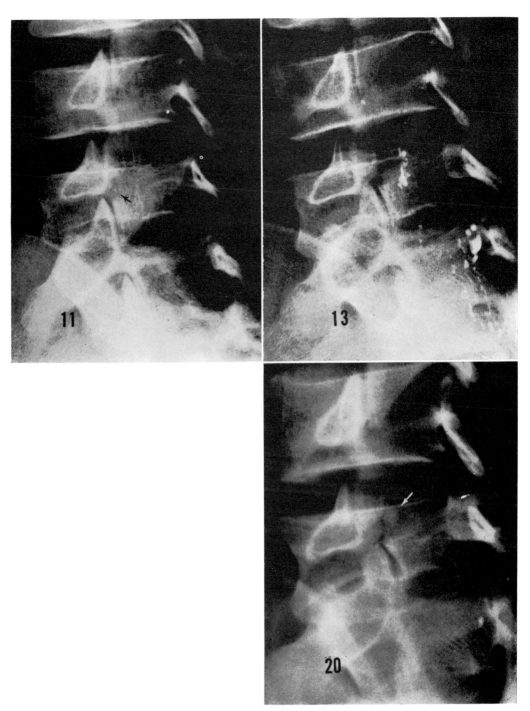

a wide break in the neural arch and no healing of the spondylolisthesis. Reexamination at the age of twenty revealed the spondylolisthesis unchanged in degree but with early thinning of the lumbo sarcal disc. At that time the tip of the articular process of the sacrum had become rounded off by pressure against the remnant of the 5th arch and a separate ossicle (*white arrow*) had developed. The patient was active in athletics and essentially symptom free. (Courtesy of Dr. Homer C. Pheasant, Los Angeles, California.)

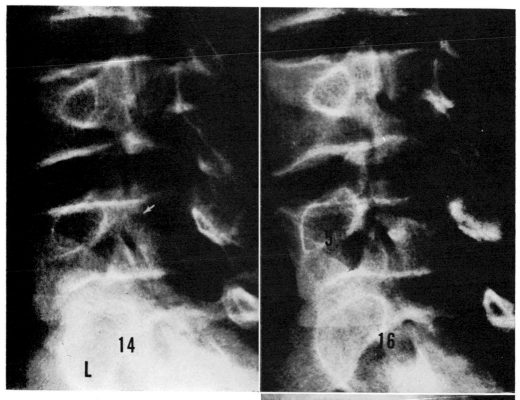

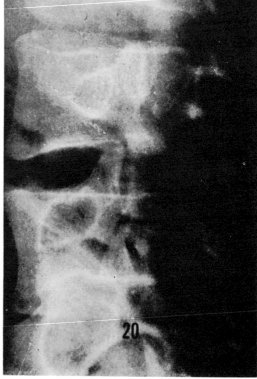

Fig. XIII:10. Stress fracture developing in a normal right arch incidental to a defect on the opposite side. The patient was first examined at fourteen years following a bicycle collision. There were six lumbar segments, the lowermost sacralized on the left. The right 5th pedicle appeared normal but there was a possible slight infraction thru the slender left 5th isthmus (*white arrow*). Two years later back pain had become increasingly severe with spasm and limitation of movement. The roentgenograms at sixteen years showed that a definite spondylolysis had developed on the left side during the two-year interval. The right 5th pedicle was now crossed by a zone of radiolucency (*black arrow*). This structure had apparently developed a "fatigue fracture" incidental to unbalanced stresses resulting from the defect on the opposite side. Four years later the right 4th articular process had

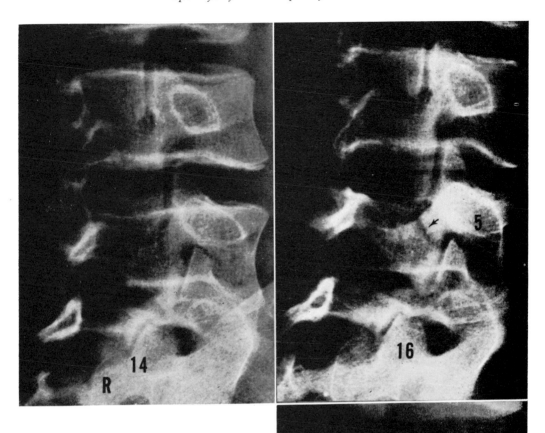

forced its way downward into the stress fracture splitting open that defect. Now, at twenty years, the remainder of the right 5th inferior articular process was hooked fast behind a somewhat eroded 6th superior process probably preventing spondylolisthesis. The condition on the left side was essentially unchanged. Symptoms at twenty years were no longer troublesome. Spondylolisthesis did not occur but a compensating hypertrophy of the lower back muscles had developed as shown on the photograph of his back taken at that time. "Exhaustion fractures" of bone have been studied by Professor C. Henschen of Basle using spectro-radiographic methods. The condition has also been studied independently by Looser, Milkman, Hartley and others. Figure IX:20 illustrates a stress fracture in Paget's disease. (Courtesy of *The American Journal of Roentgenology.*)

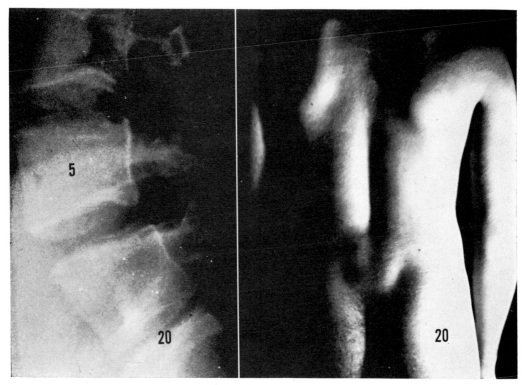

Fig. XIII:10 C.

the 5th neural arch. Shadows of a detached arch may cause some confusion (Figure XIII:17). The PA and oblique projections will usually resolve these possible sources of error.

Once the bony masses develop they seem to remain unchanged. A female patient, age thirty-four, had fallen heavily landing on the buttocks. She immediately suffered severe low back pain for the first time. When first examined six months following injury, there was lordosis, constant discomfort in the lower back, absent right patellar reflex and straight leg raising restricted to 45 degrees but no referred pain. The radiograph showed a bilateral break in the 5th neural arch with some spondylolisthesis and small bilateral bony masses. The patient was reexamined seven years

after her fall. There were no significant symptoms at that time. A comparative study of the roentgenograms showed virtually no change in the bony structure at the site of injury during this interval. Another patient followed for eight years showed little change in the bony masses during that interval (Figure XIII:13).

As mentioned earlier the usual type of spondylolysis is probably not congenital in origin. However, a congenital elongation or defect of a neural arch may occur rarely but the developmental character and disproportion of the anomaly is usually obvious. Spondylolisthesis may be present. These abnormalities occur either in the lower spine or the cervical region (Figures XIII:18, XIII:19, XIII:20 and XIII:21).

ATYPICAL SPONDYLOLYSIS

In the upper lumbar region a cleft may rarely occur in the pars interarticularis of the neural arch. Radiographically these have the appearance of a vicarious articulation with a double cortex and a radiolucent space between. They have

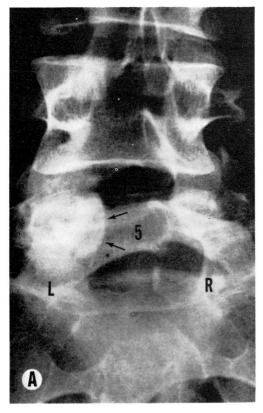

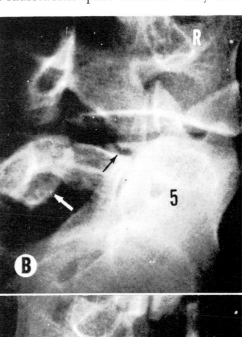

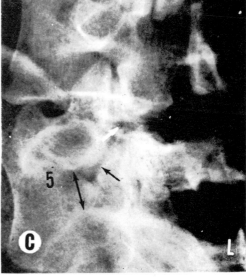

Fig. XIII:11. Male, age twenty-nine, with sciatic pain exaggerated by sneezing. Some low back pain with limitation of motion. This patient has bilateral breaks in the 5th neural arch as seen in the oblique projections. The PA view (A) shows a rounded callus-like bony mass projecting from the left side into the spinal canal (*black arrows*). In the right oblique projection (B) this same bony mass is seen extending from the left lamina forward into the canal (*white arrow*). The left oblique projection (C) visualizes the break in the 5th neural arch (*white arrow*). No forward slipping was visualized upon the lateral film but the plane of the 5th posterior articulation is seen well posterior to that of the 4th in both of the oblique studies. The oblique views also show compensatory stabilizing bony impingements. The right oblique shows the stabilizing impingement between the 4th articular process and the lamina of the 5th neural arch. (*black arrow on B*). While on the left side the contact is between the 5th pedicle and the sacral articulation (*single black arrow on C*). The left oblique projection also shows constriction of the foramen between the 5th pedicle and the ala of the sacrum (*double headed arrow*). (Courtesy American Journal of Roentgenology.)

usually appeared in the 2nd and 3rd lumbar arches and are probably congenital in origin. Specimens have been examined by Nathan and by Jones. The latter found a movable joint lined by articular cartilage. In all of the cases seen by this author as well as the specimens above mentioned there were present small additional ossicles or stabilizing bony masses (Figures XIII:22, XIII:23, XIII:24 and XIII:25). Friberg studied 280 cases of neural arch defect. In this whole group there was one female infant of one year with multiple congenital anomalies involving the extremities and the entire spine. The lateral roentgenogram revealed sharply delineated clefts crossing the isthmuses of all neural arches from T_{11} to L_5 inclusive. These had the appearance of joint spaces not unlike the atypical spondylolysis seen in Figure XIII:23.

PSEUDOSPONDYLOLISTHESIS

We have seen how a forward slipping of the vertebra may occur without arch defect in those patients with a congenitally long isthmus. Spondylolisthesis without a break in the neural arch may likewise occur in those patients with degeneration and thinning of the intervertebral disc accompanied by a partial destruction of the posterior articulation. This constitutes the so-called pseudospondylolisthesis, described by Junghanns in 1930. It usually occurs at the 4th lumbar disc level but may develop in the cervical region or elsewhere. The partial loss of the lowermost anterior element of the articulation destroys the stabilizing effect of that structure and allows the vertebra to subluxate forward encroaching upon the intervertebral foramen Figures XIII:26, XIII:27, XIII:28 and XIII:29 also XIV:40B and VII:21.

RETROSPONDYLOLISTHESIS

If the disc becomes thinned by degeneration and the posterior articulations remain intact the uppermost vertebra is likely to become displaced backward, the so-called retrospondylolisthesis. Certain active factors, i.e., traction of the erector spinae muscles and elastic tension of the ligamentum flavum probably play a part

---

Fig. XIII:12. Female, age forty-nine. There was no history of injury obtainable. She complained of pain in the lower back radiating down the right lower extremity. The P.A. and oblique roentgenograms showed bilateral bony masses projecting medially and forward into the spinal canal from the region of the neural arch of the 5th lumbar vertebra (*arrows*). Note the anterior flattening of the mass seen on the right oblique roentgenogram. There is no evidence of arch defect. Myelography failed to reveal any disc protrusion and the bony mass did not distort the sac. The myelogram (M) was made with the patient supine. Fortunately for this study, some of the opaque medium entered the epidural space and lay between the dura and the bony mass on the right side. The position of the 5th right lumbar nerve root is indicated by the slender column of opaque material (*arrows*) which accompanies that structure. It will be seen that, as the nerve sweeps downward and laterally toward the intervertebral foramen, it is impinged upon and deflected medially by the bony mass. Oil is also seen along the first right sacral root. Pressure may be exerted upon a nerve root by bony masses of this type. These are probably old healed fractures occurring early in life. (Courtesy of *Journal of Bone Joint Surgery*.)

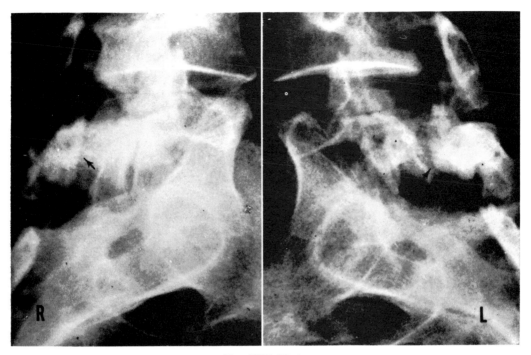

Fig. XIII:12 A.

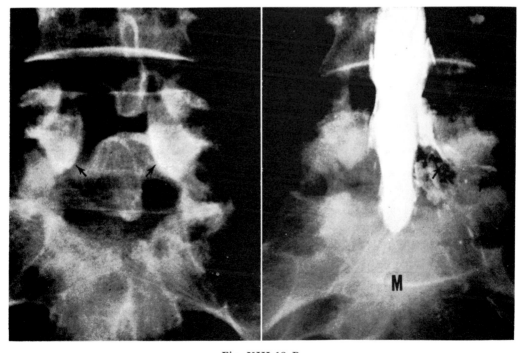

Fig. XIII:12 B.

in the backward movement. Also, in the lower lumbar region the planes of the posterior articulations are inclined at an angle and tend to force the upper vertebra backward as it moves downward incidental to thinning of the disc. In the middle and upper lumbar region, however, the planes of the posterior joints are more nearly vertical so that this wedging effect by the joint surfaces is less of a factor. In fact, the joint surfaces may be separated in the upper lumbar region placing a stress upon the capsules of the joints (Figures XIII:30, XIII:31 and XIII:32, also XIV:12).

An important feature of retrospondylolisthesis is the resultant foramen encroachment. The lower posterior margin

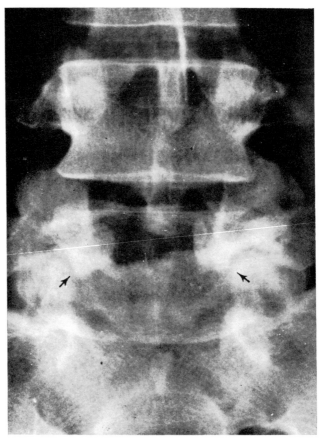

Fig. XIII:13. Male, age twenty-two. He had previously fallen sixteen feet, landing on his back. He stated that his lower limbs were paralyzed four hours at that time. For the next four or five years he had recurrent attacks of weakness and loss of power in the lower extremities. There was local pain in the back during this time but no sciatica. The roentgenograms, made sixteen months after injury, revealed breaks in the arch of the 5th lumbar vertebra with bony masses (*arrows*) projecting into the spinal canal on each side. There was a first degree spondylolisthesis. Reexamination of this patient eight years after injury no longer showed motor disturbance of the lower limbs. The Achilles and patellar reflexes were normal. The patient did complain of periodic muscle spasm in the lumbar region. The roentgenographic reexamination showed the bony condition of the neural arch of the 5th lumbar vertebra essentially unchanged. (Courtesy of *The Journal of Bone and Joint Surgery.*)

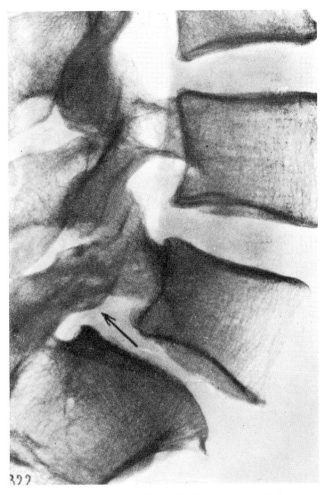

Fig. XIII:14. Radiograph showing spondylolisthesis in a sixty-eight year old man. The neural arch is elongated, fusiform, and with a cortex and the spongiosa irregular in texture (*arrow*). The condition probably represents an old healed fracture. Illustration taken from Schmorl and Junghanns' *Die Gesunde und Kranke Wirbelsaule im Roentgenbild*. Edition I, 1932. (Courtesy of Georg Thieme, Verlag.)

of the upper vertebral body moves backward into the foramen while the superior articular process from the vertebra below moves upward and forward into the opening. Usually there is also some herniation of disc substance backward into this space. Flexion-extension studies are likely to reveal an instability at the degenerated disc level (Figure XIII:36).

It is necessary to use meticulous care in positioning the patient, otherwise a false appearance of retroposition may appear on the radiograph when no displacement is actually present. Also, one must bear in mind that the AP diamenter of the sacrum is slightly less than that of the undersurface of L$_5$. However, the important consideration at this level is the relative position of the contiguous posterior margins of the 5th vertebra and the sacrum. If the former is subluxated posterior to the sacrum a condition of

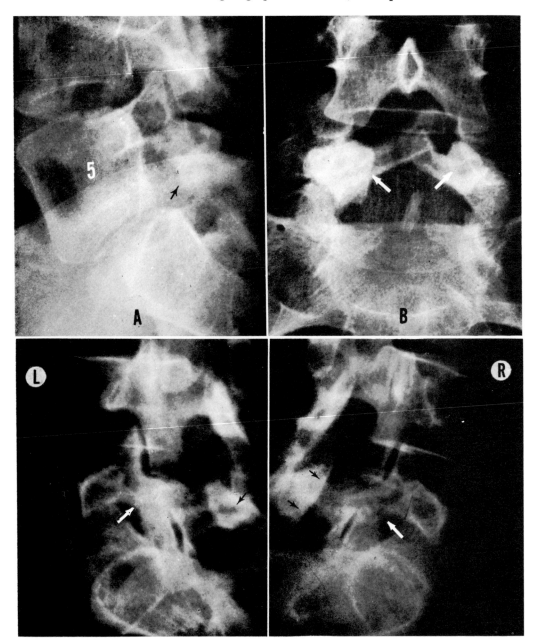

Fig. XIII:15. Female, age forty-four. No history of injury was obtainable. The lateral projection (A) showed minimal spondylolisthesis of the 5th lumbar vertebra and increased density, at the neural arch *(arrow)*. The P. A. roentgenogram (B) revealed callus-like bony masses on both sides, larger and more dense on the left *(white arrows)*. The left and right oblique roentgenograms (L and R) revealed the neural arch of the 5th lumbar vertebra to be intact on both sides *(white arrows)*, but the bony masses were seen posteriorly bulging into the spinal canal *(black arrows)*, that on the left side (right oblique projection) being flattened in front *(double black arrows)*. These masses are probably due to old healed fractures occurring early in life. (Courtesy of *The Journal of Bone and Joint Surgery*.)

retrospondylolisthesis is present. Retro-spondylolisthesis may also occur in the cervical region with resultant foramen encroachment (Figure XIV:14).

ROTARY AND LATERAL SPONDYLOLISTHESIS

Rarely a rotary type of subluxation, with or without a lateral slipping may result from a unilateral arch defect. Direct observation of the back with the patient standing will reveal an asymmetrical rotation of the pelvis in relation to the torso. There is a resultant imbalance in the stresses and the stabilizing structures of the lower lumbar area somewhat similar to that present with scoliosis. Various types of rotation occur. With one of the posterior articulations serving as a fixed point and center of movement the superjacent vertebra may become rotated either forward or backward. With a defect in the isthmus the rotation is likely to be forward (Figure XIII:33). With a widening of the posterior joint the rotation of the vertebra is backward (Figure XIII:34). There may or may not be a lateral displacement in cases of rotary spondylolisthesis (Figure X:17).

THE WEDGE DISC

Of considerable clinical significance is the wedge shaped lumbosacral disc. Normally this structure may be somewhat thicker in front than posteriorly. However, with wedging, as the name implies, the sacrum becomes tipped on a transverse axis and the posterior margin of the disc becomes thinned. As a result, the bony margins of the 5th vertebra and the sacrum are nearly in contact. It can be demonstrated experimentally that pressure between the posterior margins of vertebral bodies forces the disc substance backward (Figures XIII:32, VIII:2 and XIV:34). Tipping of the sacrum and wedge formation may result from a break in the neural arch. Figures XIII:35 and XIV:36.

INSTABILITY STUDIES

Films made at the full limits of flexion and extension in cases of forward spondylolisthesis or of the retro subluxated type, reveal disc distortions and gliding movement between the vertebral bodies at the involved level. This corresponds essentially to the observations of Knutsson who described a condition of praeternatural mobility in patients with degenerated discs (Figures XIII:36 and XIII:37).

As mentioned earlier the vertebral displacement causes some distortion and bony encroachment of the intervertebral foramina (Figures XIV:29 and XIV:32). Further constriction is produced by the herniation of disc material backward into the opening (Figures XIII:38 and XIII:39).

Usually patients with a unilateral break in the neural arch do not develop spondylolisthesis. However, the forward and downward stress from the pedicle of the intact side is carried across the neural arch to the inferior articular process of the deficient side. Because of this increased stress upon the arch that structure may develop a compensatory increased density (Figure XIII:8).

In cases of bony arch defects the unsupported stresses are partly borne by various ligamentous structures. The iliolumbar ligaments extending from the 5th transverse processes to the iliac crests are especially important and serve somewhat as a sling in helping to stabilize the 5th lumbar vertebra (Figure XII:7).

Does the slipping increase? This is unusual but does occur and has been reported. However, the tissues ordinarily develop certain compensatory stabilizing factors. Bony bridging, eburnation and various bony impingements across the deficient zone of weakness gradually occur. Later, a bony shelf forms upon the anterior surface of the sacrum to support the displaced fifth vertebra (Figures XIII:40 and XIII:41).

The amount of slipping is registered as first degree or 25 per cent if the forward displacement of the 5th vertebral body upon the sacrum amonuts to one-

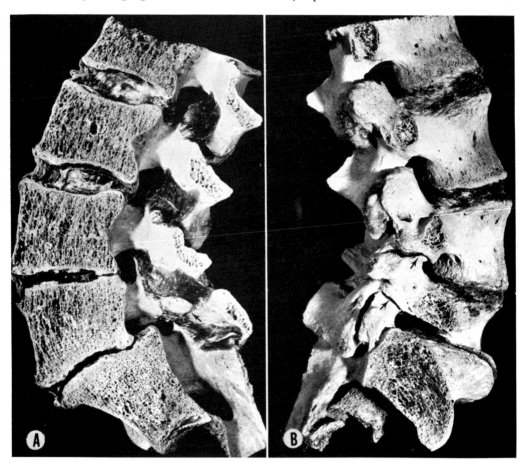

Fig. XIII:16. Sagittal section from the cadaver of a male, seventy-two years old with spondylolisthesis. Photograph (A) shows an ossicle 7 x 12 millimeters within the ligamentous tissue bridging the neural arch defect (*arrow*). Photograph of the lateral surface (B) reveals the stabilizing impingments which have developed beneath the 4th and 5th pedicles (*arrows*). The radiographs (C and D) made before section of the specimen show the bony mass bulging medially and forward into the spinal canal (*arrows*). Impingement of the 5th superior articular process beneath the 4th pedicle is seen on each radiograph. Projection D is the left oblique and shows the impingement on the left side. (Courtesy of the publisher ot *The Journal of Bone and Joint Surgery*.)

fourth the AP diameter of its articulating surface. A fourth degree spondylolisthesis therefore results in a complete displacement of the 5th vertebra forward and entirely off from the supporting sacrum (Figure XIII:42).

In this chapter certain observations have been presented which have a bearing upon matters still considered controversial. No attempt has been made to either prove or disprove them but only to present the facts observed. Nor has this author attempted to completely exhaust the subject of neural arch deficiencies and their resultant displacements. There is a voluminous literature on the subject already available.

REFERENCES

Albright, F., and Reifenstein, E. C., Jr.: 1948, *Stress Fracture Parathyroid Glands and Metabolic Diseases,* Williams & Wilkins Co., Baltimore.

Bailey, W.: 1947, *Rad., 48:*107–112, Etiology.

Barr, J. S.: 1955, *J. Bone J. Surg., 37A:*878–880, Editorial.

Batts, M., Jr.: 1939, *J. Bone J. Surg., 21:*879–884, Atypical defect.

Brandt, G.: 1941, *Erzebn. d. Chir. u. Ortho., 33:* 1–59; Abs. Year Book *Rad.,* 1941, p. 35, Stress Fracture.

Chandler, F. A.: 1931, *Surg. Gyn. Obst., 53:* 273–306, Anatomy.

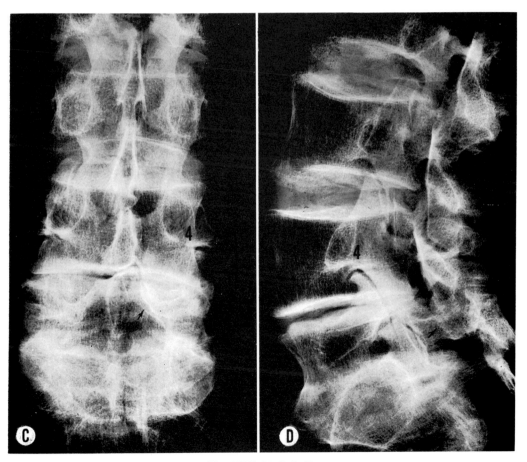

Fig. XIII:16 C & D.

Congdon, R. T.: 1932, *J. Bone J. Surg., 14:*511–524, Anatomy.

Fletcher, G. H.: 1947, *J. Bone J. Surg., 29:*1019–1026, Retrospondylolisthesis.

Friberg, S.: 1939, *Acta Chir. Scand.,* Supp. 82, *55:*1–140, Atypical.

Gallucio, A. C.: 1944, *Rad., 42:*143–158, Anatomy.

Ghormley, R. K., and Kirklin, B. R.: 1934, *Am. Jor. Roent., 31:*173–176, Technique.

Gill, G. G., *et al: J. Bone J. Surg., 37A:*493–520, Anatomy.

Gill, G. G.: Personal Communication, Bony Masses.

Hadley, L. A.: 1955, *J. Bone J. Surg., 37A:*787–797, Bony Masses.

Hagelstam, L.: 1949, *Acta Chir. Scan. Supp., 143:*1–156, Retrospondylolisthesis.

Hartley, J. B.: 1943, *Brit. Jor. Rad., 16:*255–262, Stress Fracture.

Henschen, C.: Quoted by Hartley and by Brandt, Stress Fracture.

Hertzmark, M. H.: 1960, *Bull. Hosp. Joint Dis., 21:*50–64, Operated a bony mass.

Hitchcock, H. H.: 1940, *J. Bone J. Surg., 22:*1–16, Development.

Jones, M. D.: 1960, *J. Bone J. Surg., 42A:*1076–1078, Atypical.

Kleinberg, S.: 1934, *J. Bone J. Surg., 16:*441–444, Development.

Knutsson, F.: 1944, *Acta Rad., 25:*593–609, Instability.

Looser, E.: 1930, *Deutsche Ztsch. f. Chir., 152:*210–357, Stress Fracture.

Macnab, I.: 1950, *J. Bone J. Surg., 32B:*325–333, Pseudospondylolisthesis.

Melamed, A., *et al:* 1947, *Am. Jor. Roent., 58:*307–328, Retrospondylolisthesis.

Meschan, I.: 1945, *Am. Jor. Roent., 53:*230–243, Movements.

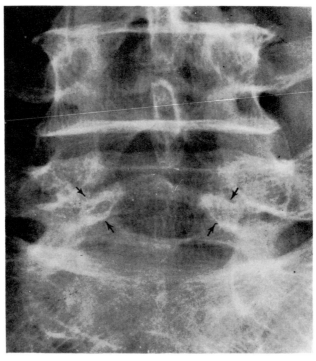

Fig. XIII:17. Confusing shadows but not bony masses in a male, aged 64. There was a break in the neural arch of the 5th lumbar vertebra with a first-degree spondylolisthesis. The oval shadows enclosed by the arrows are formed by the cortex of the detached posterior portion of the neural arch. They are posterior and medial to the cortices of the corresponding pedicles. In order to produce such a shadow of the cortex, the roentgen ray must pass through, parallel to the surface of the bone at that point. These shadows are not to be mistaken for those of the bony masses described in this chapter. (Courtesy of *Journal of Bone and Joint Surgery*.)

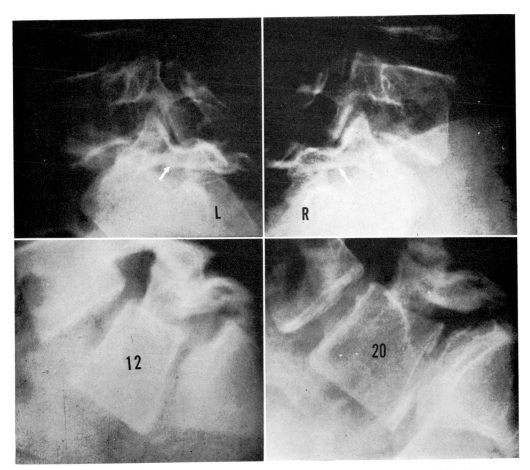

Fig. XIII:18. A case of first-degree spondylolisthesis with lordosis in a young girl without any break in the neural arch. The right and left oblique studies made at twelve years show a long pars interarticularis with intact cortex on each side (*white arrows*). The 5th posterior articulations lie well behind the plane of the fourth. There was considerable increase in the lumbar curve. When she was reexamined eight years later at the age of twenty the fifth neural arch was still intact. The spondylolisthesis was unchanged but the lordosis had lessened somewhat as she became older. This was probably a case of congenitally long isthmus with resultant spondylolisthesis and lordosis. On the lateral study at twelve years the vertebral bodies are accentuated by retouching. (Courtesy of *American Journal of Roentgenology.*)

Meyerding, H. W.: 1933, *Rad., 20:*108–120, Anatomy.

Milkman, L. A.: 1934, *Am. Jor. Roent., 32:*622–634, Stress Fracture.

Mitchell, G. A. G.: 1934, *J. Bone J. Surg., 16:* 233–254, Anatomy.

Nathan, H.: 1959, *J. Bone J. Surg., 41A:*303–320, Atypical defect.

Oppenheimer, A.: 1942, *Rad., 39:*98–100, Atypical defect.

Pheasant, H. C.: Personal Communication, Bony Masses.

Reinhardt, K.: 1957, *Jor. de Rad. et d Electro., 38:*905–915, Rotary.

Roche, M. B., and Rowe, G. G.: 1951, *Anat. Rec., 109:*253–259, Atypical.

Rowe, G. G., and Roche, M. B.: 1953, *J. Bone J. Surg., 35A:* 102–110, Etiology.

Schmorl, G., and Junghanns, H.: 1959, *The Human Spine in Health and Disease* (English

Edition), Grune & Stratton, New York.

Schneider, C. C.: 1957, *Rad., 69:*863–866, Development.

Scott, W. G.: 1942, *Am. Jor. Roent., 48:*491–509, Technique.

Smith, A. D.: 1934, *J. Bone J. Surg., 16:*877–888, Retrospondylolisthesis.

Stewart, T. D.: 1935, *J. Bone J. Surg., 17:*640–648, Pseudospondylolisthesis.

Taillard, W.: 1957, *Les Spondylolisthesis* (Original French), Masson et Cie Editeurs, Paris; or 1957, *Die Spondylolisthesen* (German Translation), Hippokates Verlag, Stuttgart.

Fig. XIII:19. Congenital deficiency of the 5th neural arch with a third-degree spondylolisthesis. This young man of twenty-two years complained of low back pain referred down the left leg. The roentgenograms revealed long slender asymmetrically developed lamina for the 5th neural arch, not united in the mid line (*arrows*). There was a complete spina bifida with the sacral canal open throughout. The lumbosacral disc was practically destroyed. Because of the displacement of L_5, an erosion of the posterior margin of the upper sacral surface had developed to allow space within the neural canal. The rare distortions of this type in the shape and development of the neural arch need be considered only as congenital anomalies.

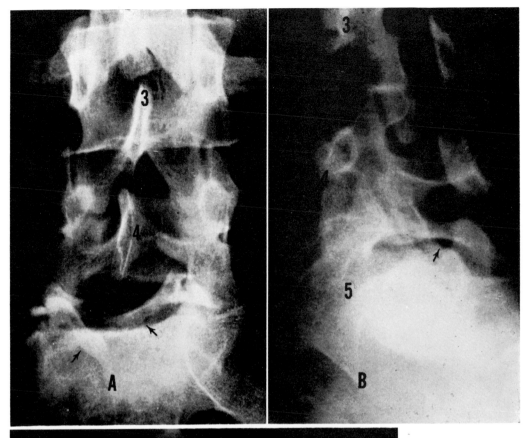
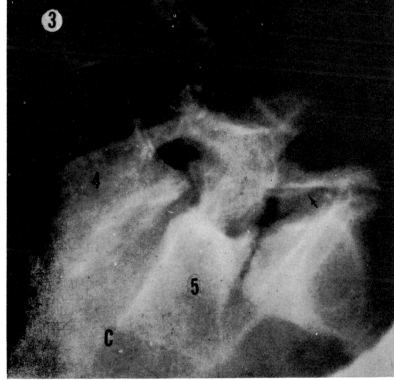

Fig. XIII:20. Congenital elongation of the 6th cervical neural arch with first degree spondylolisthesis in a male of sixty-one years. The oblique projections (A and B) clearly demonstrate the elongated pedicles *(black arrows)* and there is a congenital incomplete closure
of the 6th neural arch visualized on D *(white arrow)*. The intervertebral disc and the posterior articulations are of normal thickness rather than destroyed as seen in Figure XIII:29.
(Courtesy of Dr. K. L. Mitton, Schnectady, N. Y.)

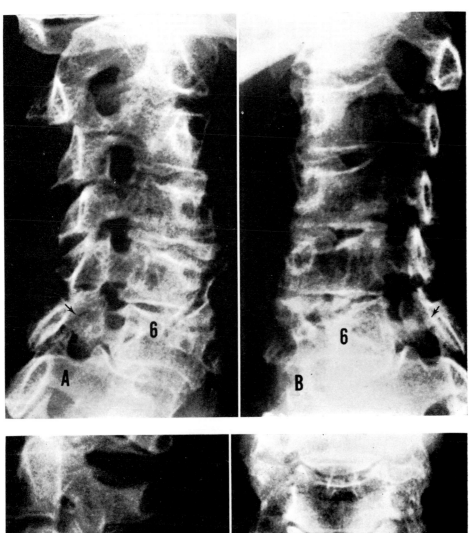
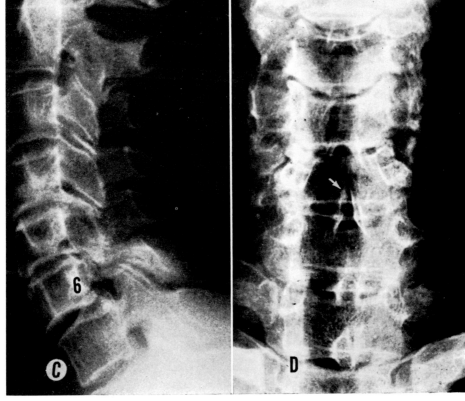

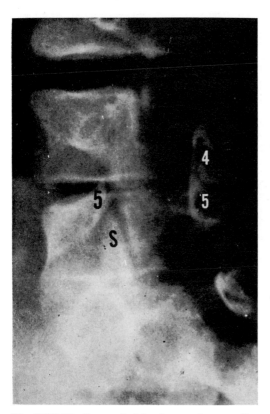

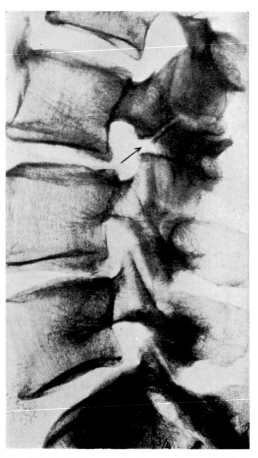

Fig. XIII:21. Congenital lumbosacral anomalies in a female of fifteen years. The 4th and 5th neural arches are fused (*white digits*) . From this mass a large articular process projects downward to articulate with the sacrum and with a process projecting upward from the 5th pedicle.

Fig. XIII:22. The atypical type of spondylolysis occurring in the upper lumbar region. Sagittal view, half lumbar spine of a sixty year old male showing a cleavage through the pars interarticularis of the 3rd lumbar vertebra. Copied from Schmorl and Junghanns Edition I, 1932, this figure shows the dehiscence sharply indicated and bordered by narrow zones of increased cortical density (*arrow*). The appearance is suggestive of a joint structure. (Courtesy of Georg Thieme - Publisher.)

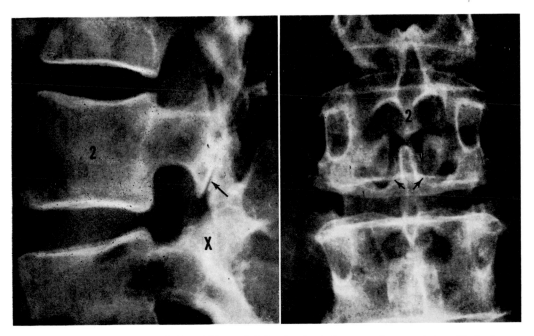

Fig. XIII:23. Female, aged sixty. Bilateral defect in the isthmus or the pars interarticularis of L₂ (*long arrow*). This appears almost like an articulation between the pedicle and the lamina of the neural arch, but the normal articulation between L₂ and L₃ occurs at X. In the P. A. projection separate ossicles (*paired arrows*) appear medial to the defects in the arch of L₂. This individual is characteristic of an atypical group observed by this author and others having a cleft formation in a second or third lumbar arch usually with the formation of separate ossicles along side. Oppenheimer, Nathan, Schmorl and Junghans, and Batts as well as Roche and Rowe have all reported studies which indicate that atypical spondylolysis in the upper lumbar region is doubtless congenital. A congenital dehiscence of this type in the isthmus of a lower lumbar arch has not been observed by this author. However in Friberg's case which was undoubtedly congenital there were joint-like clefts in all of the lumbar vertebrae as well as in T₁₁ and T₁₂. (Courtesy of *The American Journal of Roentgenology*.)

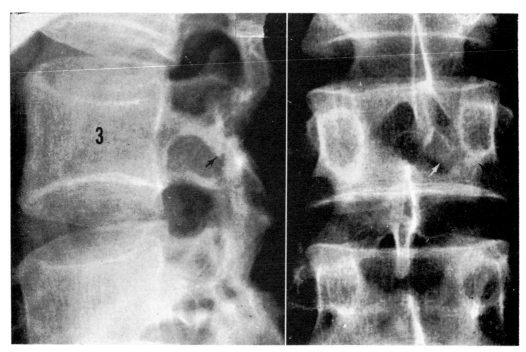

Fig. XIII:24. Male, age twenty-five, with unilateral defect in the isthmus of the left 3rd lumbar vertebra *(black arrows)*. The small size of the neural arch on this side compared with the right would seem to indicate that the condition was either congenital or developed very early in life. A separate ossicle is visualized medial and adjacent to the defect *(white arrow)*. Steroscopic studies show this ossicle entirely anterior to the spinous process and lying at the plane of the neural arch. Such studies also reveal the defect more clearly.

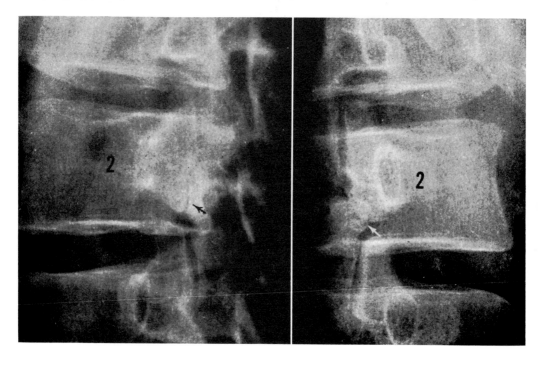

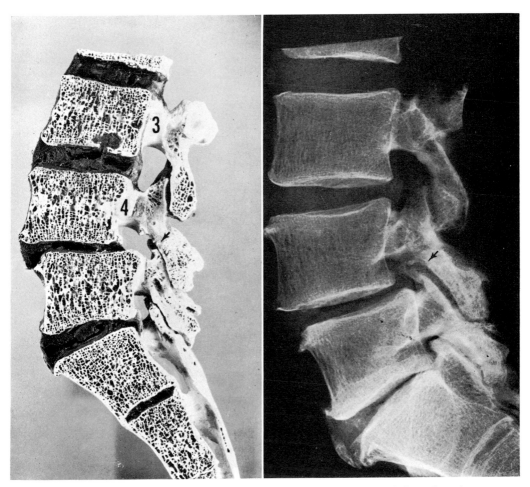

Fig. XIII:26. Specimen No. 6014 Pseudospondylolisthesis in a male of sixty-nine. A combination of 4th disc degeneration and partial destruction of the 4th posterior articulation has resulted in a subluxation forward of the 4th vertebral body even without any break in the neural arch (*arrows*). Some foramen distortion has resulted. The Schmorl's node in L$_3$ does not cast a radiographic shadow in this case. L$_4$ is the usual level for pseudospondylolisthesis.

Fig. XIII:25. Male of forty-five years, no suggestive symptoms. There is a bilateral defect in the pars interarticularis of the second lumbar vertebra (*black arrow*). On the right side a small ossicle lies within the deficiency but apparently did not produce symptoms (*white arrow*). At this level the planes of the vertebral bodies are fortunately horizontal and there is little shearing stress to produce subluxation.

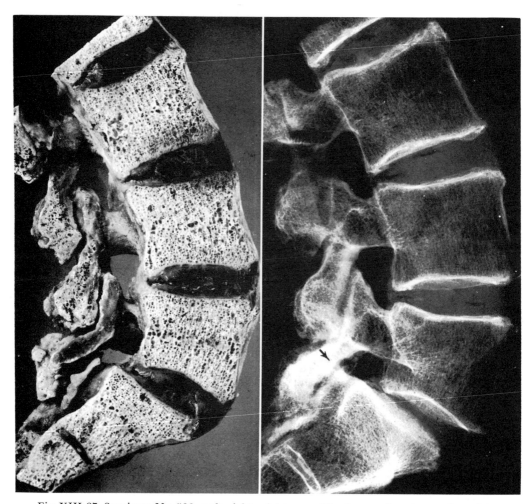

Fig. XIII:27. Specimen No. 536, male eighty-eight years. Nearly complete destruction of the lower element of the 5th articulation (*arrows*) has allowed a first degree subluxation forward of the 5th vertebral body even without disc degeneration or a break in the neural arch. Considerable bone sclerosis and foramen encroachement has resulted.

Fig. XIII:28. Female, age sixty. Low back pain - limited motion. (A) Lateral view showing pseudospondylolisthesis of L_4 forward on L_5. There is no break in the neural arch. The oblique view (B) shows the 4th posterior articulation partially destroyed. The tip of the 5th articular process (*above black arrow*) has become almost completely eroded. (Courtesy of *American Journal of Roentgenology*.)

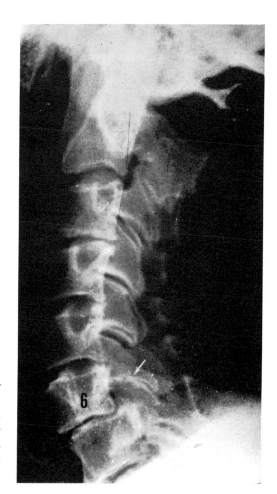

Fig. XIII:29. Pseudospondylolisthesis of C_6 forward on C_7 with thinning of the disc and some destruction of the posterior articulations. This sixty-one year old man had fallen striking on the head, neck and shoulders four months before. The condition appears to have been of long duration but trauma may have played a part.

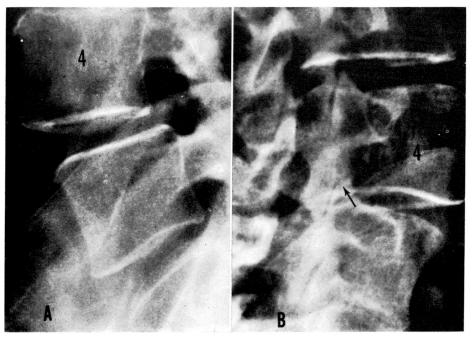

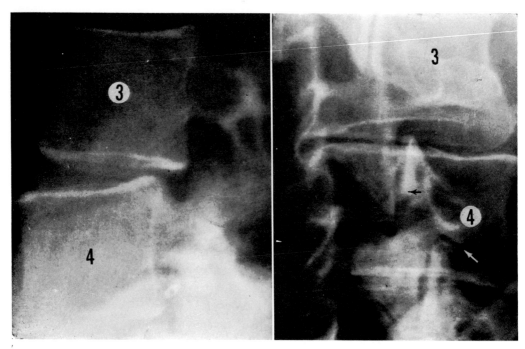

Fig. XIII:30. Retrospondylolisthesis in a male of forty-five years. There was a history of lumbar pain, intermittent for many years, referred down the left leg but no history of injury. The lateral projection shows displacement of L_3 backward upon L_4. The intervertebral disc is thinned by degeneration and the corresponding foramen is encroached in both the cephalo-caudad and the anteroposterior diameters. A telescoping of the posterior articulation has occurred as indicated by the distance between the black arrows, in the oblique projection. Each arrow indicates the lower margin of a joint surface. They should be opposite of each other. There is some impingement of the 5th superior articular process beneath the 4th pedicle (*white arrow*).

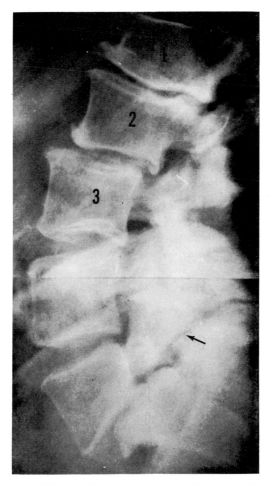

Fig. XIII:31. Retrospondylolisthesis in a male of sixty-three with lordosis, limited lumbar movement, right sciatica and diminished Achilles reflexes. The film reveals degeneration and thinning of the 1st and 2nd lumbar discs, but with intact posterior joints. As a result, backward displacement of the corresponding vertebral bodies has occurred. This retro-spondylolisthesis has produced bony encroachment of the corresponding intervertebral formina. The arrow indicates an old defect of the 5th neural arch with a second degree forward slipping of L_5 and a compensatory bony shelf formation at the anterior portion of the lumbosacral disc. There is an advanced sclerotic reaction involving the neural arches and the posterior joints incidental to the lordosis. (Courtesy of the *American Journal of Roentgenology.*)

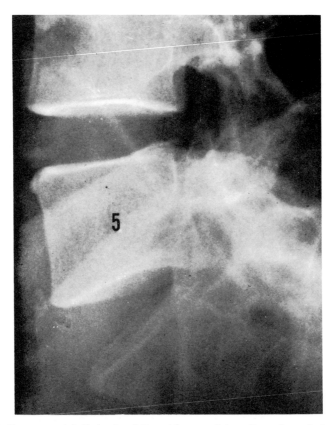

Fig. XIII:32. Retrospondylolisthesis of L$_5$ with a wedging distortion of the lumbosacral disc. As the sacrum becomes rotated upon its transverse axis its upper surface is tipped forward and the articular processes are thrust upward and forward to encroach upon the 5th intervertebral foramina. These openings are constricted not only by the sacral articular processes but also by the posterior margin of the 5th vertebra and the disc substance which herniates backward into the foramina (see Figure XIV:34).

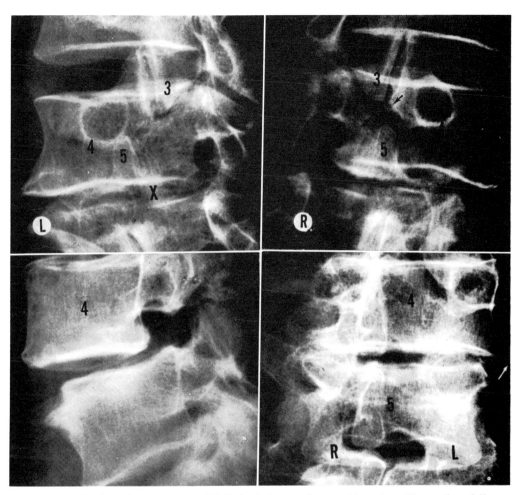

Fig. XIII:33. Anterior rotary spondylolisthesis in a male, age thirty-nine. The patient fell off a load of hay onto his back at twelve years of age. He now has pain and paresthesia down both legs. Upon direct observation the right side of the pelvis is seen to be rotated backward. The left and right oblique studies *(above)* reveal a break in the 4th neural arch on the right side *(black arrows)*. There is a wide deficiency with smooth margins between the tips of the right 3rd and 5th articular processes. The 4th and 5th apophyses seem to be intact on the left side so that the 4th left posterior joint becomes the axis of rotation (at X). The lateral and A. P. projections (below) show a rotation of the 4th vertebral body forward and toward the left side *(white arrow)*. This explains the apparent backward displacement of the pelvis on the right which was noted during the preliminary examination. There may also be a certain degree of side slipping due to the thinned 4th disc. The history of severe injury seventeen years before with smoothness of the wide neural arch defect and the degenerative changes in the 4th disc indicate probable chronicity of the process. (Courtesy of *American Journal of Roentgenology.*)

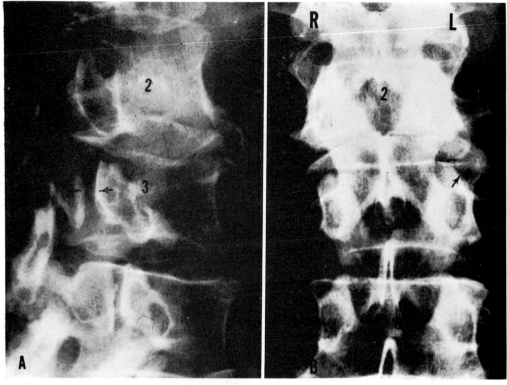

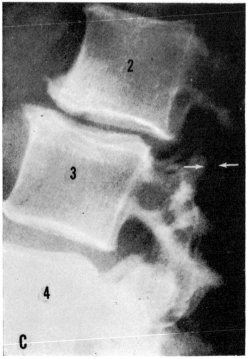

Fig. XIII:34. Posterior rotary spondylolisthesis. A falling accident resulted in twisting the back of this fifty-three year old female. She complained of pain in the right lumbar region. The 45 degree oblique radiograph (A) shows a widening of the 2nd right posterior articulation (*black arrows*) indicating a ligamentous injury to the capsule of this joint. This condition together with the laxity due to the degenerated state of the 2nd disc has allowed the second vertebral body to rotate backward and toward the right side upon the vertebra below. This constitutes a rotary reverse spondylolisthesis on a traumatic basis. Note the lateral displacement (*black arrow*) of the 2nd vertebra toward the right side on the A. P. projection (B). The posterior subluxation is visualized on the lateral film (C) and the widened posterior joint appears between the two white arrows.

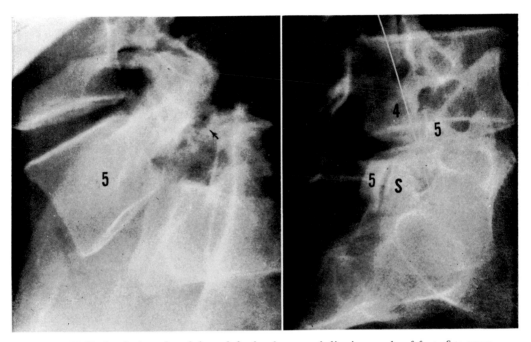

Fig. XIII:35. Lordosis and wedging of the lumbro sacral disc in a male of forty-five years. He complained of low back pain worse with fatigue. There was marked lordosis with protective muscle spasm and he carried his back with a list toward the right side. The radiograph shows a wide defect in the 5th neural arch (*arrow*) with an extreme degree of lordosis. Note that the sacrum is horizontal with its anterior surface directed downward and slightly backward. In spite of the wide dehiscence in the neural arch there is no spondylolisthesis although wedging distortion of the lumbosacral disc has occurred. This is because the sacrum is tipped. In the oblique projection the 5th posterior articulation with the sacrum is seen to lie well behind the 3rd and 4th posterior joints (*white line*). Normally the 5th joint is beneath or even anterior to the plane of the 4th. Lordosis with a break in the 5th neural arch places additional stress upon the suspensory ligament between the 5th transverse process and the iliac crest (Figure XII:6). Lordosis also places a telescoping stress upon the posterior articulations and their capsules in the lower lumbar region.

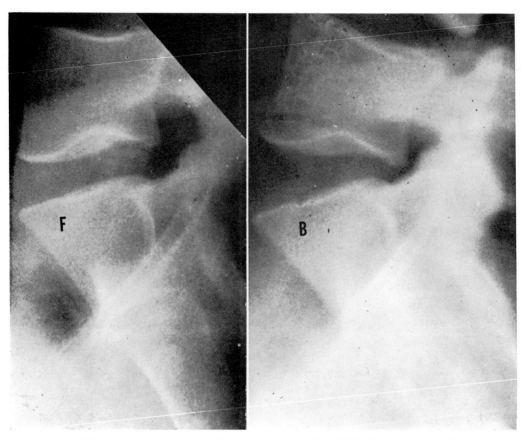

Fig. XIII:36. Flexion-extension studies demonstrating instability in a patient with retro-spondylolisthesis. Male, age thirty-one. The forward bending (F) projection shows a reverse spondylolisthesis with only minimal encroachment upon the intervertebral foramen. The surfaces of the 5th vertebra and the sacrum are parallel. Upon backward bending (B) the reverse spondylolisthesis is increased, the lumbosacral disc is wedge shaped and the encroachment of the foramina is considerably increased.

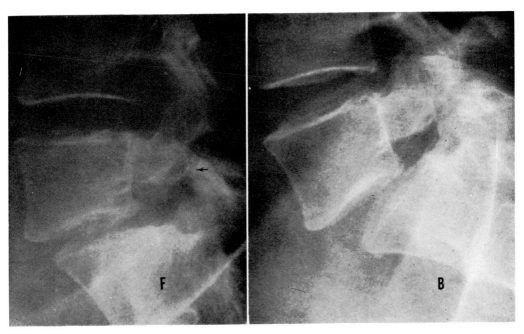

Fig. XIII:37. Flexion-extension studies showing instability in a patient with first degree forward spondylolisthesis. This male of thirty-three years complained of constant dull ache in the low back referred down the left leg to the knee. This was relieved by forward bending but exaggerated by backward bending. He could not work with the hands above his head. A radiograph made with the patient bending forward (F) shows a break in the neural arch (*arrow*) and a first degree spondylolisthesis. The contiguous surfaces of the sacrum and the 5th vertebra are parallel but with some loss of disc substance. The anterior diameter of the 5th intervertebral foramen of each side is increased. The film (B) made in the backward bending position reveals an increase of the spondylolisthesis. There is a wedging of the lumbosacral disc. This will normally force disc substance posteriorly. The diameters of the 5th foramina are materially lessened in the backward bending position. This observation partially expains the increased pain upon backward bending. The detached portion of the 5th neural arch was later removed with gratifying improvement of symptoms but some increase of the spondylolisthesis.

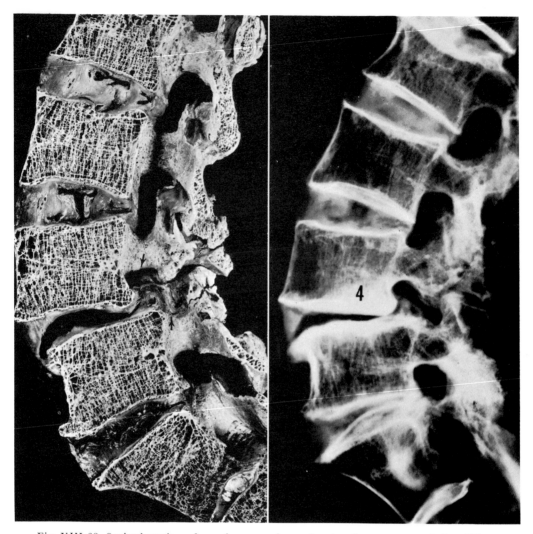

Fig. XIII:38. Sagittal section of a cadaver specimen showing foramen constriction. There is a false joint in the 4th neural arch with disc degeneration and spondylolisthesis of the 4th lumbar vertebra forward on the 5th. The disc substance bulges into the foramen, and the nerve, still in situ, is being compressed into a small thin ribbon *(between the arrows)*. The roentgenogram of this specimen shows the spondylolisthesis and the foramen constriction. The constriction however is always actually much greater than revealed by the radiograph since it is partially caused by the displaced soft tissues. (Courtesy of *American Journal of Roentgenology.*)

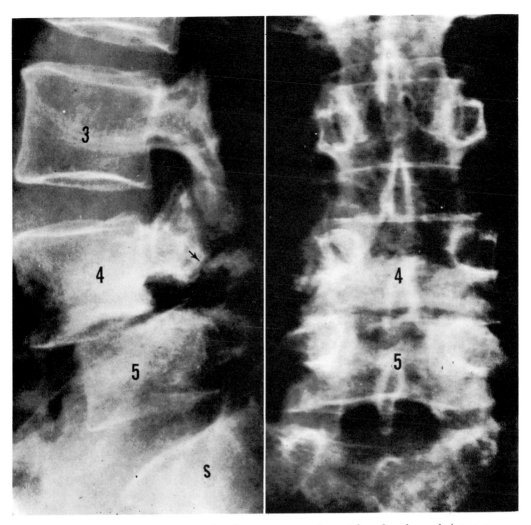

Fig. XIII:39. Spondylolisthesis causing foramen encroachment in a female aged sixty-two. She had complained of pain in the legs since falling from a horse at the age of 16. The roentgenogram shows a break in the 4th neural arch (*arrow*) with spondylolisthesis of L_4 forward on L_5 and with distortion of the intervertebral foramen. Compare with the roentgenogram in Figure XIII:38. In the A. P. projection (pedicles retouched) the foramen diameter is materially reduced in a cephalo-caudad direction because of the thinned badly degenerated 4th disc. (Courtesy of *American Journal of Roentgenology*.)

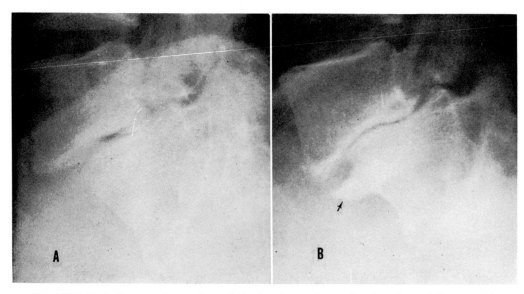

Fig. XIII:40. Follow up observations of the lumbosacral junction in a forty-eight year old hockey player. The patient had been subjected to repeated injuries. There was a history of low back pain with recurrent sciatica of eight years duration. (A) The original examination revealed a break in the 5th neural arch with spondylolisthesis and marked encroachment upon the intervertebral foramen. There was disc degeneration, apparently with vacuum formation and a sacralized 6th lumbar segment. (B) Reexamination ten years later. Although there was some stiffness the sciatica had not been present for the previous seven or eight years. There was now a complete loss of the 5th disc with eburnation of the adjacent vertebral body surfaces and development of the S curve described by Schmorl. A stabilizing bony shelf had formed upon the anterior surface of the sixth segment (*arrow*), partially inclosing the displaced disc substance. The 5th intervertebral foramen was almost completely obliterated. These observations illustrate the compensatory adaptation of the body structures and the frequently observed gradual subsidence of symptoms incidental to degenerative arthrotic changes.

Fig. XIII:42. Twenty-three year old housewife with 4th degree spondylolisthesis, pregnant at term. In spite of the fact that the 4th and 5th vertebral bodies occupy a position within the pelvis in front of the sacrum (S), this patient was able to spontaneously deliver herself of three living children. There was no history of injury. The films showed an extreme degree of lordosis and the impinging spinous processes had developed articulations at their points of contact.

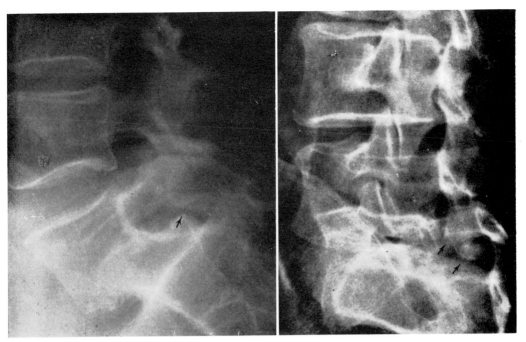

Fig. XIII:41. Late healing stage of a 2nd degree spondylolisthesis in a female patient of sixty-one years. She complained of vague, low back discomfort but could give no history of serious injury. The lateral radiograph shows an ankylosed second degree spondylolisthesis. In both the lateral and the oblique projections one is able to visualize a massive fusiform enlargement of the neural arch (*arrows*). The foramen although distorted in shape, appears to be adequate in size. Compare with Figures XIII:14 and XIII:19.

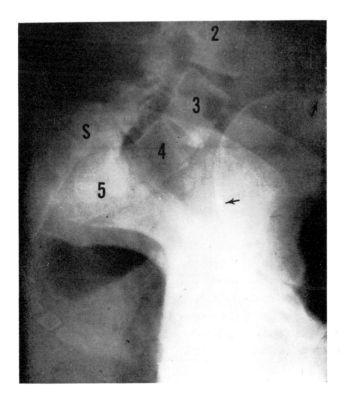

Chapter XIV

Intervertebral Foramen and Spinal Nerve Studies

THE IMPORTANCE of the intervertebral foramen lies in the fact that except for C_1 and C_2 each peripheral nerve must pass through one of these openings. Any pathology involving this "crossroads" between the nervous system and its skeletal support must be considered in evaluating the symptoms of nerve root compression.

In the cervical region there is a close five-way interrelationship between the foramen, the nerve root which passes thru it, the vertebral artery contacting the root in front, the covertebral joint anteriorly and the posterior cervical articulation in back.

Degenerative and arthrotic changes involving these structures play an important part in the production of intervertebral foramen constriction.

THE COVERTEBRAL ARTICULATIONS

Bony projections or lips, variously termed the uncinate or lunate processes extend upward from the lateral margins of the upper surfaces of the lowermost 5 cervical vertebrae. These articulate with the vertebral bodies above and promote lateral stability of the cervical spine. Von Luschka in 1858 called them intervertebral half joints and described them as true synovial structures. They are mentioned also as uncovertebral joints, neurocentral joints or Luschka joints. More accurately they are fissure spaces resulting from degeneration of disc substance as seen in older individuals. They are not true joints and are not present in the newborn. Observe Figure I:16.

Normally the interval between the upward projecting lips and the vertebra above are only about one-third the thickness of the disc. Soon after degenerative thinning of the disc begins, these projections impinge upon the superjacent vertebra. As disc thinning continues,

these processes are forced outward and laterally like the clinching of a horseshoe nail or a paper stapler. This results in the formation of laterally directed spurs or osteophytes. These are often shaped like the head of a bird. They project either toward the invertebral foramen posterolaterally or more forward toward the vertebral artery in the transverse foramen (Figures XIV:1, XIV:2, and XIV:3).

Intervertebral disc thinning with covertebral spur formation is more commonly encountered in the mid and lower cervical region. This is where the greater amplitude of anterior-posterior disc gliding occurs.

Degenerative thinning of the disc also results in a telescoping of the posterior joints. With telescoping, the uppermost articular processes tend to subluxate backward and downward upon the opposing surfaces below with resultant foraminal encroachment.

THE POSTERIOR APOPHYSEAL ARTICULATIONS

The flat, transverse planes of the posterior joints allow a generous amplitude of anterior-posterior gliding movement. The elastic ligamentum flavum is prolonged laterally into that part of the joint capsule adjacent to the intervertebral foramen. These articulations are subject to the various conditions which may affect any diathrodial joint: trauma, arthritis or degenerative and arthrotic changes.

Acute arthritis may involve one or more of the posterior articulations accompanied by local pain and limitation of motion. Because of their proximity to the intervertebral foramina, radicular pain may also be present. The sharpness of the roentgen image is blurred and a well-delineated shadow of the arthritic joint may not be seen. Care must be taken to compare this joint with those above and below, bearing in mind that a con-

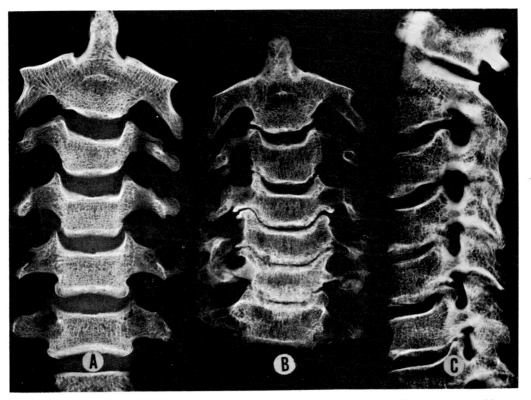

Fig. XIV:1. A, Transverse section from the cervical spine of a man, fifty-four years old showing proximity of the uncinate processes to the undersurfaces of the superjacent vertebrae. Compare this interval with the thickness of the normal disc.

B: Section from the cervical spine of a woman, eighty-nine years old. Impingement is just beginning in the upper cervical region, while advanced degeneration has involved the lower three cervical discs with eburnation of the adjacent bone surfaces. Beak-like osteophytes have developed laterally as a result of the covertebral impingement.

C: Oblique section from the cervical spine of a man, eighty-one years old, showing normal intervertebral foramina above. The lower foramina are encroached upon by osteophytic spurs projecting posterolaterally from the covertebral articulations. (Courtesy of the *Journal of Bone and Joint Surgery*.)

siderable asymmetry and variation in the planes of the joints is normal. With recovery the normal sharpness of the joint shadow may return. The condition may become chronic with degenerative or arthrotic changes (Figures XIV:4, XIV:5 and XIV:6). If there is disc thinning ankylosis may result. Serial studies will show the progressive development of these changes. A destructive arthritis of the posterior joints may allow forward subluxation of the vertebral body like the pseudospondylolisthesis occurring in the lower lumbar region (Figure XIV:7).

Bony spur formations about the margins of the posterior articulation gradually increase in size. They may eventually become sufficiently large to be palpable laterally or even to impinge upon the under-surface of the transverse process causing bony encroachment of the intervertebral foramen. Such a condition may likewise result in pressure of the spur against and deflection of the vertebral artery. Encroachment upon the intervertebral foramen may result in distortion of the nerve root.

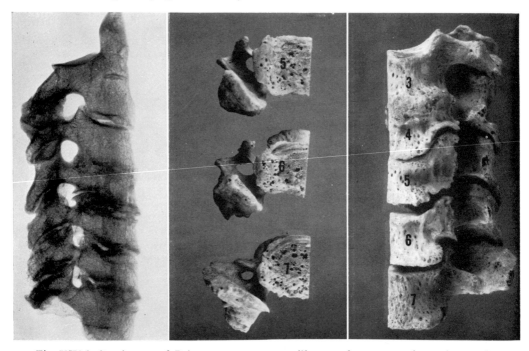

Fig. XIV:2. Specimen and P.A. roentgenogram to illustrate how a spur formation at the covertebral joint may cause bony encroachment of the intervertebral foramen. There is ankylosis between C_3 and C_4, probably acquired but of long duration with, in this case, a smooth oval intervertebral foramen. The foramina below this are encroached upon.

In the center photograph the top view of the fifth cervical body shows the covertebral spur overhanging the foramen for the vertebral artery. Spurs on the upper margins of C_6 and C_7 encroach upon the intervertebral foramen more posteriorly at the site of the cervical nerve root. In the frontal view (right) with part of the transverse processes removed, the vertebral bodies are seen placed slightly apart to better visualize the chicken-head shaped spur formation at the covertebral joints. Pressure of these spurs against the sympathetic plexis surrounding the vertebral artery is said to be at least in part responsible for the bizarre symptomatology of the Barré Lieou syndrome characterized by vasomotor disturbances about the head and face. Of these may be mentioned: lacrimation, salivation, flushing, vertigo, tinnitus and paroxymal deep or superficial pain.

TECHNIQUE

Roentgenograms of the cervical region made in three planes are essential. The postero-anterior projection is made with the patient lying face down upon the Bucky table and with the forehead supported by a small sandbag. The central ray is aligned with the occiput and the undersurface of the mandible. By means of this technique all of the cervical discs and covertebral articulations can be visualized. If impingements of the posterior articulations beneath the transverse processes are present, they are seen laterally in this roentgenogram (Figure XIV:7). The supine A.P. chewing technique is also useful.

In the lateral roentgenogram the impingement of the superior articular process beneath the transverse process may be visualized as a line crossing the vertebral body in the anterior posterior direction. These lines must not be mistaken for fracture lines. A somewhat similar line or shadow may be cast by covertebral osteophytic impingements. Differentiation between these two is made by the postero-anterior projection (Figure XIV:8).

In the lateral roentgenogram also, one may visualize a projection backward of the posterolateral covertebral osteophytes. This has somewhat the appearance of disc substance bulging backward into the spinal canal, but it is directed more laterally toward the intervertebral foramen (Figure XIV:8A disc 5 and 8C foramen 5 white arrow). In the oblique roentgenogram one is able to visualize encroachment of the intervertebral foramina, anteromedially by vertebral body marginal spurs and posterolaterally by spur formation from the superior margins of the posterior articulations (Figures XIV:9, XIV:10 and XIV:11).

In the cervical region the foramina are directed downward, laterally and forward about 45 degrees to the sagittal plane and are properly visualized by the oblique view. The 45-degree posterior-anterior cervical roentgenogram is best made with the patient sitting upright, spine erect, chin up, the occlusal plane of the teeth horizontal, and the shoulder of the side to be visualized resting against the vertical plate holder. The latter should be at such a height that the upper end of an eight by ten inch cassette is level with the patient's ear. Use a measuring triangle of thin wood with angles of 45 degrees-90 degrees-45 degrees about eighteen inches long on each of the two short sides. By sighting across the long edge of the triangle downward from above the patient, arrange the transverse plane of the shoulders and the sagittal plane of the skull each 45 degrees to the plane of the film. The head may be steadied by a small block of balsa wood between the cheek and the plate holder. The target of the tube is directed toward the mid-cervical region and angulated 10 degrees downward, using a target film distance of six feet.

This method visualizes all of the cervical foramina of that side next to the film beginning with that beneath the second vertebra. There is, of course, no intervertebral foramen beneath the first vertebra where the second cervical nerve leaves the spinal canal. The oblique roentgenogram can also be made with the patient lying upon the Bucky table, well supported by sandbags, but this technique is somewhat more difficult.

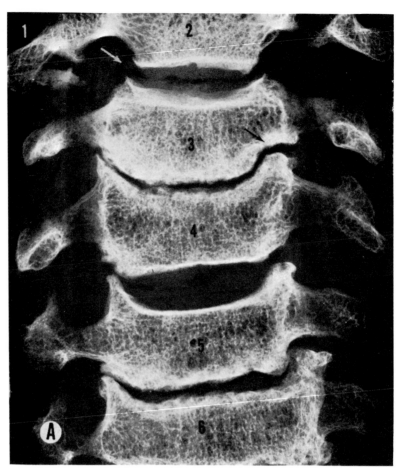

Fig. XIV:3. A, Roentgenogram of a coronal section one-fourth inch thick from the cervical spine of a seventy-one year old male. The C_2 and C_4 discs are essentially normal in thickness. They are much thicker at the mid-point than laterally at the covertebral joints. These latter structures soon develop bony impingement when degeneration of the disc occurs. The third and fifth discs exhibit advanced degenerative changes with thinning. Eburnation has developed beneath contacting vertebral bony surfaces uncushioned by adequate disc substance. The white arrow indicates the source of the upper section, B; black arrow indicates the covertebral joint, section C.

B: (*Above*) A normal covertebral joint (X7) at the left end of the second disc. While there is a fissure of the disc cartilage, as usually seen in specimens from older individuals, these are not true joint spaces. The disc material is still thick enough to prevent bony impingement at the covertebral joints.

C: (*Below*) Impinging covertebral joint, C_3 (X7), with loss of cartilage, eburnation and spur formation which bulges against and deforms the side of the vertebral artery seen at the right side of the section (*longer arrow*). It must be remembered that the vertebral sympathetic passes along side this artery upward into the cranial cavity. Additional new bone is being laid down in the fibrocartilage covering the spur (*short arrowhead*).

$\longrightarrow$

THE NORMAL OBLIQUE CERVICAL ROENTGENOGRAM

A roentgenogram of the cervical spine made according to the 45-degree oblique technique reveals the intervertebral foramina in their normal shape and symmetrical position. The topmost or second cervical is oval and those below this point are shaped, as Schmorl has described, somewhat like the "sole of a shoe." The second and seventh are directed more laterally than those intervening. Each foramen is bounded above and below by a pedicle, in back by a poster-

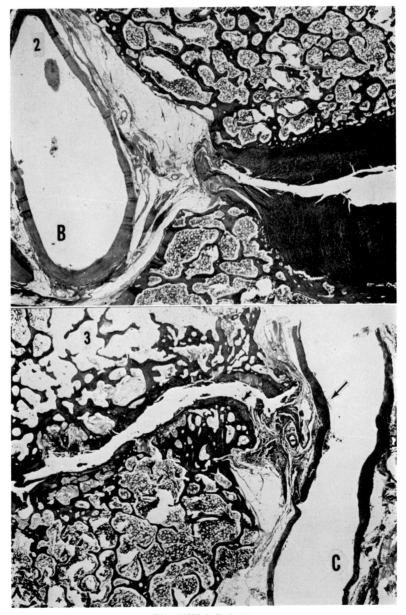

Fig. XIV:3 B & C.

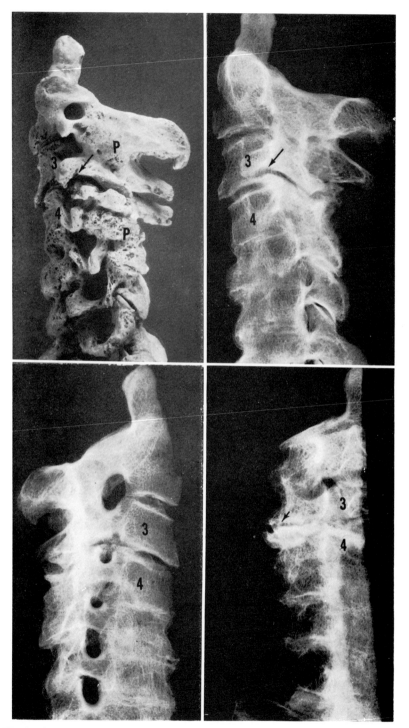

Fig. XIV:4. Photograph and radiographs of specimen from an eighty-five year old male showing impingement beneath the third transverse process. There is marked forward hyperplasia of the posterior C_{3-4} articulation. The spur formation upon the superior articular

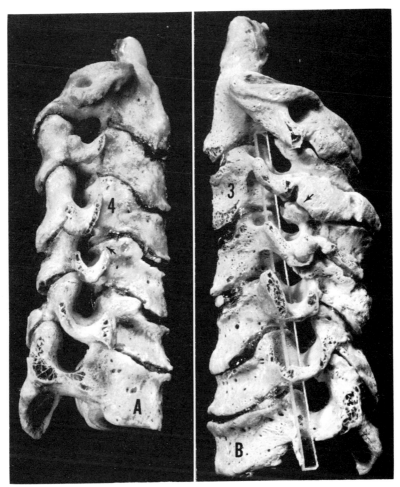

Fig. XIV:5. A, Right side of the cervical spine from a man seventy-eight years old, showing covertebral spur encroachment anterior to the fourth intervertebral foramen (*black arrow*).

B: Arthrotic hyperplasis of the third posterior articulation on left side of the cervical spine from a woman sixty-four years old. There is impingement beneath the third transverse process and encroachment upon the intervertebral foramen from behind (*arrow*). A plastic rod in the transverse foramina indicates the position of the vertebral artery. This courses immediately anterior to and in direct contact with the cervical nerve roots. (Courtesy of the *Journal of Bone and Joint Surgery*.)

process of C_4 is so large that it projects forward to articulate with the under-surface of the third transverse process (*long arrows*). The corresponding foramen is substantially decreased in size by this spur as shown by the oblique radiograph on the extreme left. On the P. A. projection note the spur formation laterally from the third posterior joint (*arrow*).

ior articulation and in front by vertebral bodies and the intervertebral disc. Shadows of the gargoyle-shaped transverse processes may partially overlie these openings.

Close to the posterior border of the foramina the laminae of the same side of the arch are seen in section, that is, their cortex in profile. Those for the second and seventh arches are oval and larger than the intervening third, fourth, fifth and sixth laminae which are smaller and more flattened. The posterior articulations are visualized between and partially overlapped by the shadows of the laminae.

In the oblique view of the normal cervical spine, all arches, as well as the foramina, pedicles and vertebral bodies appear in a smooth, sweeping, symmetrical curve about equidistant from each other. Any mal-alignment in this curve or irregularity in the spacing of the sec-

tions indicates a disturbance in the structure or the articulation of those cervical units.

The arch of the first vertebra may normally appear just slightly anterior to the curve of the other laminar sections. The spinous processes in this view should be just visible at their tips behind the spine and the angle of the jaw usually crosses the second vertebra.

The articulation between the first and second bodies, extending transversely, is seen just above the second foramen. It is not abnormal for the edges of the articular surfaces of this joint to be slightly out of alignment with each other.

The cortices of the pedicles on the side opposite to the visualized foramina, that is, the side farthest from the film, appear as a curved line of small equidistant oval shadows. If correct angulation has been used in making the roentgeno-

---

Fig. XIV:6. Male, fifty-five years of age. Acute arthritis posteriorly at C_2 on the left side with evidence of recovery. Flexion-extension studies showed fixation of movement between the upper cervical segments. The original lateral roentgenogram (A) in extension shows an erosion of the second posterior cervical articulation (*arrow*). The arthritic process seems to have destroyed the articular surfaces. While there is evidence of a reaction within the bone, both above and below the joint, one does not see the sclerotic eburnation characteristic of a degenerative arthrosis. Neck pain referred to left trapezius muscle with limitation of motion had been present for five or six weeks without radiation to the arm or hand.

The patient was reexamined twenty-two months later. The acute symptoms had subsided after about two months. There was some residual discomfort and occasional pain of less severe character. Flexion-extension studies still showed fixation of movement between the second and third segments. There was a unilateral ponticulus posterius on the left side only (*white arrows*).

The patient was again reexamined at the age of sixty-three; there had been no recurrence of the early symptoms. The comparative lateral radiograph (B) made eight years after film (A) showed complete healing of the acute arthritic process at the second posterior articulation. The joint had become fused and surrounded by bony masses projecting posteriorly, anteriorly and laterally (*black arrows*) on radiographs B and C, the second intervertebral foramen was encroached upon. Arthritis of a posterior cervical joint most commonly occurs at C_2. This is in contrast with disc changes which develop at the mid and lower cervical levels where the amplitude of anterior-posterior neck movement is greater.

gram, this line of pedicle shadows will overlie the shadows of the vertebral bodies near their anterior surfaces. The vertical interpediculate distance represents the size of the foramen.

CERVICAL FORAMEN ENCROACHMENT

There are various ways in which intervertebral foramen encroachment may occur. The first is physiological. The foramen is constricted by normal dorsal extension movements, or by a permanent lordosis increasing the normal cervical curve and causing the superior articular processes to become thrust upward and forward into the upper portion of the foramina. Dorsal kyphosis causes a compensatory exaggeration of the cervical curve.

In the cervical region the extremes of lateral flexion, dorsal extension or

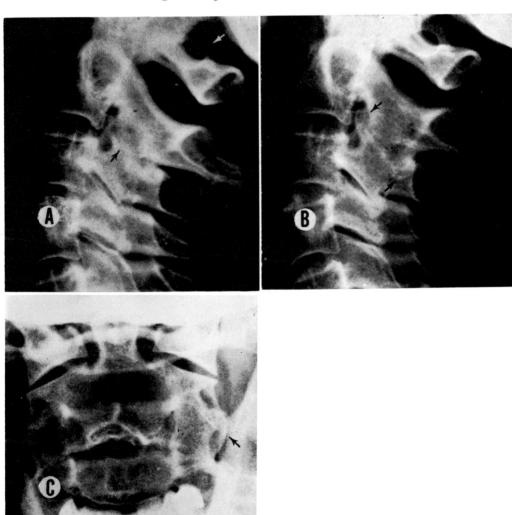

rotation may normally decrease the size of the foramen by as much as one-third on the side toward which the movement occurs with a corresponding enlargement on the opposite side. Pain in the arm and shoulder from brachial root pressure may be aggravated by dorsal extension of the neck or by rotation or flexion toward the affected side. These patients hold the cervical spine straight, thereby eliminating its normal anterior curve. The normal physiological movements are of diagnostic value and may be utilized in evaluating or eliciting the symptoms of nerve root pressure.

As mentioned above, bony exostoses projecting forward from the posterior joint may cause foramen encroachment. Likewise the bony spurs from the covertebral joint project laterally and backward into the foramen. The encroachment is much more extensive than it appears on the roentgenogram because ligamentous tissue is also displaced into this opening from the posterior joint capsules or the longitudinal ligament. The opening may be partially or even completely occluded by these masses.

Constriction of the intervertebral foramen may be caused by a posterior joint telescoping and by wedging of the superior articular processes forward. En-

croachment also results from a decrease in the anterior-posterior diameter of the opening when the vertebral body above becomes displaced backward.

Any abnormal constriction in the size of a normal intervertebral foramen if not actually causing nerve root pressure, nevertheless decreases the reserve safety cushion space surrounding that nerve and may predispose to pressure. The subsequent development of radiculitis, edema, hemorrhage, additional disc pressure or movement of adjacent structures may be sufficient to produce radicular symptoms.

Trauma, either fracture or dislocation, may be a factor in the production of foramen encroachment. Most displacements are forward and these tend to enlarge the opening. Backward displacement of a cervical vertebra however, very definitely produces constriction of the intervertebral foramen (Figure XIV:12).

Studies of the cadaver specimens indicate that intervertebral disc degeneration is the most common cause of foramen encroachment.

Upon microscopic section one finds the nerve occupying about one-fifth to one-fourth the diameter of the normal cervical foramen, which is a complete bony ring. The remainder of the space

---

Fig. XIV:7. Female, seventy-one years of age, complained of radicular pain to the right thenar eminence and the first three fingers. The P. A. projection (A) reveals extensive arthrotic change involving especially the 3rd and 4th pairs of posterior articulations with spur formation extending laterally (*arrows*). The lateral projection (B) shows the arthrotic process involving the 2nd, 3rd and 4th posterior articulations. At the C_3 level the spur formation extends forward and impinges beneath the 2nd pedicle (*arrow*). Compare with Figure XIV:4. The degenerative change of the 4th posterior joint has allowed forward subluxation of the corresponding vertebral body. This is a pseudospondylolisthesis in the cervical region. The right oblique projection (R) reveals complete obliteration of the 3rd and 4th intervertebral foramina by the spur formation (*arrows*). While on the left side (L) there is marked encroachment upon the 3rd foramen (*arrow*). The 2nd, 5th and 6th openings appear to be essentially normal in size and shape on both sides.

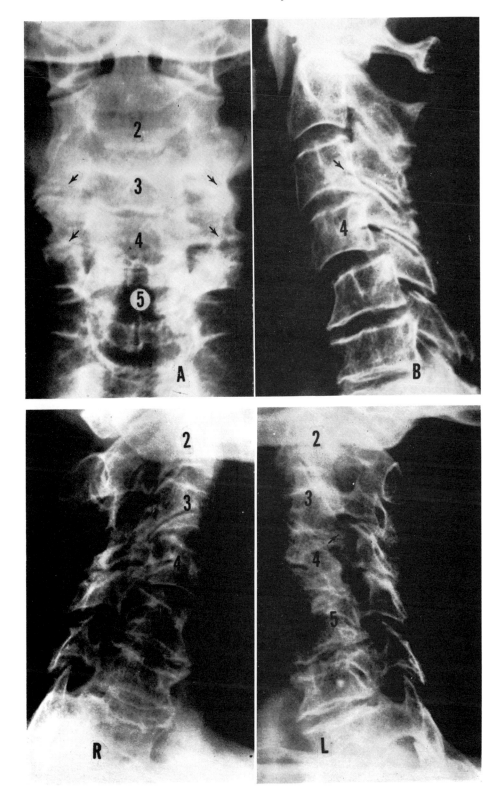

is taken up by lymphatics, blood vessels, areolar and fatty tissue. This constitutes a compressible saftey cushion space which allows the physiological encroachment caused by dorsal extension to occur without nerve root compression (Figure XIV:13). At levels of congenital non-segmentation, where movement between adjacent vertebral segments has never occurred, no cushion space is necessary. There the foramen is smaller than normal, round or oval in shape, smooth in contour and the nerve may fit the opening more closely (Figure XIV:14).

In the cervical region where the nerves leave the cord and the spinal canal in a horizontal direction the nerve root is found in the lower part of the intervertebral foramen. This is in contrast with its position in the upper part of the lumbar foramina where the nerves are more vertical (Figures IV:2 and XIV:26). Bony or fibrous tissue encroachment may reduce the size of the foramen, crowding the nerve still further into the lower portion of the opening. It may become flattened in a ribbon-like manner or greatly reduced in size (Figure XIV:15). In examining cadaver material the nerve can usually be separated within the foramen by blunt dissection but in some cases of foramen encroachment it is adherent because of the fibrosis surrounding the nerve. Under these circumstances it is removed with some difficulty by cutting dissection. Microscopic study of such foramina shows the increased mass of fibrous tissue surrounding the nerve root bundles.

Patients with foramen encroachment often complain of local pain, tenderness, muscle spasm, and limitation of neck motion. They frequently suffer also from

---

→

Fig. XIV:8. Female, eighty-four years of age with cervical and occipital pain for years and with restricted movement of the neck. The radiographs reveal advanced degenerative, sclerotic and hyperostotic changes with foraminal encroachment and impingement of the posterior articular processes. The long black arrows indicate the bony impingement between the hyperplastic superior articular processes and the undersurfaces of the corresponding transverse processes (see Figure XIV:4). On the left oblique projection (C) the 3rd and 4th intervertebral foramina are seen to be encroached upon by enlarged posterior articular processes projecting forward from the posterior joints (small black arrows). While the 5th foramen, because of advanced disc degeneration at that level, is constricted above and in front by a spur projecting backward from the arthrotic covertebral joint (*white arrow*). In the lateral projection (A) the impingement of the enlarged posterior articular processes beneath the corresponding 3rd and 4th transverse processes are seen as curvilinear shadows crossing the middle of the corresponding vertebral bodies (*black arrows*). These lines are of course continuous with the posterior articulations behind. However, the line crossing the 5th vertebra on A just below the digit 5 is not continuous with the posterior articulation. This curved line is caused by the covertebral impingement at the 5th disc level. These lines crossing a cervical vertebral body are a common finding and must not be mistaken for a fracture following trauma. In the P. A. projection (B) are seen the 3rd and 4th arthrotic posterior articulations with large spurs projecting laterally (*black arrows*). Immediately above the O is faintly seen the covertebral impingement and spur which is responsible for the encroachment of the left 5th intervertebral foramen (*white arrow on projection C*). The right side of the unclosed first cervical arch is higher than its fellow on the left side (*white arrows projection B*). These are seen entirely separate in the lateral view (A).

the referred pain of radiculitis. In the cervical region this condition is characterized by pain or paresthesia referred to the occiput, shoulder, arm or hand and corresponds in distribution to that of the involved nerve roots. It is frequently aggravated by increased intraspinal pressure as by coughing, sneezing

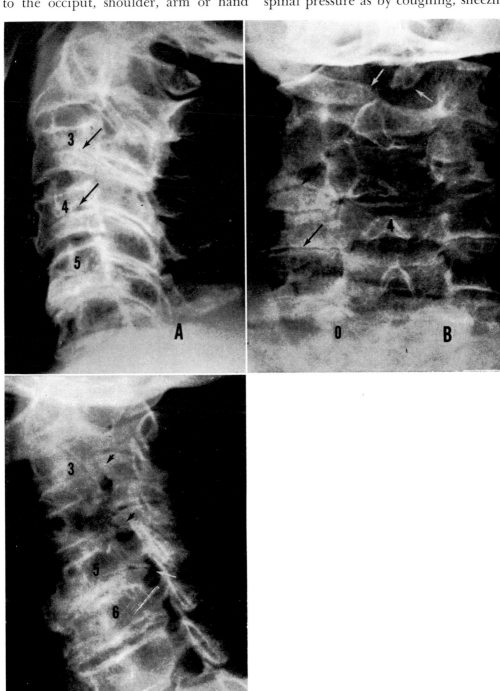

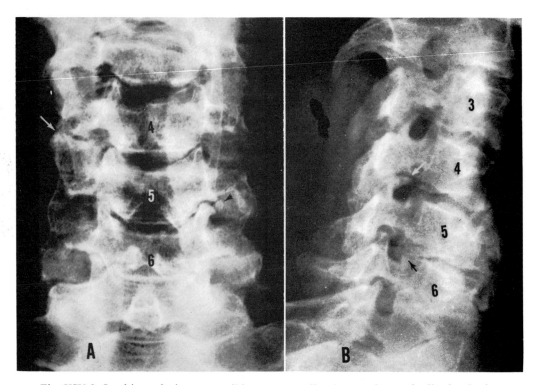

Fig. XIV:9. In this study it was possible to personally observe the gradually developing clinical picture of chronic degenerative arthrotic change in the spine over a period of years. The most consistent observation was the periodicity of the symptoms with the exacerbations gradually fading again into complete remission. There was chronic localized neck pain and tenderness to deep pressure over the right midcervical region, aggravated by flexion or rotation toward the right. Painful muscle spasm occurred on the right side from time to time. Subsequently the symptoms gradually became less troublesome, but recurred occasionally. The A. P. projection (A) reveals an arthrotic process involving the right fourth posterior articulation *(white arrow)*. In the right oblique view (B) the bony spur from this joint is seen encroaching upon the fourth intervertebral foramen *(white arrow)*. There is minimal covertebral spur encroachment of the 5th intervertebral foramen *(black arrow)*. The second, third, sixth and seventh foramina are normal in shape and size. Note the small unusual intercalary ossicle visualized on the A. P. projection (A) at the tip of the left fifth covertebral spur *(black arrowhead)*. This is the characteristic bird's head shaped covertebral spur formation.

→

Fig. XIV:10. Progressive encroachment upon the intervertebral foramina by covertebral spur formation over a period of twenty years. A, was made at fifty-four years of age and B at seventy-four. During this interval there was a degenerative thinning of the 3rd, 4th and 6th intervertebral discs with shortening of the cervical spine. Note the impingement and sclerosis of the covertebral joints with resultant spur formation *(arrows)*. These osteophytes projected backward constricting the size of the foramina. There was also some arthrotic change of the 2nd posterior joint which caused encroachment upon that opening. The 5th and 6th segments were previously fused into a block vertebra so that no change occurred in the size or shape of the 5th intervertebral foramen. The patient suffered from recurrent attacks of pain and paresthesia of the shoulder, arm and hand. Later the symptoms became less troublesome. (Final examination by courtesy of the University Hospital.)

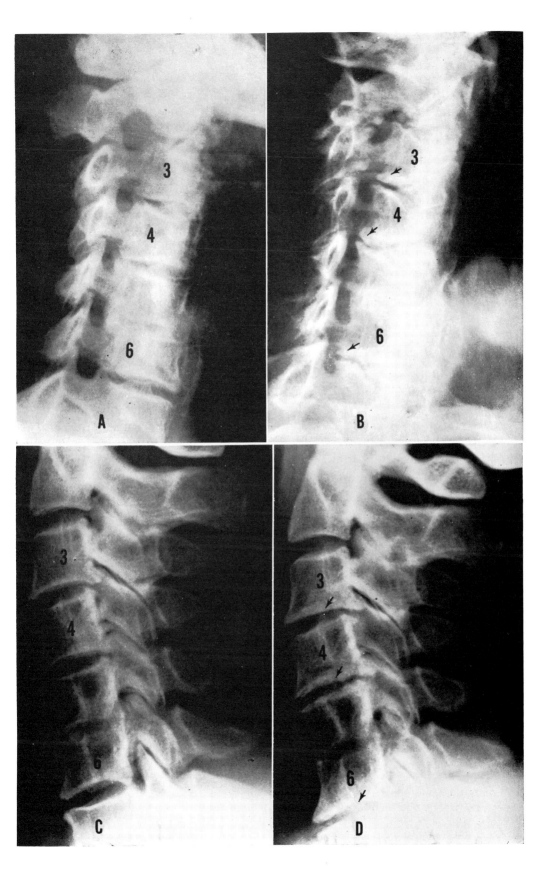

or bearing down, the so-called Dejerine sign. The pain is increased by rotation or flexion of the neck toward the painful side or by dorsal extension. The arm and forearm reflexes may be diminished and the patient may later develop weakness or atrophy of the forearm or hand muscles. Not all patients, however, suffering from radiculitis exhibit foramen encroachment on the roentgenogram. Also certain patients with bony foramen encroachment may not complain of radicular symptoms at the time of the roentgenographic examination. The condition is characterized by recurrences and remissions.

In addition to the local and referred pain these patients may suffer from a group of bizarre symptoms the so-called chronic cervical syndrome. The following have been described: paroxysmal deep or superficial pain in various parts of the head, face, ear, throat or sinuses; sensory disturbances in the pharynx; vertigo and tinnitus with diminished hearing. Certain vasomotor disturbances are also included as a part of this syndrome, namely; sweating, flushing, lacrimation and salivation.

THORACIC REGION

Since the thoracic roots are relatively small, compression of these structures does not occur in the formina of this region. The arthrotic changes incidental to degenerative processes in the costovertebral articulations may prove never the less to be a real cause of symptoms.

Even in the absence of spondylitis deformans patients frequently complain of pain and tenderness to deep pressure posteriorly in the thoracic region. Intercostal pain, referred around to the anterior chest wall may cause apprehension, especially if it is on the left side.

The relatively large intervertebral foramina lie just above the level of the intervertebral discs. They provide a generous perineural cushion space for the thoracic nerves which are much smaller than those either in the cervical or lumbar regions.

The posterior joints of this area are

Fig. XIV:11. Progressive encroachment upon the intervertebral foramina by posterior joint spur formation, (A) at forty-two and (B) at sixty-five years of age. Since there was little degenerative thinning of the intervertebral discs (except for No. 3), covertebral spur formation with resultant foramen encroachment from that cause did not occur. The arthrotic process with spur formation originally (A) involved the 2nd and 5th posterior articulations. Twenty-three years later (B), considerable additional encroachment had occurred (*arrows*). The position of the patient was practically identical at both examinations. Minimal kyphotic angulation at the 3rd disc level was visualized upon both the original radiographs (A and C). During the interval there was some thinning of the anterior portion of the 3rd disc and as a result the kyphosis increased while the 3rd and 4th spinous processes separated more widely (*white arrows D*). In the final, lateral study (D) observed the sclerosis of the arthrotic 2nd, 4th and 5th posterior articulations (*black arrows*). Also note the generalized demineralization which had developed during this twenty-three year interval.

The patient had complained of recurrent pain in the neck with remissions throughout this period. The bony hyperplasia about the posterior articulations in the upper cervical region later became easily palpable. These areas were tender to pressure.

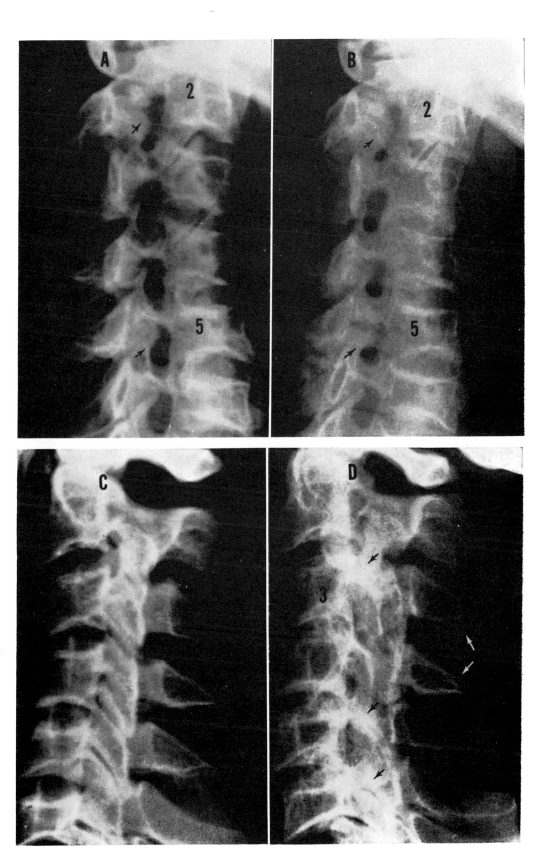

subject to degenerative arthrotic changes with loss of cartilage, eburnation and spur formation. This may result in marked foramen encroachment. But even if the opening is reduced to less than a fourth of its normal size the nerve will not be compressed because of its smaller diameter Figure XIV:16.

In addition to the posterior articulations each segment presents two pairs of joints for the ribs (Figure XIV:17). Any or all of these three pairs of joints may develop arthrotic changes.

The first, eleventh and twelfth ribs articulate with the transverse process and centrum of the corresponding vertebra. From the second to the tenth vertebra inclusive the rib head articulates at the disc with its own segment as well as with that of the vertebra above.

The intervertebral nerve upon leaving the foramen after giving off a small branch to the sympathetic plexus divides into an anterior and a posterior branch. The latter dips backward between the transverse process and the rib below to penetrate the chest wall. The anterior division, passes postero-laterally between the tubercle articulation and the lower portion of the transverse process to become the intercostal nerve. It lies in close proximity to the tubercle joint and might conceivably be affected by hyperplastic spur formation at that point (Figure XIV:18).

Patients with pain in the thoracic region, often with paravertebral tenderness to deep pressure, may show radiographically a hyperplastic spurring of the costo-transverse articulations (Figure XIV:19). This is a common finding in patients past middle life.

LUMBAR FORAMINA

The larger lumbar foramina, as in those vertebrae above, are bounded in front by the vertebral bodies and the posterolateral surface of the disc between them, while above and below are the pedicles. Posteriorly occur the superior and inferior articular processes united by the lateral prolongation of the liga-

----

Fig. XIV:12. Male, sixty-five years of age. Automobile accident in which the patient was thrown forward striking the forehead on the windshield. There was pain in the cervical spine, shoulder and arm with paresthesia of the forearm and hand. The neck was supported by a cast for two months. The retouched lateral roentgenogram (A) made twenty months after injury shows backward displacement of C_4 (both the vertebral body and its neural arch) on C_5 (*long arrow*). This retrosubluxation has thrust the 5th superior articular processes upward and forward into the foramina. The right oblique projection (R) reveals the 4th foramen on that side to be completely obliterated, while on the left side (L) there is a substantial constriction of the 4th opening (*small arrows*). Thinning of the 4th disc also contributed to this encroachment. The A. P. diameter of the spinal canal is narrowed between the C_4 vertebral body and the C_5 arch as indicated by the length of the long arrow in the lateral projection (A). The symptoms were more aggravated on the left side, where the occlusion of the C_4 foramen was not complete. Note the congenital nonsegmentation of the 2nd and 3rd vertebral bodies and their arches. The decreased mobility at this block vertebra may have been a factor in producing this injury when the head was forced backward. The A. P. projection thru the mouth shows the atlas displaced toward the left with its right lateral mass rotated posteriorly upon the axis. This backward rotation is also visualized on the right oblique roentgenogram (R) at the white arrow.

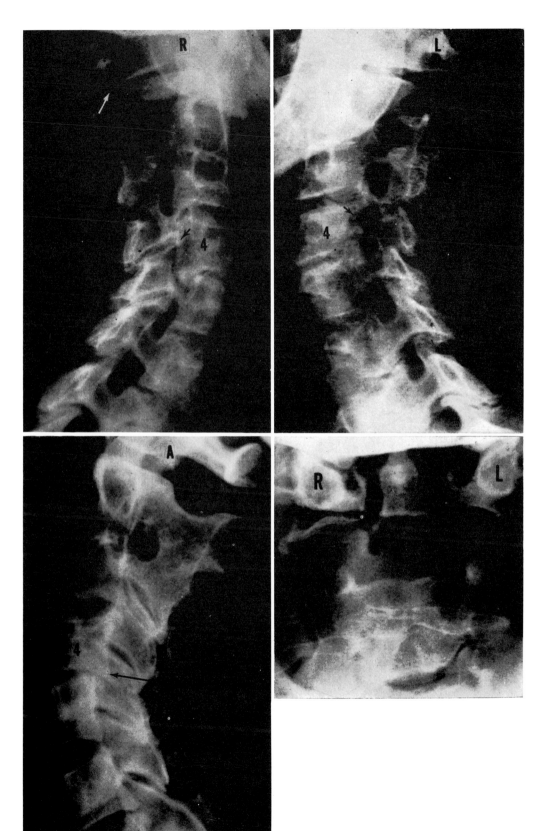

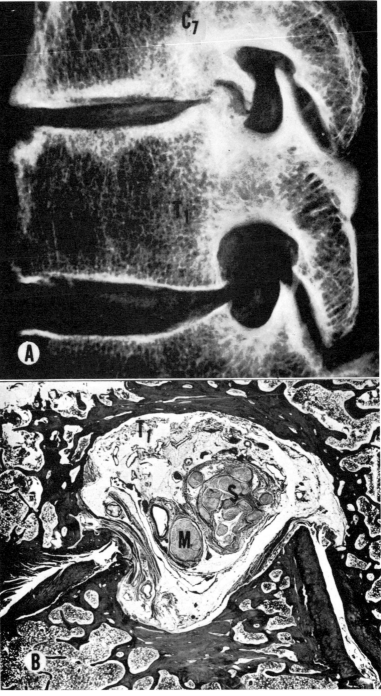

Fig. XIV:13. Radiograph A (X3) of a one-fourth inch thick section at the cervicodorsal level of an eighty-five year old male. The first thoracic foramen, is essentially normal. At the C_7 level, however and incidental to the degenerated disc, the covertebral joint has developed a pair of osteophytes which encroach upon the intervertebral foramen. There is also some telescoping of the posterior joint.

mentum flavum which at this point constitutes the anterior fibers of the capsule of the posterior articulation.

The nerve issues from the superior portion of the opening and passes in a spiral direction, laterally, downward and forward. The fifth foramen although transmitting the largest lumbar root is smaller than those immediately above. Its size is usually adequate, however.

Of some importance is a ligament which at times passes from the lumbosacral disc to the ala of the sacrum bridging over the fifth lumbar root. Bony formation in this structure has been found to produce nerve compression (see Figure XII:7).

SPINAL MOVEMENTS

In the lumbar, as in the cervical region, a physiological encroachment results upon the side toward which lateral bending occurs. There is a corresponding

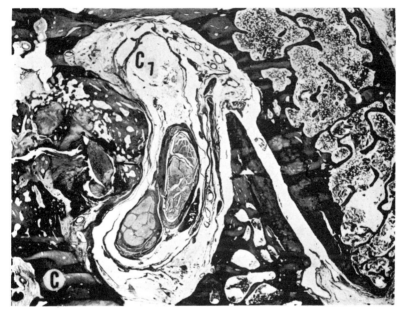

The section B showing the first thoracic foramen (T_1) (X7), reveals ample cushion space surrounding the sensory and motor nerve roots. There is also ample space for the many blood vessels, areolar and fatty tissues. The sensory nerve (S) consists of many bundles and is larger than the motor nerve (M) which lies anterior and below it. A small bony spur is visualized projecting into the foramen from the disc region on the left. This intervertebral foramen is essentially normal. Compare with roentgenogram A.

C, Section of the seventh cervical foramen (X7). The covertebral osteophytes are seen encroaching upon the anteromedial (*left*) margin of the foramen. A small mass of extruded disc substance is entrapped between the two spurs (*arrow*). This is also visualized as a clear space on the radiograph. It is not attached and in some of the sections it fell out leaving an open space (area indicated by dots). Much has been written about "herniations of the cervical disc causing foramen encroachment." However, in our experience it is the osteophyte formation at the covertebral joints which usually causes the cervical foramen encroachment medially. This small unusual mass of herniated disc is entirely surrounded by the bony spur formation as seen on both the section and the radiograph. The nerve roots of C_7 show fibrotic thickening of the perineurium. Compare them with the normal root section in T_1 (B). Courtesy of the publisher of the *Journal of the Bone and Joint Surgery.*

enlargement of the opening on the side away from which the movement takes place. Anterior flexion results in a substantial enlargement of all lumbar foramina while dorsal extension produces the opposite effect (Figures XIV:21, XIV:22, XIV:23, and XIV:24). Contralateral list of the lumbar spine away from the side of a sciatica indicates a protective attempt to enlarge the foramen of exit of a painful nerve root. In one patient studied, this contralateral list was lost when the foramina became enlarged by anterior flexion. As the patient bent forward his body swung towards the midline, i.e., the painful side, until the spine was in a symmetrical position. As he straightened up the reverse movement occurred. He gradually reassumed his contralateral list away from the painful side upon again reaching the vertical position.

Homolateral list toward the side of a sciatica indicates an attempt to lessen ten-

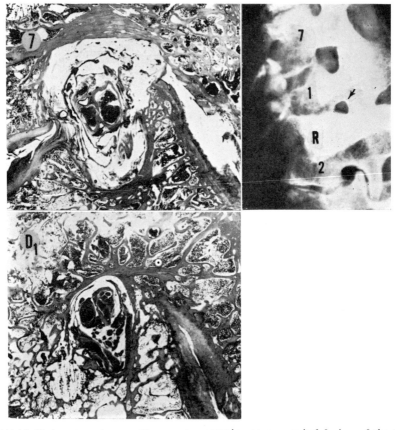

Fig. XIV:14. Cadaver specimen with non-segmentation or congenital fusion of the 1st and 2nd thoracic vertebrae. The radiograph shows the head of the first rib (R) articulating with this block vertebra. The 7th cervical intervertebral foramen above is the site of movement and is normal in shape and size but the non-segmented foramen where no movement is present is small and round (*arrow*). A section (X5) taken from the 7th foramen reveals the adequate cushion space surrounding the nerve at the movable level. In the section below, however, the nerve occupies relatively more of the space in the small T_1 foramen. Here no cushion space is necessary, since there is no movements between the segments of the block vertebra. (Courtesy of the *American Journal of Roentgenology*.)

sion upon the involved nerve. A patient may maintain a combination of homolateral list and forward flexion, thereby attempting to relax the nerve tension and at the same time enlarging the foramen of exit.

Homolateral and contralateral scoliosis may alternate in the same patient.

A patient with lumbar foramen encroachment and with root pain may obtain relief from pain by maintaining a position of forward flexion but the pain will be aggravated upon dorsal extension. This was marked in the patient reported in Figure XIV:25, whose spine remained fixed in ventral flexion, even during painful heroic attempts at backward bending.

TECHNIQUE

Roentgenograms of the lower portion of the spine are routinely made in the P. A. prone projection rather than with the patient supine. When the patient is lying face downward, the anterior lumbar curve allows the central ray to pass through more nearly parallel to the plane surfaces of nearly all of the vertebral bodies. Also the sacrum is not foreshortened. Depending somewhat upon the curvature of the spine, the distance between the lumbo-sacral junction and the film may be no greater when the patient is prone than it is when he is supine, because in the latter instance the part is elevated away from the table by the buttocks and the mid-thoracic portion of the spine.

The oblique view is very important. For this the patient first lies on his back and then rolls up onto his side until the transverse plane of his body forms an angle of between 45 and 60 degrees with the table top. The central ray is centered just below and anterior to the anterior superior iliac spine. With the left side lowermost, one may see the articulations and the pars interarticularis of the left side, while posteriorly appear the laminae of the right side.

In the lumbar region, the foramina at each side of the spinal canal overlie each other in the lateral view. To separate them it is necessary to turn the patient slightly. In order to visualize the fifth lumbar foramen, the patient should be placed on the side to be studied but turned 10 degrees toward the prone from the true lateral position. The central ray is angulated 10 degrees toward the feet and centered just above and behind the iliac crest. Stereoscopic studies with transverse shift will show the fifth lumbar foramen enface through the lower most iliac bone. This is a special 80 degrees lateral lower lumbar foramen technique. Since the tissues within the foramen are less dense than the intervertebral disc, it is not at all unusual to visualize that structure bulging backward into the opening.

A comparison of the cephalocaudad diameters of different foramina can be made from the anteroposterior view by noting the distance between the pedicles of adjacent vertebrae, although, this gives only an idea of the antero-posterior diameter of the openings. The 45 degrees lumbar film (prone or supine) gives an excellent visualization of the posterior articular processes and the joint between them. Here the foramen is not seen en face but, as in the antero-posterior view, its size can be judged from the interpedicular distance. For the fifth lumbar, this is measured from the cortex of the ala of the sacrum upward to the undersurface of the fifth pedicle.

LUMBAR FORAMEN CONSTRICTION

Intervertebral disc thinning and trauma, either fracture of the vertebral body, fracture of its arch, or dislocation of one vertebral body upon another, may cause encroachment or even obliteration of the foramen.

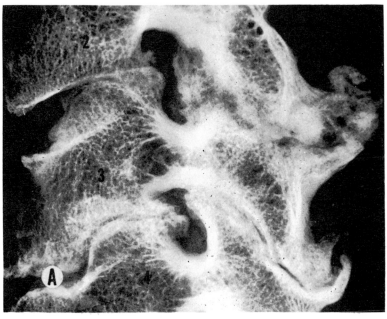

Fig. XIV:15. Foramen encroachment, nerve distortion and perineurial fibrosis. The oblique radiograph (A) (X2.5) shows parts of the C_2, C_3 and C_4 vertebrae with the interposed second and third foramina. There is advanced arthrosis of the posterior articulations with spur formation. Also disc cartilage destruction is present with large osteophytes projecting backward from these covertebral joints into the inter-vertebral foramina. The third disc is completely destroyed with a large osteophyte at the covertebral joint projecting backward into the third foramen. There is resultant bony encroachment of both foramina.

B: Shows a section of the second foramen (X7), bounded above by the dense sclerotic pedicle of C_2. The large rounded bony mass projecting into the foramen from the posterior articulation has flattened the normally round or oval nerve root into a ribbon-like structure, slightly curved on section (*arrow*).

C shows a section of the third foramen (X7). The marked encroachment of this foramen is primarily by the bony spur projecting backward from the covertebral joint on the left side. New bone is being laid down in the fibrocartilage covering this structure (*arrow*). There is a thickened section of the longitudinal ligament which has been pushed into the foramen by this spur. Secondly, a spur has become thrust forward into the upper portion of the foramen from the posterior joint. Lastly, from thinning of the disc the third and fourth pedicles are closer than normal so that the cephalocaudad diameter of the foramen is decreased. The nerve root is much smaller than normal and it has become displaced downward onto the floor of the foramen. It has developed a dense fibrosis of the perineurium, especially of its inferior portion. The blood vessels are much fewer in number throughout this foramen than normal. To appreciate the amount of constriction of this opening and its nerve root please note that it is shown at the same magnification as the section of a normal foramen in Figure XIV:13B. (Courtesy of the *Journal of Bone and Joint Surgery*.) ────────→

Somewhat related to dislocation are cases of spondylolisthesis. Some of these show foramen encroachment and some do not (Figures XIV:28 and XIV:29).

Reverse spondylolisthesis is a very definite entity and produces foramen encroachment. This results when the articular process from below becomes subluxated forward and upward into the foramen, a condition usually resulting from disc degeneration, or tipping of the vertebral body (Figures XIV:30, XIII:30, and XIII:31).

As the degeneration and disc thinning occur the vertebral bodies approach more closely and a sclerosis of their plane surfaces develops. This type of bony reaction results from the irritation of pres-

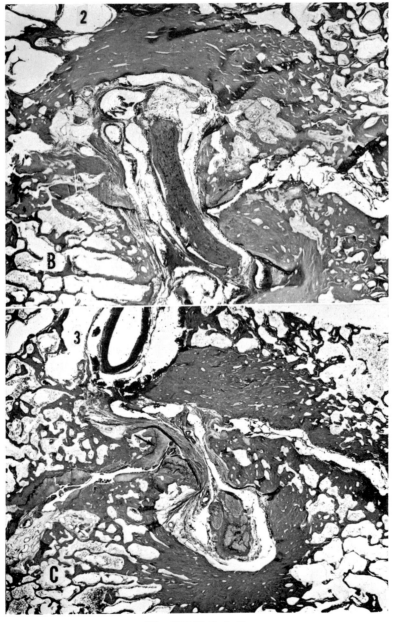

Fig. XV:15 B & C.

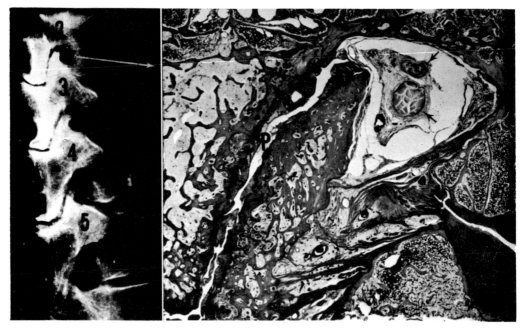

Fig. XIV:16. Specimen Male seventy-two: Advanced degenerative arthrosis of the posterior joints in the upper thoracic level. The 5th foramen is about normal in size but the second foramen is only one-fourth of the normal diameter. The photomicrograph (X8) shows this constricted foramen with its posterior articulation (P) devoid of articular cartilage. The thoracic nerves are relatively small (*arrows*) as compared to the cervical roots. For this reason there still remains an adequate cushion space surrounding the nerve in spite of the marked foramen encroachment. All of the throacic nerves are much smaller than the cervical or the lumbar nerves.

sure between two bone surfaces uncovered by articular cartilage and is greatest at the point of greatest pressure (Figures XIV:31 and XIV:32). Sclerosis is also noted in telescoping or imbrication of the posterior articulation when impingement occurs between the tip of an articular process and the pedicle above or the lamina below. This degenerative or wearing out process commonly termed "osteoarthritis" is in no sense an inflammation of the joint and therefore may be more properly termed an arthrosis (Figures XIV:33 and VII:21).

An arthritic process of the posterior articulations ordinarily is capable of causing root pressure but an osteoarthritis of the Marie-Strumpell type which may progress to complete ankylosis of the posterior joints may, in the absence of disc thinning, leave the foramina normal in size and shape (Figure IX:7).

As a result of disc degeneration and thinning, the foramen diameter may become decreased in several ways: The pedicles are brought more closely together decreasing the cephalocaudad diameter. Thickening or buckling of the ligamentum flavum often takes place. This ligament may even become ossified (Figures XIV:34 and XIV:35). Because of the inclined plane of the posterior articulation, the lower vertebra may become wedged forward as the disc undergoes thinning. This reverse spondylolisthesis causes a decrease in the antero-posterior diameter of the foramen. The superior articular process from below subluxates upward and forward into the foramen, constricting the size of that opening (Figure XIV:36).

If imbrication of the posterior articulation becomes sufficiently pronounced, a bony impingement occurs between the tip of the superior articular process and the pedicle or transverse process above. There may also occur an impingement between the tip of the inferior articular process and the lamina of the arch below.

With this impingement there may develop a new articulation with fibro-cartilage bumper formation. Erosion and sclerosis of the underlying bone occurs, usually with hyper-plastic bone spurs about the joint margin. These impringements are painful and the foramina are encroached upon (Figure XIV:37).

The vertebral bodies are not connected by a strong longitudinal ligament at the plane of the pedicles so that herniation of a weakened disc, may occur backward and laterally into the fixed

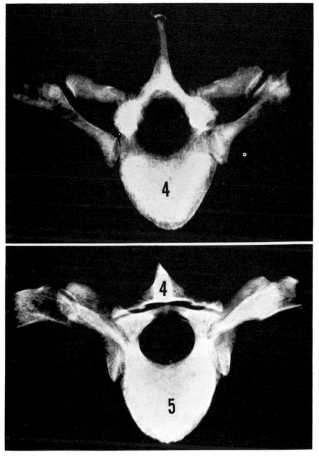

Fig. XIV:17. Specimens from a male of sixty-nine years: Radiographs of the 4th and 5th thoracic vertebrae at slightly different angles to show the three pairs of joints for each segment. On the 4th is seen the two articulations for each rib while number 5 is tipped forward to visualize the almost transverse plane of the posterior articulations between adjacent segments. The sharp triangular shadow posteriorly is a small section detached from the 4th arch.

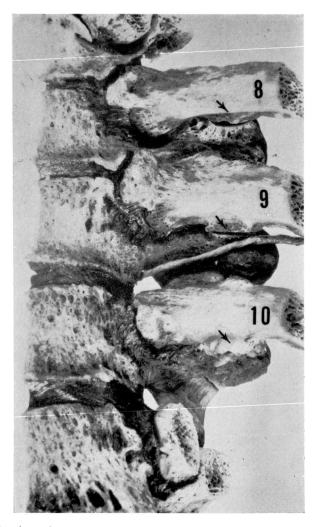

Fig. XIV:18. Specimen from a male of sixty-one years showing the proximal ends of the left 8th, 9th and 10th ribs articulating with the vertebral bodies and the corresponding transverse processes. Except for T_1, T_{11} and T_{12} the head of each rib bridges the intervertebral disc and articulates both with the vertebra above and below. The head of the rib with its slightly rotary respiratory movement has here developed arthrotic changes at its articulation with the adjacent vertebral bodies. There are also hyperplastic joint changes at the tubercle-transverse process joints (*arrows*) where a slight rocking movement normally occurs. The nerve root upon leaving the intervertebral foramen supplies a small branch to the sympathetic plexus before dividing into its anterior and posterior branches. The latter encircles the posterior articular process as it dips backward between the transverse process above and the rib below. The anterior branch continues in a postero-lateral direction beneath the rib as the intercostal nerve. On this specimen a cord was placed to show the course of this intercostal branch and its close proximity to the arthrotic tubercle-transverse joint. The anterior branch of the nerve is well separated from the arthrotic process at the head of the rib. The posterior branch approaches rather closely to the apophyseal articulation in back.

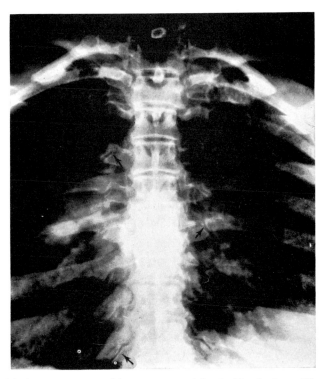

Fig. XIV:19. This forty-seven year old woman complained of backache, stiffness and tenderness to deep pressure along the paraspinal region of the thorax. Patients with paraspinal tenderness frequently show evidence of arthrotic change in many of the costotransverse articulations such as noted in this individual (*arrows*).

bony ring of the foramen. This herniation of the disc into the foramen constitutes still another type of encroachment which merits recognition (Figure XIV:38).

NERVE CHANGES INCIDENTAL TO FORAMEN CONSTRICTION

Macroscopically the compressed nerve may show some alteration in its shape, such as a flattening, concavity or triangulation incidental to the external pressure (Figure XIV:39). Bulging disc substance, exostoses or subluxation of a posterior joint may produce pressure upon the root. In each case, since the foramen is a complete bony ring, counter pressure is exerted by the remaining circumference of the opening. In certain cases there is a marked fibrosis and thickening of the epineurium which surrounds the entire nerve, firmly attaching the root to the foramen walls and extending inward between the different nerve bundles as the perineurium. In a study of the cadaver material it was always necessary to remove such a nerve by sharp dissection in contrast to the normal nerve surrounded by its cushion space which was easily removed from the foramen by blunt dissection.

Microscopically, various morphological changes with stages of nerve degeneration and regeneration were noted.

Certain nerve bundles and ganglion cells were found flattened. Many Schwann tubules outlined by the neurilemma were empty of myelin and axones where the macrophages had removed these degenerated elements. In other sections of the

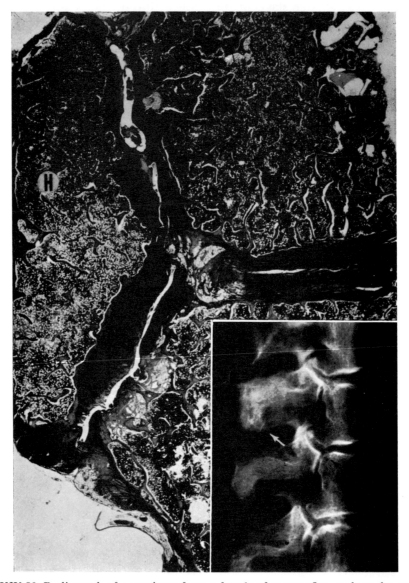

Fig. XIV:20. Radiograph of a specimen from a female of seventy-five to show the articulation of the head of each rib with the vertebra above, the one below and the disc between them. The tubercle of the rib articulates with the transverse process of the lower of these two vertebrae (*white arrow*). Exceptions are the first, eleventh and twelfth thoracic segments wherein the rib does not articulate with the vertebral body above. The photomicrograph (X11) thru the rib head (H) and the two vertebrae was taken from the middle articulation (*black arrow*). The disc and the two cartilage covered articular surfaces on the rib radiate from a common central point devoid of cartilage. Costal movement incidental to respiration produces slightly rotary movement at this joint. Hyperplasia of the joint margins is usually noted in older individuals.

same nerve bundle, these tubules were seen already filled with muliple rods of Schwann protoplasm and nuclei. This is said to represent a later stage in the process of nerve regeneration. Some evidence of edema of the endoneurium was observed. Haemorrhage beneath the perineurium was found involving numerous roots in one specimen having adhesions about those structures. Sclerosis of arteriols within the nerve bundle was also observed (Figures XIV:40, XIV:41, and XIV:42).

DISCUSSION

Patients presenting the clinical picture of recurrent low back pain and nerve root pressure are too often and without adequate study diagnosed as "herniated disc." This picture has come to be termed the "ruptured disc syndrome." These symptoms result in part from nerve root pressure or irritation. They may or may not be increased by bearing down, the Dejerine sign, which increases the intraspinal pressure. This is more dependable than the cough test which also causes movement of the low back. The pathological condition is usually sought within the spinal canal while the less accessible intervertebral foramen may be inadequately explored. Herniation within the canal may exert

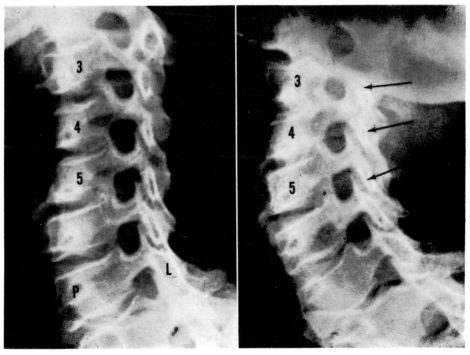

Fig. XIV:21. Female, twenty-three years of age. Physiological foramen constriction from movement. Oblique films were made at the limits of forward and backward neck movement. (Second foramen retouched). It will be noted that dorsal extension (film on the right causes a physiological constriction of the midcervical foramina (*arrows*). There is a symmetrical curved alignment produced by the various structures; the foramina, pedicles and lamina (L) on the side next to the film and the pedicles (P) on the side farthest from the film (Figure IV:6).

pressure upon a lower nerve root while producing adjacent foramen encroachment. For instance, the cadavers in Figures XIV:39 and XIV:40 showed herniation of the fourth disc backward into the spinal canal. In both cases the fifth root was displaced and there would have been a filling defect upon the myelogram. In each, the fourth foramen was encroached upon. Removal of the intraspinal hernia alone would not have relieved the foramen encroachment. Successful operative treatment necessitates not only removal of the hernia for distal

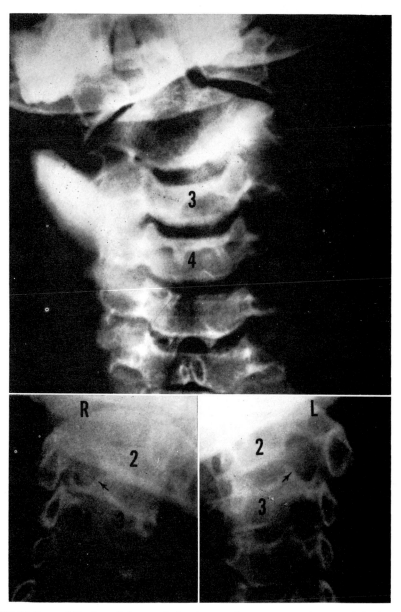

Fig. XIV:22. Lateral flexion of the cervical spine causing an encroachment of the intervertebral foramina. With the second and third cervical bodies tipped toward the right there is a dynamic constriction of the opening upon that side.

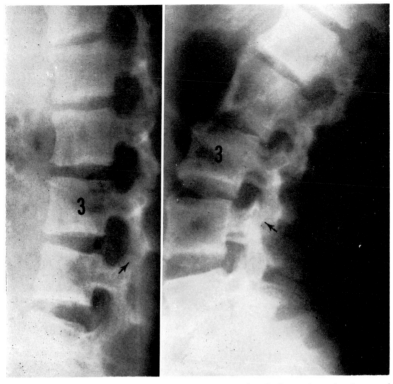

Fig. XIV:23. Flexion-extension studies of the lumbar spine in lateral projection to show the normal change in size and shape of the foramina, also the wedging of the intervertebral discs incidental to the usual physiological movements. The arrows at the third posterior joints indicate the gliding movement of these structures. Upon full anterior flexion only the tips of the articular processes are in contact. (Courtesy of the *American Journal of Roentgenology.*)

root pressure, but also proper attention to the adjacent foramen constriction. The cause of nerve root pressure may be disc herniation into the spinal canal or, among others, radiculitis, trauma, tumor, malignancy, extradural abscess, osteomyelitis, edema and as shown above, constriction of the intervertebral foramen. Duncan has shown that gradual constriction of a nerve in young animals destroyed the myelin about the axone but did not completely destroy its function or produce paralysis. However, after six and a half months there was a significant decrease in the size of the limb muscles and a reduction in the number and size of the nerve fibers below the constriction.

In cases of nerve root compression the cause must be sought not only as a herniated disc within the spinal canal but also the importance of intervertebral foramen, even to its most lateral limit, as apparent in properly evaluating radicular symptoms.

Preliminary conservative management is most important and should be given a thorough trial before subjecting the patient to operative interference. If that becomes necessary, it is imperative that the surgeon consider, not alone the spinal canal, but also the intervertebral foramen, even to its most lateral limit, as a possible site of the root pressure.

Various surgeons have relieved patients suffering from nerve root pressure by decompressing the intervertebral foramen. Some of the patients were previously unrelieved by disc operations within the spinal canal. Disc substance bulging into the foramen may be left undisturbed if the root is decompressed. Currettement of the disc is to be avoided

since that leaves the structure thinned and results in further constriction of the foramen. At any operation to relieve nerve root pressure, a very careful search within the intervertebral foramen even to its most lateral limits is always indicated. Removal of a herniated disc from the canal alone may not be sufficient but successful relief of the nerve root pressure may require at least a partial facetectomy.

REFERENCES

Adkins, E. W. O.: 1955, *J. Bone J. Surg., 37B:* 46–62, Spondylolisthesis pressure.

Allen, K. L.: 1952, *J. Neurol. Neurosurg. Psych., 15:*20–36, Spurs.

Boreadis, A. G., *et al:* 1956, *Rad., 66:*181–187, Luschka joints.

Brain, R.: 1954, *Ann. Int. Med., 41:*439–446, Cervical spondylosis.

Briggs, H.: 1945, *J. Bone J. Surg., 27:*475–478, Foramenotomy.

Bucy, P. C., *et al:* 1948, *J. Neurosurg., 5:*471–492, Disc compression.

Clark, E., *et al:* 1956, *Brain, 79:*483–510, Spondylosis cord pressure.

Danforth, M. S., and Wilson, P. D.: 1925, *J. Bone J. Surg., 7:*109–160, Sciatica.

Davis, D., *et al:* 1948, *New Eng. J. Med., 238:* 857–866, Radiculitis.

Duncan, D.: 1948, *J. Neuropath. exp. Neurol., 7:*261–273, Experimental.

Epstein, J. A., *et al:* 1951, *Surg. Gyn. Obst., 93:* 27–38, Spondylosis-compression.

Frykholm, R.: 1951, *Acta Chir. Scand.,* Supp. 160, Clinical Investigation.

Gayral, L., *et al:* 1954, *New York State J. Med., 54:*1920–1926, Barré-Lieou Syndrome.

Gillespie, H. W.: 1946, *Brit. Jor. Rad., 19:*420–428, Anatomy.

Gunther, L., *et al:* 1929, *Arch. Int. Med., 43:* 212–248, Spondylitis-radiculitis.

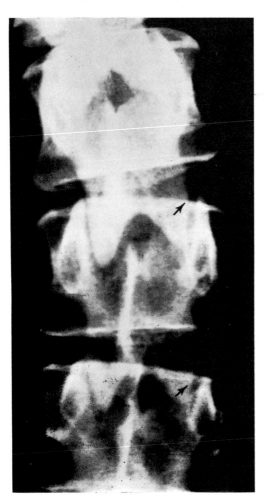

Fig. XIV:24. The lumbar spine, held in lateral flexion shows the normal physiological wedging of the intervertebral discs. Note the resultant telescoping of the articulations on the concave side with the opposite relationship of the joint surfaces on the right. Also the upper margins of the posterior joints separate on the convex side *(arrows)*.

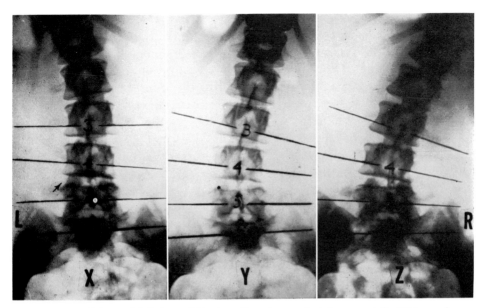

Fig. XIV:25. Right and left lateral flexion. Female, aged eighteen, while lifting a heavy weight she felt a sudden pain down the left leg. Thereafter she maintained a forward stooped position with a list to the right away from the painful side. The diagnosis, confirmed by operation, was a herniated disc, left side, 4th lumbar foramen. These films were made in the standing position. The lines indicate the corresponding transverse planes of the vertebral bodies in each of the radiographs. There was a normal flexion toward right side (Z). It will be seen that the foramen (axial interpedicular distance) becomes greater in a caphalo- caudad direction on the side away from which the bending occurs and smaller on the concave side. In attempting to stand upright, (Y) the patient held the spine with a list away from the left or painful side keeping the 4th foramen as large as possible. Upon attempted left lateral flexion (X) the lower lumbar spine was held rigid. The L_4 disc (*arrow*) was wedgeshaped, indicating a reflex attempt to hold the corresponding foramen as large as possible. This was done in order to avoid root pressure at the site of the herniated disc. It must be remarked that lateral flexion studies of a patient, with other localized lumbar pathology may show this restricted movement but without the accompanying clinical picture of nerve root pressure. (Courtesy of the *J.A.M.A.*)

Hanfly, S. S.: 1943, *Arch. Surg., 46*:652–663, Compression pain.

Hasner, E., *et al:* 1952, *Acta Rad., 37*:141–149, Movements.

Holmes, W., and Young, J. Z.: 1942, *J. Anat., 77*:63–96, Nerve regeneration.

Josey, A. I.: 1949, *J.A.M.A., 140*:944–949, Occipital pain.

King, R. B.: 1962, *J. Neurosurg., 19*:986–999, Cervical spondylosis.

Kovács, A.: 1955, *Acta Rad., 43*:1–16, Deformed posterior joints.

Lindblom, K.: 1944, *Acta Rad., 25*:195–212, Foramen encroachment.

Lindblom, K., and Rexed, B.: 1948, *J. Neurosurg., 5*:413–432, Anatomical studies.

Lyon, E.: 1945, *J. Bone J. Surg., 27*:248–253, Covertebral joints.

Lyon, E.: 1942, *J. Bone J. Surg., 24*:805–811, Intercalary bones.

Munro, D.: 1956, *New Eng. J. Med., 254*:243–252, Compression radiculitis.

Nathan, H.: 1959, *Anat. Rec., 133*:605–618, Anatomy.

Neuwirth, E.: 1954, *New York State J. Med., 54*:2583–2590, Covertebral joints.

Nugent, G. R.: 1959, *Neurol., 9*:273–281, **Spon**dylosis.

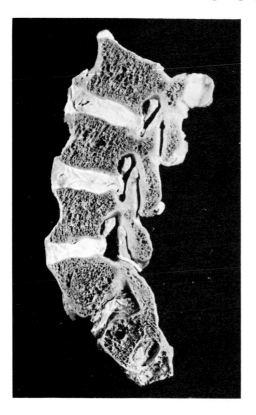

←——————————

Fig. XIV:26. Sagittal section of the lower three lumbar bodies and sacrum showing the ligamentum flavum forming a part of the posterior wall of the invertebral foramen. Here we see in the lumbar region the relationship between the size of the normal foramen, the disc thickness and the diameter of the nerve. Also note the exit of the nerve thru the upper portion of the foramen in contrast to the cervical region where the intervertebral nerve issues from the middle or lower part of the opening.

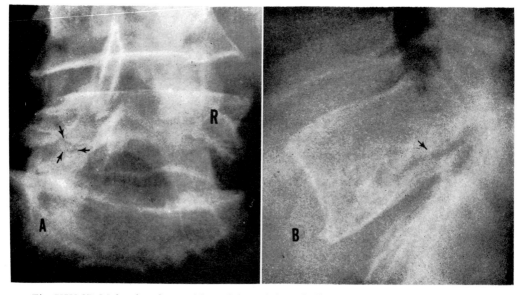

Fig. XIV:27. Male, sixty-four, with wedging of the 5th disc, encroachment of the foramen and a sulcus for the lumbar artery. The P. A. projection (A) shows thinning of the lumbosacral disc on the left side. The 5th vertebra is also slightly wedgeshaped. Telescoping of the 5th left posterior articulation has caused a constriction of the cephalo-caudad diameter of the 5th intervertebral foramen. The small black dashes on the left oblique film (C)

——————————→

Pool, J. L.: 1943, *Bull. New York Acad. Med.,* *29*:47–58, Cervical disc syndrome.

Rosenheck, C.: 1925, *J.A.M.A.,* *85*:416–418, Meralgia Paresthetica.

Schlesinger, P. T.: 1955, *J. Bone J. Surg., 37A:* 115–124, Anatomy.

Schnitker, M. T.: 1957, *J. Neurosurg., 14:*121–128, Pressure on root.

Smyth, M. J.: 1958, *J. Bone J. Surg., 40A*:1401–1418, Root irritability.

Stern, W. E., *et al:* 1954, *Neurol., 4*:883–893, Disc disease.

Teng, P.: 1960, *J. Bone J. Surg., 42A*:392–407, Root compression.

Whiteleather, J. E., *et al:* 1946, *Rad., 46*:213–219, Hernia cervical disc.

Williams, P. C., *et al:* 1933, *J. Bone J. Surg., 15*: 579–590, Facetectomy.

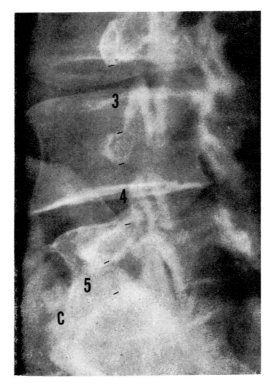

indicate the cortices of the pedicles which limit the boundaries of the foramina. The 3rd and 4th openings are normal in size. The lowermost foramen, however, as limited by the 5th pedicle and the ala of the sacrum is considerably narrowed. This patient has a sulcus eroded on the left side of the 5th vertebra indicated by the points of the three arrowheads in (A). Compare with Figure XIV:28, whereon the arrows are placed in the same relative positions as they are on this radiograph. On the oblique projection (C) the sulcus shows only faintly below the pedicle. On the lateral projection (B) the arrow indicates the sulcus which was at first mistaken for a fracture until seen on the P. A. projection. It is adjacent to the undersurface of the pedicle.

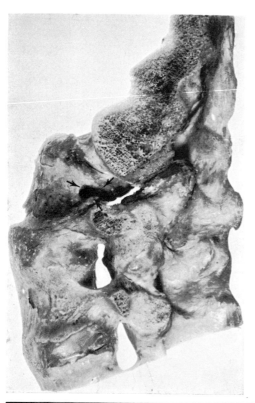

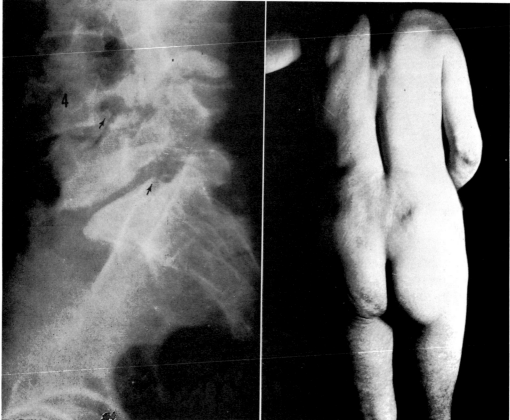

Fig. XIV:28. Specimen of spondylolisthesis showing almost complete obliteration of the 5th foramen. A compensatory sulcus for the lumbar
artery and fifth nerve has become eroded on the
lateral surface of the fifth vertebral body passing
beneath the transverse process *(arrows)*. This is
an example of adaptation to slowly changing
conditions. For other examples of sulcus formation see Figures IX:1 and XIV:33.

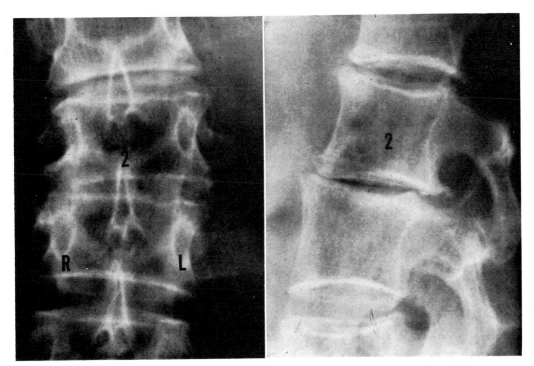

Fig. XIV:30. Female, seventy-seven. Pain in the right hip, thigh and knee referred down to the ankle. Patellar reflex absent on the right side but normal on the left. Both Achilles reflexes weak. The A. P. roentgenogram shows the second lumbar disc thinned on the right side with encroachment of the corresponding intervertebral foramen. The degenerated disc has allowed backward subluxation of the second lumbar vertebra. Additional foramen encroachment also resulted from the bony spur formation projecting backward into this opening.

←————————

Fig. XIV:29. This sixty-two year old male had complained of sciatica in the gluteal area referred down the right leg to the calf for the past six weeks. The right Achilles reflex was absent. Both patellar reflexes and the left Achilles were active. The patient supported his weight on the left side with the right knee flexed. The right gluteal fold was flattened and the 4th spinous process prominent. The roentgenogram reveals breaks in both the 4th and 5th neural arches with forward spondylolisthesis of these two vertebrae. Impingment of the neural arches and spinous processes has attained some degree of stabilization. The 4th disc is completely destroyed. Disc thinning together with the vertebral displacement has resulted in a marked distortion and encroachment of the intervertebral foramina *(arrows)*. The condition, obviously of long standing, antedates the present attack of sciatica and suggests the contributory role of other factors in precipitating the attack.

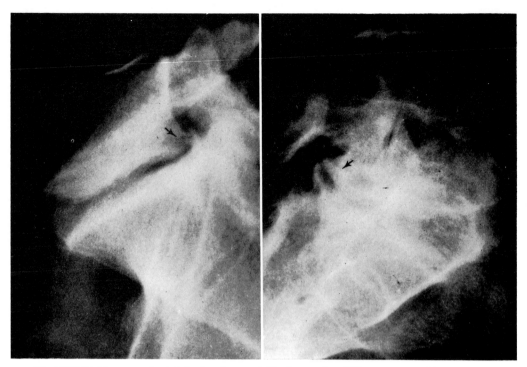

Fig. XIV:31. Degeneration of the lumbosacral disc in a male of fifty-one years. The resultant bony reaction and hyperplasis of the disc margins have resulted in osteophyte production encroaching upon the 5th intervertebral foramen (*arrows*). There was a history of low back pain of twenty years duration but the patellar and Achilles reflexes were normal.

Fig. XIV:33. Male cadaver, aged seventy-five. Had complained of pain in the right leg. Serial sections of the right 4th and 5th foramina. X, medial section with the articular process from the sacrum subluxated upward into 5th foramen which is encroached upon. Fourth and fifth discs thinned with sclerosis of adjacent vertebral bone as a result of pressure uncushioned by disc substance. Y, middle section. Note impingement of the sacral articular process against the undersurface of the 5th pedicle with bony sclerosis at this point (*arrow*). Z, lateral section. Impingement and foramen constriction extends completely to the lateral plane of this vertebra and its foramen. This is a final stage of disc degeneration. As a result of the constriction a sulcus for the nerve and artery developed on the lateral surface of the 5th vertebral body. A roentgenogram of section Y appears as Figure VII:21. (Courtesy of the *American Journal of Roentgenology.*)

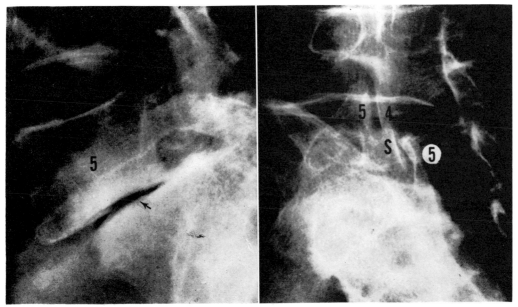

Fig. XIV:32. Male age sixty-four years. Right sciatic pain exaggerated upon bending backward. Bilateral defects in the 5th neural arch and complete degeneration of the lumbosacral disc allowed a second degree spondylolisthesis of the 5th lumbar vertebra forward and downward on the sacrum. Encroachment of the lowermost intervertebral formania with nerve root pressure resulted. Direct bony contact between the 5th vertebra and the sacrum, uncushioned by disc substance, has stimulated sclerotic changes in the bone. Compare the eburnation of these adjacent surfaces with the normal condition visualized at the fourth disc above. Complete degeneration of the fifth disc with fissure formation has allowed the development of a so-called vacuum disc (*arrow*), a not uncommon finding in advanced degeneration of the intervertebral cartilage.

The oblique projection shows the unusual character of the defect in the left side of the fifth neural arch. Because of the wide break in the pars interarticularis the superior and inferior articular processes of L_5 are widely separated. As a result the articular processes of L_4 and S_1 are closely approximated within this deficiency.

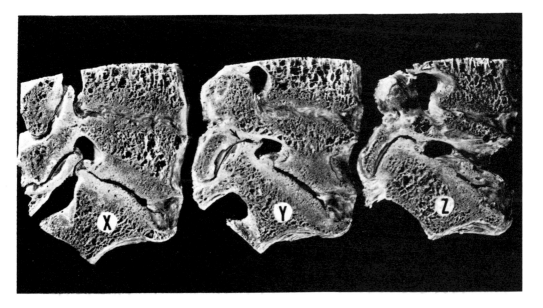

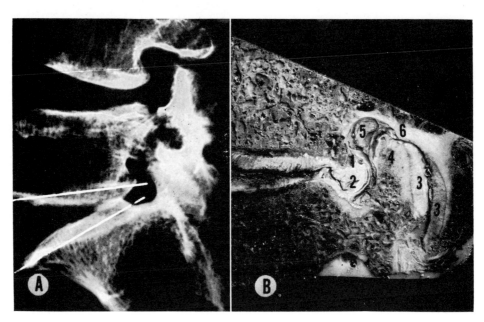

Fig. XIV:34. Radiograph (A) of a specimen with tipping of the sacrum on its transverse axis and wedging of the lumbosacral disc. Compare the encroached 5th intervertebral foramen with the normal size 4th foramen above. Photograph of the fixed tissue block (B) taken from this specimen at the L_5-S_1 level shows subluxation of the 5th vertebra backward on the sacrum (1) and herniation of disc substance backward into the foramen (2). There is imbrication or telescoping of the posterior joint so that its two articular surfaces (3) no longer register exactly opposite of each other. From the telescoping and the tipping of the sacrum the superior articular process of that structure (4) has become thrust upward and forward into the foramen to impinge against the undersurface of the pedicle where result-ant eburnation has occurred at (6). These four changes have so constricted the foramen that the nerve (5) has become distorted in shape and compressed into the small space above. Since the constriction results in part from disc herniation and ligamentum flavum buckling the radiograph does not truly depict the full extent of the encroachment. This confirms the repeated observation that abnormal changes in morphology encountered upon direct examination of the tissue are invariably more advanced than they appear to be on the radiograph. (Courtesy of the *Journal of the American Medical Association,* the *American Journal of Roentgenology,* and the *Journal of Neurosurgery.*)

→

Fig. XIV:36. Male, seventy, with pain in the lumbar region. This patient has intervertebral foramen encroachment from retro displacement of the vertebral bodies at both the second and third lumbar levels. The third disc is also wedge-shaped with the 4th vertebra tipped on its transverse axis. The 3rd foramen is thus encroached not only by the reverse subluxa-tion but in addition by the 4th superior articular processes which are tipped upward and forward into the opening, similar to XIV:34. The first lumbar disc is also degenerated and thinned but since no vertebral body slipping occurred and the posterior joints did not telescope the first intervertebral foramina remained normal in size and kyphosis developed at that level. (Courtesy of the *American Journal of Roentgenology.*)

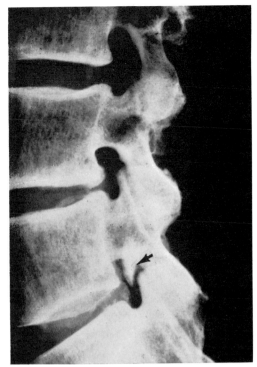

Fig. XIV:35. Encroachment of the 5th lumbar intervertebral foramen by calcified ligamentum flavum projecting downward into the opening. These have been reported by Hilel Nathan as para-articular processes.

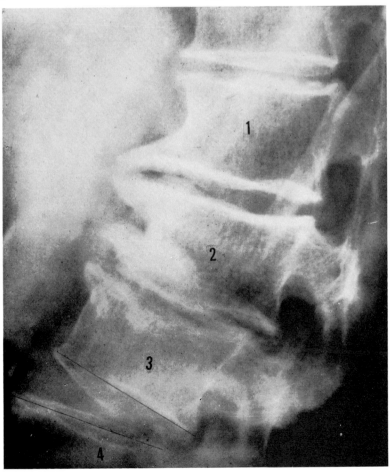

——————————————→

Fig. XIV:37. Lumbar spine studies of the author showing 4th lumbar foramen encroachment. There had been recurrent low back pain with decreasing mobility for many years after heavy lifting. Pain was present in the right hip for one month, six years before the present examination. Then, one week after backstrain and upon sudden twisting a severe pain with muscle spasm occurred in the right thigh and gluteal region. This was disabling and lasted for about one week. The right hip though painful was found to be normal upon x-ray examination and there was no loss of cartilage space, spur formation, eburnation or cystic formation. Later, weakness developed in the right quadriceps muscle with transient, localized, painful spasm of those muscles supplied by the femoral nerve. The patellar reflex was lost and muscle atrophy developed in the thigh. There was also loss of superficial pain sensation in the lower leg and paresthesia behind and below the right knee. Meralgia paresthetica was localized to a small area on the lateral surface, mid portion of the right thigh. The right quadriceps developed a sense of heaviness, weakness and easy fatigability. Transient pain occurred in the region of the right trocaonter anteriorly and posteriorly, especially after walking. There was some return of muscle power subsequently.

The lateral projection (A) shows degenerative thinning of the 4th disc with encroachment of the corresponding foramen *(arrow)*. The 3rd foramen immediately above it is normal in size. The A. P. projection (B) reveals the thinned 4th disc to be wedge shaped with its greater thickness on the left side. As a result the 4th and 5th pedicles *(retouched)* on the right side are somewhat closer than they are on the left. Note the impingement of the 4th and 5th spinous processes *(arrow)* (see Figure IX:5). In the original 80 degrees oblique projection (C) to visualize the right foramina, the openings are normal in size at the 3rd and 5th levels but the 4th foramen is constricted as a result of the thinned disc *(arrow)*. In the same projection (D) the foramina have been accentuated to better demonstrate this difference in their shape and size.

The fourth lumbar root has two main divisions. One of them joins the second and third roots to form the mixed femoral nerve passing downward beneath the inguinal ligament and supplying the anterior portion of the leg. The lower division of the fourth root descends in front of the 5th transverse process to join the 5th root and the sciatic plexus thus supplying motor and sensory innervation to the buttock and posterior leg region.

When present, all of the above mentioned symptoms occurred in various degrees of severity. At times they were only a discomfort, at other times they were most distressing.

These personal observations as well as those reported under Figure XIV:9 were recorded only to illustrate in detail: 1, the insidious onset of symptoms due to degenerative changes; 2, the part played by trauma, even minor injury; 3, the varying degree of severity; 4, the tendency to recurrence and 5, the complete absence, at times, of all symptoms whatsoever. Individuals with roentgenographic evidence of extensive degenerative changes may be entirely asymptomatic at the time of examination. Unfortunately there is no assurance that they will remain in that comfortable condition.

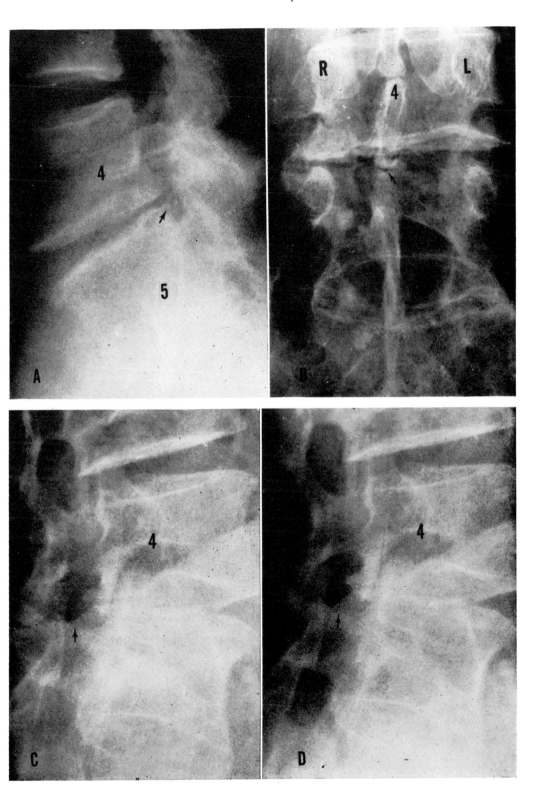

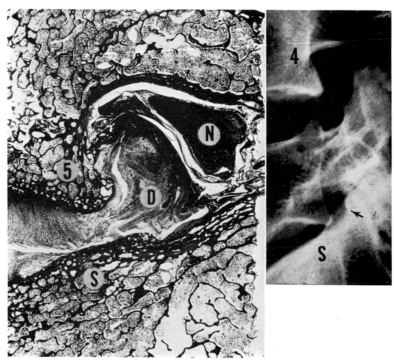

Fig. XIV:38. Enlarged section of an L$_5$ intervertebral foramen. Degeneration of the lumbo-sacral disc with thinning of the structure has allowed approximation of the posterior margin of L$_5$ to the upper surface of the sacrum (S). As a result of pressure at this point a mass of disc substance (D) has been forced backward into the intervertebral foramen. The nerve section (N) has completely lost its surrounding cushion space and has become triangular as a result of pressure from three directions. The original radiograph before section shows the thinned lumbosacral disc with the encroached foramen *(arrow)*. Compare with the normal 4th disc and foramen above. (Courtesy of the *Journal of the American Medical Association,* the *Journal of Neurosurgery,* and the *American Journal of Roentgenology*.)

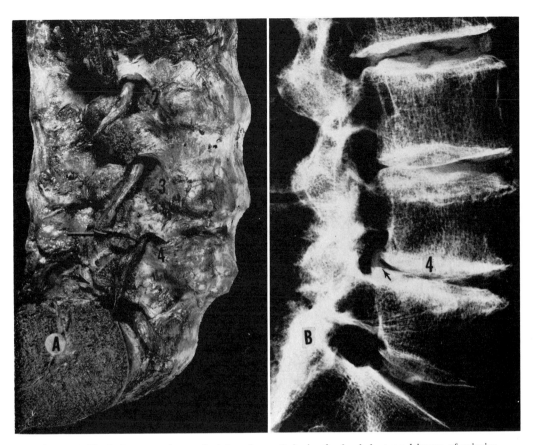

Fig. XIV:39. Cadaver, male, aged eighty-three. Pain in the back but no history of sciatica obtainable. (A) The numerals indicate the posterior portion of each intervertebral disc. This man had a subluxation of the L_4-L_5 posterior articulation with disc encroachment of the 4th foramen. Impingement of the 5th superior articular process against the under-surface of the 4th pedicle is indicated by the large arrow. Articulations and foramina above this point were normal. At the 5th posterior joint there is impingement of the sacral articular process against the undersurface of the 5th pedicle with a small separate intra-articular ossicle as indicated by the small arrowhead. Nerve roots 2, 3 and 5 appear normal and are surrounded within the foramen by a generous cushion space. Nerve root 4, however, is compressed and flattened by a decrease in the size of the foramen incidental to the posterior joint subluxation as well as a posterior herniation of the disc seen just above and behind the numeral 4. Examination of the spinal canal at this level, showed a bulging of the 4th disc substance backward into the canal, displacing the 5th lumbar root. A postmortem myelogram revealed a corresponding filling defect in the oil column. (B) Radiograph of this specimen showing 4th foramen encroachment and herniation of the corresponding 4th disc *(arrow)*. Since, in this individual, the 4th nerve root is distorted by herniated disc substance at the extreme lateral margin of the foramen, an intraspinal operation alone would have been inadequate to relieve the pressure upon this root. Obviously a thorough decompression of the full width of the foramen would have been necessary. (Courtesy of the *Journal of Neurosurgery* and the *American Journal of Roentgenology.*)

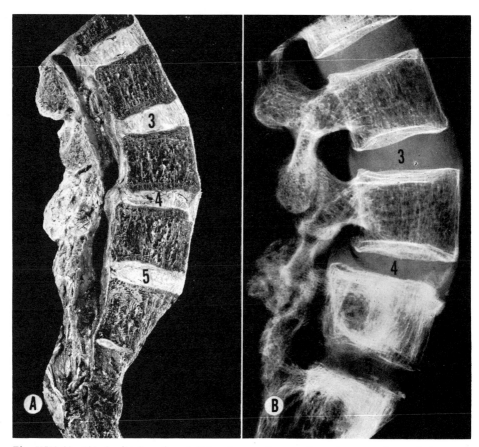

Fig. XIV:40. (A) Sagittal section, left lumbosacral area of a cadaver, male aged sixty-two. Pain in the legs for eight years before death. Bulging of the 4th disc into the spinal canal compressing the 5th lumbar nerve root and encroaching upon the 4th foramen. (B) Roentgenogram of same specimen, discs numbered. Spondylolisthesis of L_4 forward upon L_5 but no break in the neural arch. This may happen when degeneration of the disc and the posterior articulation has taken place. Constriction of the 4th foramen is present. (C) Fourth lumbar ganglion X13 compressed by the 4th foramen encroachment. Many of the large ganglion cells were flattened. (D) Fourth spinal nerve X-18 just distal to the ganglion shown in previous section but slightly greater magnification. Marked flattening of the nerve and its constituent bundles. The foramen encroachment resulted from herniation of disc substance into the opening as shown in (B). Again, operative removal of the herniated 4th disc from this spinal canal for the relief of 5th root pressure would still have left a decreased cushion space for the 4th root where it passes through the foramen. (E) Section of the left 5th lumbar root. This root was compressed between the 4th disc hernia and the dorsal wall of the spinal canal. This section, X650, shows evidence of nerve degeneration one space below the 4th disc herniation. This high power section, distal to the ganglion, shows normal nerve fibers on the right side and the lower left corner. Elsewhere there were patches of degenerative change, vacuolation, also multiple nuclei in the same

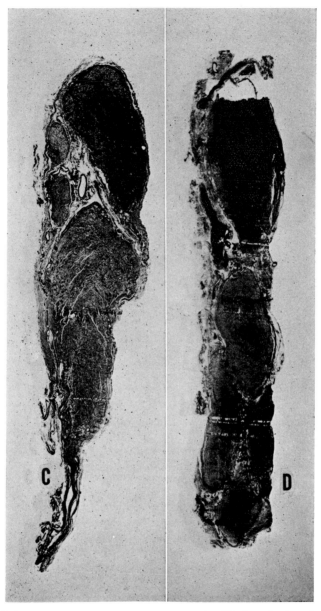

tubule. The 5th foramen was not encroached as seen in (B) but the herniated disc at L_4 pressed firmly against the 5th root. The latter was removed by sharp dissection. The patchy degenerative changes distal to the 5th ganglion here visualized may have resulted from that pressure. (F) Section through the foramina on the right side, same cadaver, showing subluxation, impingement and sclerosis of the 4th posterior articulation *(arrow)*. The 4th foramen of this side also is encroached upon with nerve root distortion while the other right foramina show ample cushion space about the nerve roots. (Courtesy of the *Journal of Neurosurgery* and the *American Journal of Roentgenology*.)

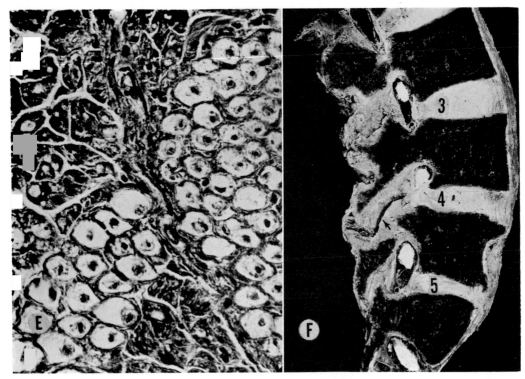

Fig. XIV:40 E & F.

Fig. XIV:41. Left lumbosacral specimen from a male of seventy-five years. This photo and the radiographs (B and C) reveal a degenerative thinning of the 2nd, 4th, and 5th discs with eburnation of the vertebral body surfaces uncushioned by disc substance. There is a resultant imbrication of the posterior articulations with impingement upon adjacent structures *(arrows)*. The 5th intervertebral foramen is encroached and the 5th nerve root was distorted and firmly attached to the vertebral walls by dense fibrous tissue. (D) X7. This section of the 5th lumbar root, removed by sharp dissection, is distal to the ganglion. It shows a concavity from pressure of the 5th intervertebral disc (arrow). Some of the nerve bundles are flattened and there is hyperplasia of the epineurium and perineurium at the upper portion of the root. (E) X48 is a somewhat greater magnification of the field indicated by the circle on section D. Note hyperplasia of fibrous tissue with marked thickening of the perineurium (P). Some of the nerves have been destroyed leaving empty Schwann tubules. A sclerotic intraneural arteriole is seen near the center of the section. (F) Greater magnification X650 of the rectangular field indicated in section E. To the left of the sclerotic arteriole appear two empty Schwann tubules outlined by their neuro-lemma. (G) X650. High power section same nerve but proximal to the ganglion showing evidence of degeneration. Many Schwann tubules are swollen, some are empty and others are filled with multiple rods of Schwann cytoplasm. In one of these tubules nine distinct nuclei are visualized. (H) Section X650 taken from the 5th left motor root lying between the ganglion and the 5th disc. Separation of nerve fibers with the endoneural spaces enlarged suggests edema of the endoneurium. These changes are similar to those reported by Lindblom and Rexed. (Courtesy of the *Journal of Neurosurgery* and the *American Journal of Roentgenology*.)

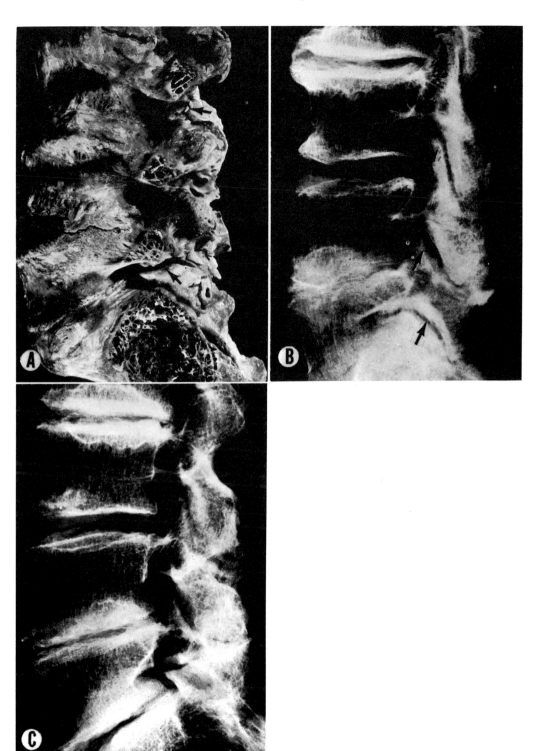

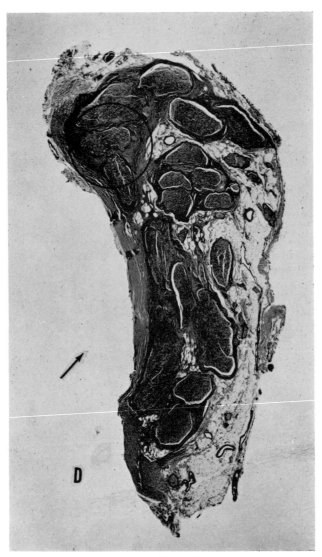

Fig. XIV:41 D.

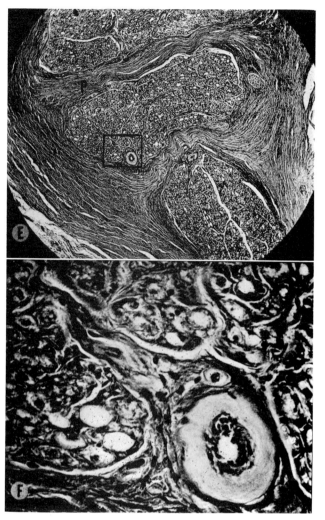

Fig. XIV:41 E & F.

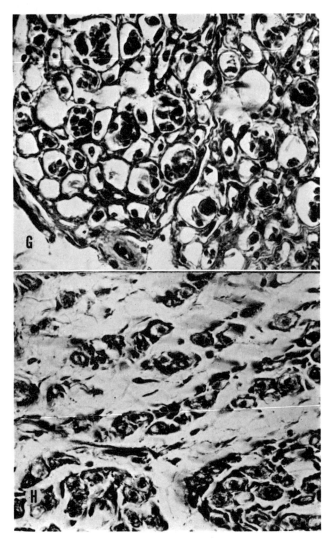

Fig. XIV:41 G & H.

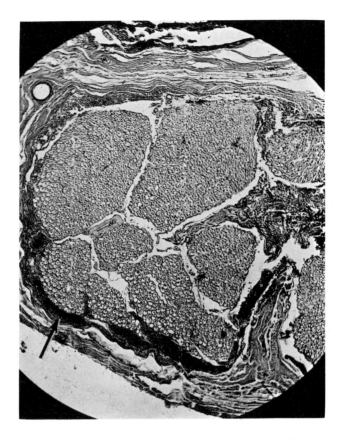

Fig. XIV:42. Male cadaver, aged eighty-five. Fibrotic changes about the nerve roots. Nerves adherent to the foramina. The section is from a lumbar nerve root, X75, showing a nerve bundle surrounded by subperineurial hemorrhage *(arrow)*. (Courtesy of the *Journal of Neurosurgery* and the *American Journal of Roentgenology.*)

Chapter XV

Dysplasias and Disturbances of Bone Formation

Various disturbances of development and nutrition involving the bony and cartilage structures are encountered in early childhood. These are to some extent interrelated and there is some overlapping of the various features ascribed to each. The terms dysplasia, meaning disordered formation and dystrophy or disordered nutrition, are used more or less interchangeably. A multiplicity of confusing synonyms and eponyms has been coined by different authors to designate these disturbances of development. The fundamental feature of the bony dysplasias is a disturbance in coordinating the various processes of bone formation. A brief review of these processes will aid in the consideration of this subject.

NORMAL BONE FORMATION

Skeletal bone may be laid down by endosteal tissue, periosteum, or by enchondral bone production at the epiphyses of growing bones. Resting cartilage cells in the epiphyseal area enlarge in size as growth occurs and become arranged into parallel columns at the epiphyseal line. Loops of blood vessels penetrate this area. Provisional calcification of these columns of cartilage then forms a supporting matrix or scaffold for the development of osteoid tissue by the osteoblasts. Subsequently this osteoid becomes ossified into true bony trabeculae and the calcified cartilage is gradually absorbed. By this process the epiphyseal line advances (Figure XV:1).

Throughout the skeleton, living bone is constantly being destroyed and replaced at all times by the coordinated activity of the osteoclasts and the osteoblasts. During bone growth this osteoclastic—osteoblastic activity produces modeling or tubulation at the metaphysis or that part of the bone adjacent to the epiphysis. This metaphyseal modeling results in the slenderizing and flare of the bone between the shaft and the wider epiphyseal end. Without modeling the end of the bone would be shaped like an Erlenmeyer flask.

The cortical bone of the diaphysis or shaft is laid down by the periosteum in the connective tissue without the interposition of a calcified cartilage matrix formation.

This contributes to increase the diameter of the shaft while enchondral bone growth at the epiphysis increases its length.

Dysplasias result from incoordination of these various processes. Certain of them may prove to be inadequate for proper bone growth. At other times a growth process may even become excessive.

Many factors influence bone formation such as: genetic, familial and hereditary tendencies, various metals and poisonous substances, diet, hormones, vitamines, enzymes, nutrition, metabolism, functional dynamic stresses, pressure, tensions and exposure to radiation.

Because of the peculiar anatomical relationships and functions of the spine, the various dysplasias and dystrophies may affect that structure somewhat differently than they do the skull or long bones.

DYSPLASIA EPIPHYSALIS MULTIPLEX
(HEREDITARY, ENCHONDRAL DYSOSTOSIS)

Multiple epiphyseal dysplasia includes as the name implies a number of different conditions characterized by disturbance of epiphyseal bone growth. Of these, achondroplasia is present at birth while Morquio's disease appears somewhat later. There is a diversity of various skeletal features but these children are all dwarfs. The bones of the extremities are short and sturdy with flaring ends and small or fragmented epiphyses. The epiphyseal zones are wide and ragged. Since the condition is caused by disturbed epiphyseal cartilage development it has been termed dyschondrogenic dwarfism. Kyphosis may be present together with platyspondylia and at times scoliosis.

The essential defect is the failure of the resting cartilage to form regular columns of maturing cartilage cells. For some unknown reason the resting chondrocytes lack either the ability or the stimulus to proliferate at the proper time and to complete their development to the stage of calcification. In addition to the disturbed arrangement of the cartilage cells into columns there are areas of cystic and mucoid degeneration the same as noted in the cartilage from stippled epiphyses, a condition which should also be included in this group (see Figure XV:6).

The shortened longitudinal bone growth results from the slow enchondral growth at the epiphyses and not from inadequate osteoblastic activity.

Periosteal bone growth does not require the provisional calcification of cartilage since the osteoid trabeculae are laid down by the osteoblasts directly in or beneath the fibrous tissue of the periostium. Periosteal growth thus increases the diameter of the bones. This accounts for the disproportionally greater diameter of the extremity bones as compared to their lengths, in these children with multiple epyshyseal displasia. In the skull the undisturbed periosteal growth in the membranous bones of the calvarium together with the restricted enchondral type of growth of the facial bones and base result in the typical large head with the saddle nose so characteristic of these dwarfs. The symptoms of this dysplasia tend to increase until puberty but may improve thereafter if the child survives.

ACHONDROPLASIA

Achondroplasia (chondrodystrophy foetalis) is an epiphyseal dysplasia of enchondral ossification of the fetal skeleton probably of a hereditary or familial character. The condition is present at birth and results in dwarfism as the child grows. This type of dwarf presents a slightly kyphotic torso of normal length, with a flattened chest, marked lumbosacral lordosis and prominent buttocks. The arms and legs are relatively short, especially the upper arms and thighs. The fingers of the so-called trident hand are short and stubby. The head is large,

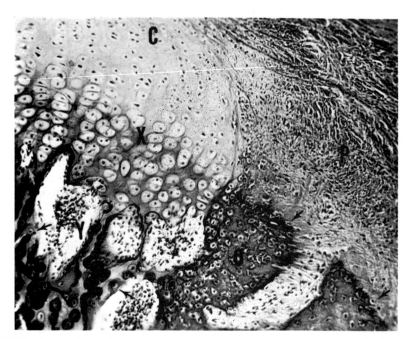

Fig. XV:1. Section from the neural arch of a newborn X160 showing both fibrous and enchondral types of bone production. The periosteum (P) on the right side of the section covers the medial side of the arch. The osteoid tissue (O) has been laid down by the periosteal osteoblasts (*black arrows*). When these cells become entrapped in the bone they constitute the osteocytes. On the left side of the section the enchondral bone production begins at the less mature cartilage cells (C). As the zone of bone growth is approached the cartilage cells become larger and are arranged in columns. Surrounding these columns is an extracellular matrix of cartilage material. This undergoes provisional calcification, shown on this section as a zone of gray with its outer margin at X. This zone of provisional calcification is responsible for the white line seen upon the roentgenogram at the epiphysis. An open space containing marrow cells and blood vessels is seen at Y. These vessels provide the calcium and the osteoblasts. When each cartilage cell reaches full maturity it disintegrates and is promptly invaded by a blood vessel. (*White arrow on extreme left margin of the section.*) Several of these disintegrating cartilage cells are visualized along the margins of the marrow spaces. Much of the calcified intercellular cartilage matrix persists as the provisional trabeculae (Z) and serves as a lattice upon which the osteoblasts lay down sheets of primary osteoid tissue. The enchondral osteoid in this section is shown as small rounded masses surrounding each osteoblast. The black arrows indicate the osteoblasts on both sides. Each side of the neural arch ossifies separately from the vertebral body. The neuro-central union is an enchondral growth center which unites at about the 4th or 5th year (See Figures I:9, I:10 and I:11).

with prominent frontal bosses, and the bridge of the nose is depressed. Four fifths of these children die during the first year but those who survive are usually intelligent and strong. They walk with a waddling gait because of the posterior displacement of the hip joints.

Radiographically, in the lateral projection, the spine presents a long kyphotic curve with marked lumbar lordosis and a horizontal sacrum. The pedicles are short because of delayed enchondral growth at the neuro-central junctions thus reducing the dorso-ventral diameter of the spinal canal to about one half its normal measurement. With the resultant intra spinal crowding, concavities develop on the posterior surfaces of the vertebral bodies.

Since achondroplasia is a disturbance of epiphyseal cartilage formation, these children have a narrow sacrum. That structure develops in width by enchondral growth from four centers at the two sides of the centrum as well as between the ala and the ilium on each side. Since the sacrum is narrow so is the fifth lumbar vertebra and those immediately above it. Normally, the transverse diameter of the spinal canal in the lumbar region increases from above downward. In the achondroplast with his narrowed sacrum however the spinal canal in this region decreases in width as it descends. Neurological symptoms may develop in these patients as a result of the spinal canal constriction in the AP and transverse diameters.

Since ossification of the cartilage plates is delayed, the vertebral bodies may be flat and proportionally smaller than the intervertebral discs. Involvement of the epiphyseal rings of the vertebra results in some distortion of the anterior corners of that structure. They may be irregular or merely rounded off. The achondroplastic spine at times resembles that of Morquio's disease. The curve of the spine, incidental to sitting upright, places additional pressure upon the anterior disc margins. This adds a further burden to the deficient growth activity of these zones and tends to promote the kyphosis. At the lumbo-sacral level likewise the lordosis is probably accentuated by the pressure upon the posterior disc margins.

The sacrum is rotated on a transverse axis passing thru its second segment thus displacing the hip joints backward and increasing the prominence of the buttocks. The body of the ilium immediately above the acetabulum is disproportionally small. This part of the bone develops at the Y cartilage within the acetabulum. As a result of prenatal aplasia at this point the ilium is small at birth and nearly quadrilateral in shape with the upper margin of the acetabulum horizontal. The pubis and ischium are elevated, a condition together with the rotated sacrum producing a constriction of pelvic inlet (Figure XV:3 black arrow). Shortening of the ilium and backward displacement of the hips results in a marked constriction of the sciatic notches.

The ends of the ribs are widened as enchondral growth lags while periosteal growth continues. This combination is likewise responsible for the short thick limb bones with flaring ends. (Figures XV:2 and XV:3).

MORQUIO'S DISEASE

This epiphyseal dysplasia described as a chondro-osteo-dystrophy probably of a familial character, presents certain features suggestive of achondroplasia. However it does not make its appearance until after the child begins to walk.

The kyphotic spine is quite characteristic. The vertebral bodies are flat and wider than normal from periosteal growth which increases their circumference. Their thickness may be even less than that of the intervertebral disc. Normally at three or four years of age the vertebral bodies are usually at least three times as thick as the discs. A bony tongue-like projection may be observed

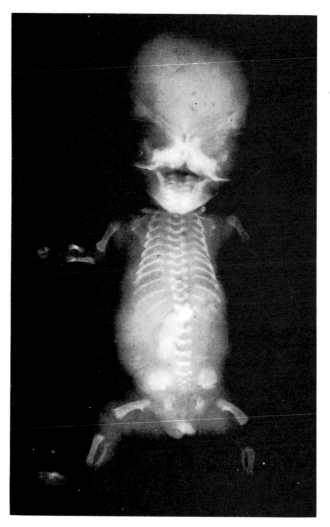

Fig. XV:2. Stillborn achondroplast monster showing the typical short extremity bones of relatively increased diameter. The vertebral bodies are flattened and the quadrilateral iliac bones show small sciatic notches.

Fig. XV:3. Achondroplasia in a female followed for a period of time. At birth (A) the disc spaces are widened. The thoracic vertebrae appear to be essentially normal but the upper lumbar segments present a projection or tongue on their anterior surfaces. The spine is straight. At one year (B) and two years (D) there was a lumbo sacral lordosis and a thoraco-lumbar kyphosis as the baby began to sit upright. Incidental to lessened enchondral growth at the neurocentral junctions, the pedicles are short with a consequent decrease in the dorso-ventral diameter of the spinal canal. Concavities have developed on the posterior surfaces of the vertebral bodies to afford increased space for the neural structures. On the AP projection made at three years (C) one notes that the spinal canal is also narrowed transversely from above downward. Normally the lower spinal canal is widest at the lumbo-sacral level. The ilia are almost quadrilateral in shape since they lack that portion of the bone just above the acetabula. The upper margins of these joint sockets are horizontal. Because the hips are on a posterior plane and the ilia are deficient,

——————————————→

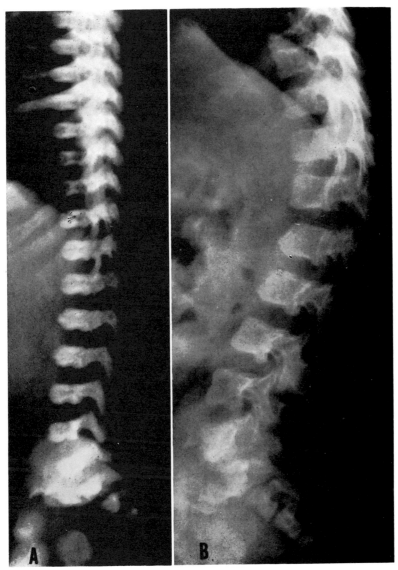

the sciatic notches are narrow *(white arrow)*. The short femoral shafts are thickened and flare widely at their ends since the periosteal bone growth is not affected in this dystrophy. At three years a reexamination showed the kyphosis to be slightly less but she had developed additional lordosis at the lumbo-sacral level.

At five years the kyphosis had completely disappeared but the lordosis and prominence of the buttocks had materially increased and the concavities had increased posteriorly on the vertebral bodies. At that time the epiphyseal development was essentially normal but with widening at the ends of the long bones. The teeth were normally developed for the age. The child had a large head with depressed nasal bridge, wide set eyes clear corneas and a large tongue. The chest was small and the extremities short and sturdy. The hands were broad and still showed the "trident" form (Inset C). The appearance of the fingers and of the ends of the long bones results from an accelerated periosteal bone growth while the enchondral bone growth at the epiphyses is delayed. (Courtesy of the Memorial Hospital, Syracuse, New York.)

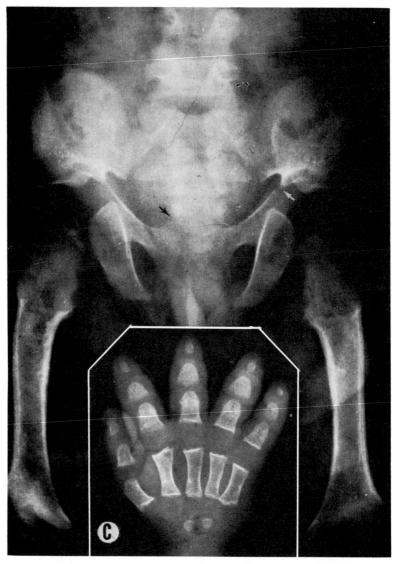

Fig. XV:3 C.

extending outward from the anterior surface of certain of the vertebrae. The kyphosis with resultant increased pressure upon the anterior margins of the vertebral bodies tends to promote an increase of the wedging. In many cases the curvature is also increased by a small vertebral body at the thoraco-lumbar level which may be displaced backward (Figure XV:4).

Pathologically the disturbance is a defective enchondral ossification at the epiphyseal line resulting in delayed bone formation. Some mucoid degeneration of the cartilage has been reported. The etiology is unknown. The marginal bony rings of the vertebral secondary ossification centers may not develop at all. Consequently if the child lives to adult life the corners of the vertebral bodies may appear notched like the preadolescent vertebrae of a normal child.

These children are dwarfed by the shortened kyphotic spine and shortened flexed extremities. The picture is that of a feeble kyphotic individual, usually of normal intelligence with head thrust foreward and narrow pigeon breast (pectus carniatum). They experience difficulty in walking. The joints may be large and stiff or in other cases the ligaments are lax allowing hypermotility. The acetabulae may be enlarged with fragmentation or irregularity of the capital epiphyses and even dislocation of the hip joints. There is coxa vara and genu valgum. The general condition is usually progressive with increasing disability (Figure XV:5).

STIPPLED EPIPHYSES

Stippled epiphyses, known as chondro-dystrophia punctata and under various other terms is characterized by multiple small calcific deposits within the

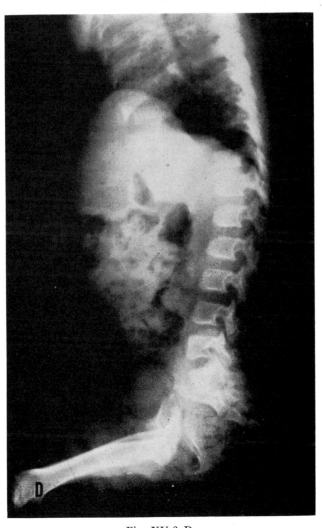

Fig. XV:3 D.

epiphyseal cartilages. The condition is present at birth but most of these children die within the first year, few reaching adolescence. In those who do survive, the calcific flecks gradually become fewer as normal ossification of the epiphyseal cartilage occurs. The vertebral bodies may be wedge shaped with a thoracic kyphosis and a lumbo-sacral lordosis. Various features of the disease suggest a relationship to achondroplasia. The dwarfism with short extremity

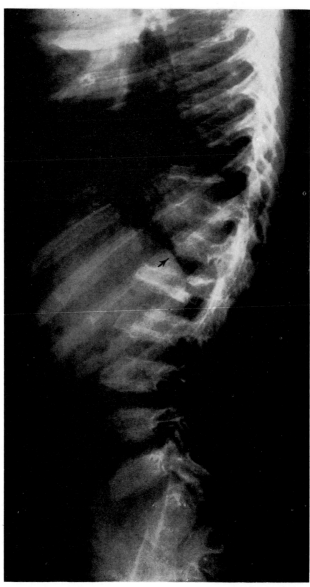

Fig. XV:4. Female five years old with Morquio's disease. The vertebral bodies are flattened but increased in their AP diameter. The discs are widened. There is a small twelfth thoracic vertebral body at the apex of the kyphosis somewhat similar to that seen in gorgoylism *(arrow)*. As in achondroplasia, there are concavities on the posterior surfaces of the lumbar vertebrae however lordosis with prominent buttocks is not present. (Courtesy of the Children's Hospital Home, Utica, New York.)

bones flaring at their ends and the cartilage destruction are suggestive of that
condition.

Harris compared the pathological
processes of achondroplasia and stippled
epiphyses. In both conditions he found

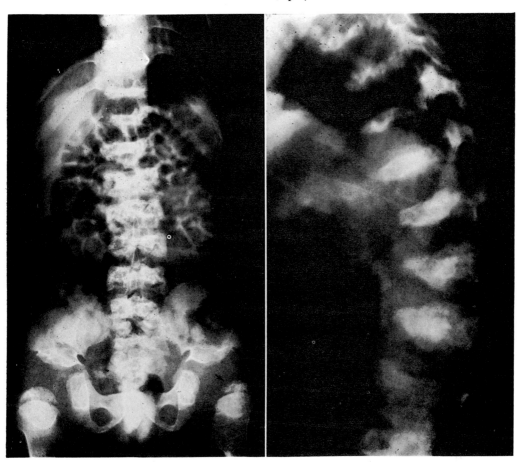

Fig. XV:5. Chondroosteodystrophy in a male showing features of both achondroplasia
and Morquio's disease somewhat complicated by the administration of steroids. The child,
only one year old, was large for his age, already showing the bone development of three or
four years. The hormone therapy had induced secondary sex changes indicative of precocious puberty.

Early appearance of the kyphosis and other symptoms together with short thighs and
arms and a large head favored a diagnosis of achondroplasia. Also this type of vertebral
body distortion may occasionally be encountered in that disease. However his flattened
vertebral bodies with large immovable joints, pectus carniatum and small buttocks were
more characteristic of Morquio's Disease. The spine and chest were rigid and resulted in
chronic lung changes which resulted in death at the age of three years.

Note the wide flattened vertebrae with a bony tongue projecting from the anterior
surface. The thoracic discs are much thicker than the centra. Wedging is present with
kyphosis. It is possible to visualize a zone of less dense bone surrounding the original more
dense vertebral bodies, the os in os. This reaction may be the result of the hormone therapy.
The acetabulae are thrust inward and distorted. The femoral epiphyses are fragmented
(*arrow*). There is narrowing of the sacrum and the pubis is elevated. (Courtesy of the
Memorial Hospital, Syracuse.)

a mucoid degeneration of the cartilage and a failure of the cartilage cells to become rearranged into linear columns as they do normally adjacent to the epiphyseal line. These patchy irregular areas of mucoid degeneration may become invaded by blood vessels and fibrous tissue or they may become calcified and undergo irregular bone formation (Figure XV:6).

Any of the cartilages may be involved, even the trachea or thyroid cartilage. The cause is unknown although various stigmata are reported. Congenital cataracts are said to be present in about thirty per-cent of the cases. There may be mental retardation, deformities and failure to thrive. The patient here reported was the victim of congenital lues.

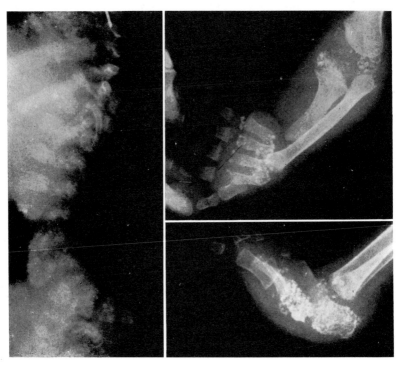

Fig. XV:6. Chondrodystrophia punctata or stippled epiphyses in an infant of eight months. There were small dense calcific deposits in all of the cartilages. The film revealed a diminutive tenth thoracic vertebral body with kyphosis and lumbo-sacral lordosis. The spinal curvatures together with the short extremities suggest a relationship to achondroplasia. The child was luetic. There were nine living siblings without evidence of similar disease. Two other siblings had died of broncho pneumonia.

The photo micrograph X52 shows a full thickness of the cartilaginous epiphysis from the pericrondrium (PC) to the bone (B). The arrows indicate areas of cartilage degeneration. On the right is an oval shaped mass of embryonal cartilage (EC). The irregular dark shadows at various points indicate calcific deposits within the areas of degenerated cartilage. On the extreme left border of the section at C, is an area of embroyonal cartilage which is undergoing calcification. The cartilage cells about this area have become slenderized and arranged into ray-like formation. The cartilage cells at the epiphyseal line adjacent to the bone (X) have not become organized into the usual columns which are normally present at zones of enchondral bone formation. None of the invading blood vessels described by Harris were identified in this specimen. (Courtesy of Dr. Howard Ferguson, Pathologist).

GARGOYLISM

Hurler's disease, gargoylism or lipo-chondrodystrophy is another form of disturbed cartilage and bone development. In this hereditary condition with a familial tendency the faulty osteogenic process is complicated by a disturbed lipoid metabolism. Lipoid deposits are found in the brain, liver, spleen, cornea, chondrocytes and other fibrous elements.

The patients are unable to metabolize compounds of high molecular weight and as a result several complex substances, lipids, polysaccharides and others are formed and become stored in the body tissues. The osteoblasts and chondrocytes become swollen, vacuolated and filled with granular material. This meta-bolic defect results in the restriction of cartilage proliferation, bone formation and the other body changes characteristic of the disease. There is likewise a faulty osteogenesis of membranous or periosteal bone.

The clinical picture of this condition is that of a kyphotic dwarf with a large head, wide spaced eyes, broad nose, thick lips and coarse heavy features (gorgoyle facies). Corneal opacities, hepato-spleno-meglia, and mental retardation usually result from the abnormal deposits of lipoid material. The limbs are of normal length but are half flexed and restricted in movement which contributes to the lessened stature.

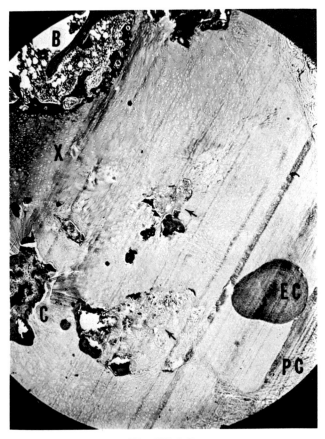

Fig. XV:6 B.

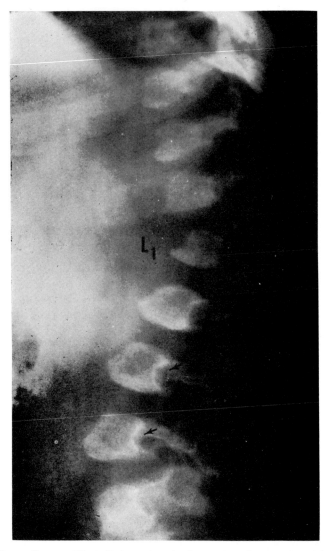

Fig. XV:7. Gargoylism or Hurler's in a female five years of age. The child showed the clinical picture of the disease. Note the backward displacement of the small L$_1$ vertebral body with the typical beak-like projection from its lower anterior margin at the kyphotic angle. The anterior longitudinal ligament is not well attached to this vertebra wherefore it is less well stabilized and becomes displaced backward.

The lower lumbar bodies are bullet-nosed and their posterior surfaces are concave like those of achondroplasia *(arrows)*. Note the widened ribs. Roentgenograms of the upper extremities indicate delayed ossification for a child of five years. Epiphyseal growth is retarded. A radiolucent area of unossified cartilage is present at the lower end of each ulna. The wrist joints are tipped toward the ulnar side. The metacarpals are widened, cystic, distorted in shape and pointed at their proximal ends. The entire appearance is that of enchondral bone growth disturbance rather than periosteal. (Compare with Figure XV:3). (Courtesy of the x-ray Department, New York State School at Rome, New York.)

————————————⟶

Most of the vertebral bodies tend to be somewhat convex on their upper and lower surfaces with the discs biconcave and not particularly increased in thickness. At the level of the kyphosis there are one or two vertebral bodies which are deficient in their upper anterior borders. These are concave in front and develop a hook-like projection from their lower anterior borders resembling in shape that of a wooden shoe. These "beaked" vertebrae are strongly suggestive of gargoylism but may also be encountered in cretinism or following heavy radiation therapy to the spinal area. The smaller vertebral body at the apex of the angle may lack stability. Because not attached to the anterior longitudinal ligament it becomes displaced backward and appears to have been squeezed out of line. Flexion-extension studies show much greater movement at this level (see Figures XV:7, XV:8, and XV:9).

Children who develop gargoylism appear normal at birth but, as in Morquio's disease, the clinical picture develops during the first year or two. Hur-

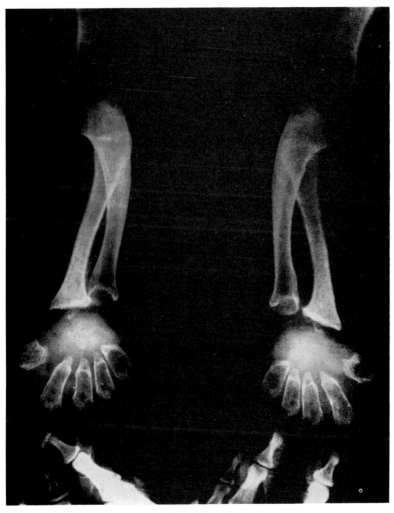

Fig. XV:7 B.

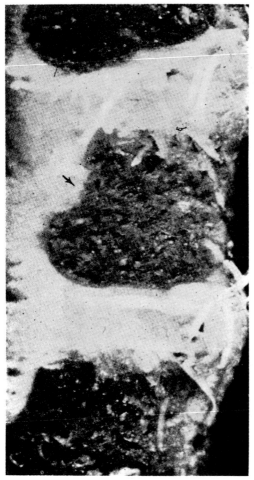

Fig. XV:8. Sagittal section of L$_2$ from a three year old female with gargoylism. There was a history of consanguinous parentage. The concavity on the anterior border was filling in with thick collagen fibers. Adjacent to the cortex was a layer of the large swollen vacuolated cells typical of Hurler's disease. These appeared to exert an osteoclastic activity, penetrating the cortex to give it the eroded concave border (*arrow*). The cartilage of the inferior epiphyseal plate extended forward beneath the under surface of the "beak." A combination of the osteoclastic activity of the vacuolated cells above, and the enchondral bone production below, tended to produce an enlargement of the beak but added little to the height of the vertebral body. This combination also partially explains the smaller size of the "wooden shoe" shaped vertebra at the apex of the spinal curve. (Compare with Figure XV:7.) (Courtesy of Dr. Lotte Strauss,

ler's is the result of defective lipoid metabolism and the severe ossification disturbance. Few of these children live to reach adulthood. There is an increased deposit of subperiosteal bone which causes an uneven thickening of the long bones and ribs. However adjacent to the spine the ribs are slender. They have been described as shaped like a canoe paddle. Unlike Morquio's the epiphyses are not enlarged but they may be tilted. The iliac bones of Hurler's and cretinism are slender with coxa valga while the pelvis seen in patients with Morquio's disease and achondroplasia presents a quadralateral shape with wide ilia and coxa vara. In all of these conditions however the metacarpals and phalanges are increased in diameter as a result of periosteal bone formation.

As mentioned above, the vertebrae subjected in early life to radiation therapy in excess of 2000r subsequently develope deformities quite similar to those noted in Hurler's disease. The spines of cretins likewise may reveal the kyphosis and wooden shoe type of deformity characteristic of gargoylism. Apparently lipid substances, radiation and hypothyroidism exert a somewhat similar deterrent effect upon the growth of these structures. Possibly disturbances of blood supply may be a factor.

The spinal augulation of the various dysplasias above mentioned as well as the "jackknife" compression fracture, seem to occur most commonly at the thoraco-lumbar level. This straight area of the spine between the thoracic and lumbar curves, unbraced by the rib structures, is apparently inadequate to withstand these unusual flexion stresses.

Mount Sinai Hospital, New York, and the *American Journal of Pathology.*

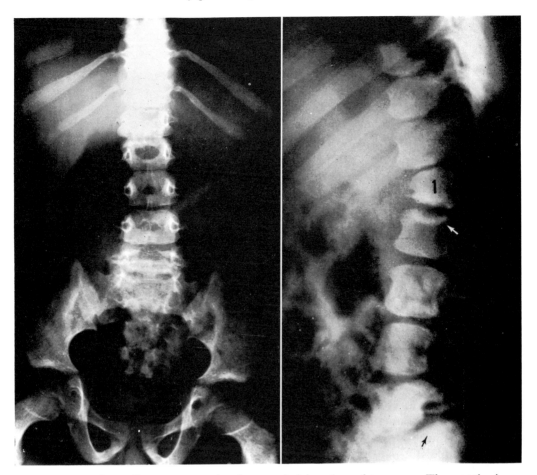

Fig. XV:9. Gargoylism at a somewhat later period in a boy of ten years. The vertebral bodies are biconvex with relatively thin biconcave discs. The L_1 vertebra at the apex of the kyphosis is small and displaced backward. The posterior surfaces of the lumbar bodies are somewhat concave. There is a reaction of the first lumbar disc involving the adjacent vertebral bodies *(white arrow),* possibly in the nature of a lipoid deposite epiphysitis. The ribs are coarse and thick but slender at their posterior margins (canoe paddle ribs). The innominate bones of the pelvis are slender and the acetabulae bulge inward slightly together with coxa valgus deformity of the hip joints. Compare these with the pelvis seen in Morquio's disease or achondroplasia Figure XV:3. In those conditions the pelvis is more quadrilateral in form. There is a break in the L_5 neural arch with spondylolisthesis *(black arrow).* (Courtesy of the x-ray Department, New York State School, Rome, New York.)

The dysplasias and dystrophies of childhood reveal a combination of various growth disturbances. Relationships exist and overlapping is present. The achondroplast shows the typical features of his condition at birth and his dwarfism is due to the lordosis and the short-ened extremities rather than kyphosis. On the other hand, Gargoylism and Morquio's disease, both kyphotic, appear in the early years of childhood. The full blown clinical picture of these two latter diseases also differs materially. However in a given individual certain features of his particular condition may be lacking and confusion may easily arise. It may be difficult or impossible to differentiate by the roentgenograms alone, making it necessary to depend upon the clinical picture and the laboratory findings.

HYPOPHOSPHATASIA

Hypophosphatasia seen at birth or in early childhood is a condition of deficient calcification of the bony structures caused by inadequate alkaline phosphatase. This enzyme is necessary to activate the calcification of the osteoid into bone. It is elaborated by the osteoblasts. In this disease these cells seem to produce sufficient osteoid tissue but they are incapable of producing adequate phosphatase, hence the deficient production of true calcified bone. The etiology is unknown but there is probably a genetic factor with some familial manifestation. If present in the new born all the bones are soft and calcified poorly or not at all. These little ones invariably succumb. When the disease appears later in infants the prognosis is better. It is then characterized by widening and irregularity of the epiphyseal lines and the cranial sutures. Angulations and infractions of the long bones develop at this time. Somewhat later there is a spotty mottled sclerosis of the small ossification centers as growth becomes established. Because of residual islands of uncalcified cartilage and osteoid tissue the metaphyses develope a mottled or streaked appearance as growth and healing occur. Premature closure of the skull sutures and loss of the deciduous teeth are features of the disease. Thoraco-lumbar kyphosis is observed. The vertebral epiphyses at first show a peculiar double layer of spotty calcification adjacent to the intervertebral discs. Later, however, the vertebral body presents a rounded bullet-nosed configuration similar to that seen in achondroplasia (Figures XV:10 and XV:11 and XV:12).

OSTEOGENESIS IMPERFECTA

Osteogenesis imperfecta or fragile bones is a condition of defective bone formation encountered in early life and characterized by soft, brittle bones which either bend or fracture easily. In about one fourth of the cases there is a familial or hereditary factor. In this group particularly, in addition to the fragility there is a high incidence of deafness and blue sclerotics. The sclera and the skin are abnormally thin.

The fundamental defect is a lack of adequate osteoblastic activity for some unknown cause. The cartilaginous matrix forms normally in this disease and provisional calcification occurs in the usual manner. However there is a paucity of osteoblasts to form the osteoid trabeculum, so that bone formation is delayed in its final stage. If osteoblasts are present in adequate numbers they remain inactive. Periosteal formation is also deficient because of the lack of osteoblasts.

There are two general types of osteogenesis imperfecta, the prenatal and the childhood or tarda variety. The prenatal type, which may even be visualized in utero, is characterized by short, thick extremity bones showing fractures in various stages of healing. It is said to be the healing of these intrautrine fractures which is responsible for the thickness of the extremity bones at this time. The

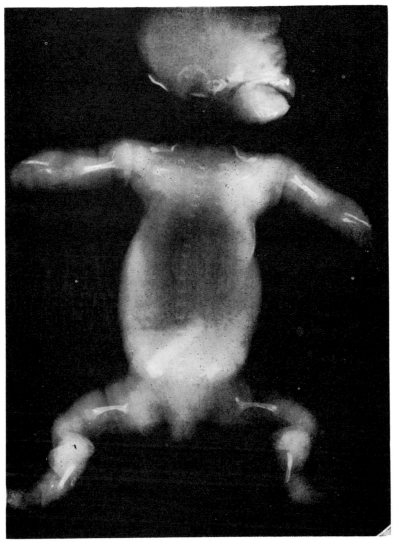

Fig. XV:10. Hypophosphatasia in a still born infant at term. Ossification centers are present for the thoracic, lumbar and sacral bodies but the neural arches and most of the cervical segments have not yet appeared. Compare with the normal fetus at ten weeks gestation (Figure I:7). Except for the frontal ossification centers the calvarium was entirely boneless and the fetus was practically without skeletal structure. Note multiple curves in the lower extremities. (This individual was mentioned as case three by Currarino and Neuhauser: *A.J.R., 78:392.* Courtesy of Dr. Paul Riemenschneider, Memorial Hospital, Syracuse, New York.)

ribs have a peculiar crinkled appearance due to the multiple healed fractures of those structures. The prenatal is the more serious type and nearly all of these children die within the first year. Those who do survive, together with others who appeared normal at birth, develope the childhood type of fragilitas ossium. This is characterized by slender, curved extremities and is the osteogenesis imperfecta tarda. This type may also be encountered in the adult. Since the epiphyseal activity is relatively normal in this condition, the extremity bones are of normal length but curved and slender in the shafts. Their ends are enlarged and because of deficient periosteal bone growth the cortex is thin and delicate. Fractures are frequent. They may be spontaneous and cause little pain, but

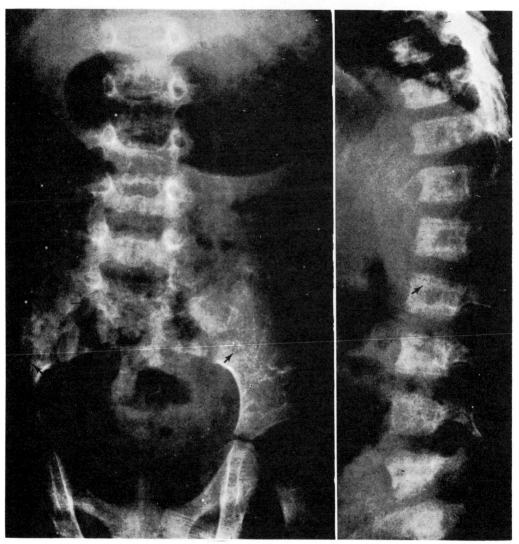

Fig. XV:11. Hypophosphatasia in a male infant one and one-half years of age. The spotty shadows at the vertebral epiphyses and the sacroiliac regions resulted from improper ossification (*black arrows*). The osteoid tissue does not form bone because of inadequate alkaline phosphatase. At this age the vertebral bodies have a mottled double-layer appearance at the epiphyses. Later they assume the rounder "bullet-nosed" configuration seen in achondroplasia. There is minimal kyposis at L_1 and the lumbosacral curve is flattened. In this child the serum calcium and phosphorus were normal but the alkaline phosphatase was diminished. Cartilage or uncalcified osteoid tissue entrapped at the ends of certain long bones during growth had produced streaks or patches of uncalcified bone (*white arrows*). At reexamination one year later the epiphyseal line had moved leaving these radiolucencies entrapped in bone farther from the epiphyses.

(Courtesy of the Memorial Hospital, Syracuse, New York.)

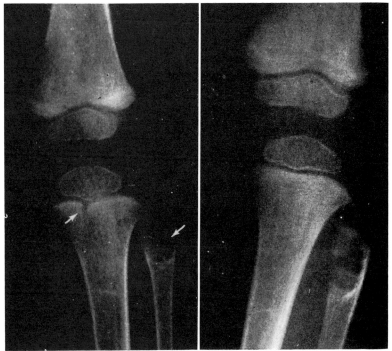

Fig. XV:11 B.

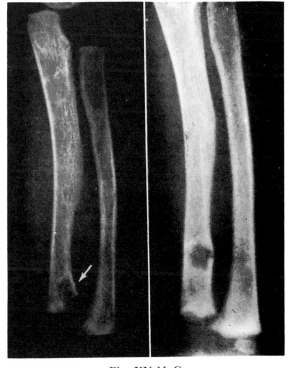

Fig. XV:11 C.

they heal readily for some unknown reason in spite of the disordered bone formation. Osteoporosis is general with decreased trabeculation. The vertebral bodies become compressed, flattened and wider than normal. Some of them may be wedge shaped and the child developes a curvature of the spine. The vertebral bodies may be actually thinner than the discs or even disappear altogether. However if the vertebral height is maintained the bulging biconvex discs expand into the osteoporotic vertebrae. Dwarfism may be caused by the shorter spine and the curved extremities with relaxed ligaments and poor muscular development (Figures XV:13 and XV:14).

MULTIPLE ENCHONDROMATOSIS
(DYSCHONDROPLASIA-OLLIER'S DISEASE)

This condition is a dysplasia characterized by masses of uncalcified hyaline cartilage within the metaphyses of multiple long bones. Ollier in 1898 considered the condition to be a primary disturbance of fetal growth with delayed ir-

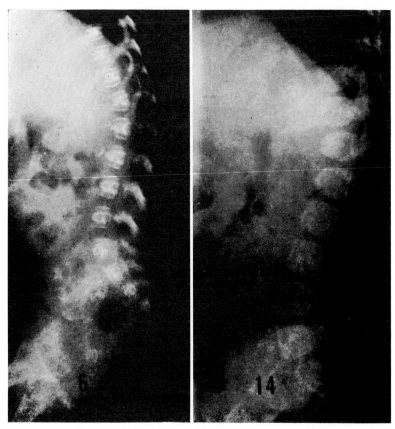

Fig. XV:12. Hypophosphatasia in a female child at six months and at fourteen months. The serum alkaline phosphatase in this child and both parents was consistently low. She succumbed at two and one half years. On the earlier film there are bands of uncalcified tissue adjacent to the zone of provisional calcification at each epiphyseal plate. Eight months later these are still faintly seen. *(arrow)*. The later vertebrae resemble those seen in the chondrodysplasias and hypothyroidism. (Courtesy of Dr. L. Luzzetti, Dr. E. B. D. Neuhauser, and the *American Journal of Roentgenology*.)

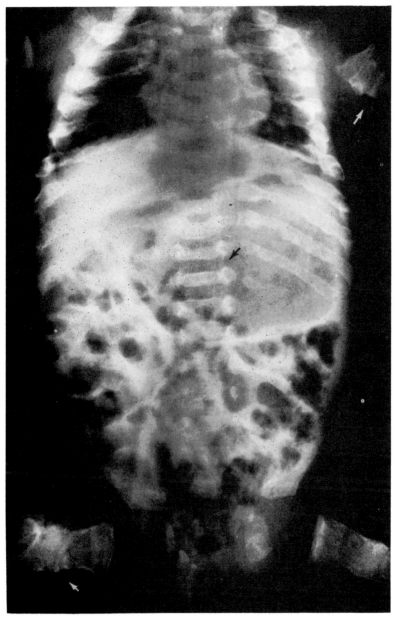

Fig. XV:13. Osteogenesis imperfecta of the prenatal type in an infant one month old. The femurs and humeri are short, thickened and wrinkled with multiple fractures *(white arrows)*. The short thickened appearance of these bones at birth differs materially from the long slender curved extremity bones noted in the "tarda" type of this disease. Multiple healed fractures of the ribs give them a crinkled appearance. The vertebral bodies are thinned, flattened and widened *(black arrow)*. The child was born prematurely with multiple fractures and a soft skull. The Wasserman test was negative but there were multiple hereditary stigmata with some question as to the child's paternity. Both the mother and grandmother were of subnormal mentality and the latter had given birth to an infant with a similar condition eight months before. (Courtesy of the Memorial Hospital, Syracuse, New York.)

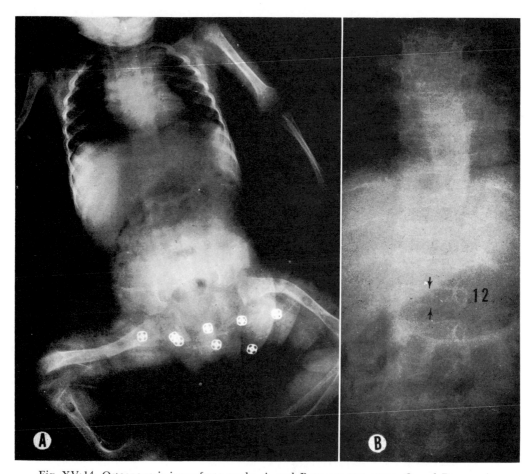

Fig. XV:14. Osteogenesis imperfecta tarda, A and B at age two years, C and D same individual at ten years of age. There was a generalized porosity of all bones with softening and multiple deformities. The child had blue sclera and platyspondylia at two years (B) with vertebral bodies and discs about the same thickness. The arrows indicate the thickness of T12 at that time. The child had a history of multiple fractures. When reexamined at ten years there was a marked bowing of the extremities. The spine length, occiput to sacrum, was only approximately the same as it had been eight years before. Note the protrusion of the hips inward *(white arrow C)*. This disease is the result of inadequate osteoblastic activity while the osteoclastic process continues. As a result the vertebral bodies are affected but not the intervertebral discs. As the child's vertebrae had collapsed the discs had expanded proportionally and the spinal canal had thus maintained its same length. In the lateral projection at ten years (D) the black arrows indicate the corresponding vertebral bodies. Some of these such as L_2, L_3, and L_4 are biconcave and considerably flattened. Others, including T12 are completely destroyed, there remaining only a white line indicating the two cortical plates in contact. Compare with the same T_{12} of eight years before as indicated by the distance between the two arrow points in B. The intervertebral discs have become tremendously enlarged proportionally, to reach a thickness in some cases many times that of the adjacent vertebral bodies. Radiographs B and D are reproduced at normal size. (Courtesy of the University Hospital and Dr. Mark Harwood, Syracuse, N. Y.)

regular ossification at the epiphyseal cartilage. New masses of cartilage, appearing as radiolucent streaks, evolve from the epiphyseal plate and extend into the marrow cavity of the diaphysis without forming true bone. This formation continues and the growth lengthens until the epiphyses close. Normal ossification is hindered for some unknown reason. The hyaline cartilage proliferates at the periphery, expanding and thinning the cortex. The cartilage masses may later undergo mucoid degeneration and subsequently show irregular speckled calcification. Even malignant changes may occur.

Usually, tho not always, the condition is unilateral, involving the long bones and producing a shortening of the extremities on one side. This shortening may even be present at birth. The skull, ribs and pelvis may be involved but the vertebrae as in this patient is only rarely the site of enchondromatosis (Figure XV:15). The condition is probably congenital and familial in character.

Various biopsy studies have shown large masses and columns of a typical unossified hyaline cartilage without evidence of the normal provisional calcification. Uncalcified osteoid or cartilage is not readily resorbed, apparently calcification is necessary for that process to occur.

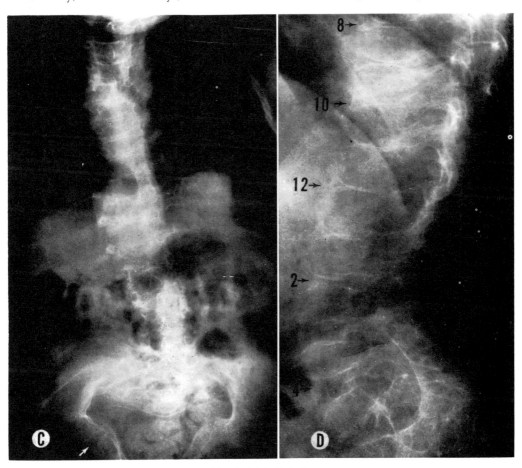

Fig. XV:14 C & D.

There is usually fibrosis of the bone marrow.

The actively growing generalized enchondromatosis has not usually shown evidence of malignant change except those accompanied by hemangiomata, the so-called Moffucci's syndrome. However the multiple as well as the solitary enchondromata may change to a chondrosarcoma.

The serum calcium, phosphorous and phosphatase levels are essentially within normal limits. Pathological frac-

tures may occur. These patients are usually of normal mentality and healthy but may suffer inconvenience from the unilateral short limbs. Cases have been observed into the sixth decade.

Familial exostoses, multiple hereditary osteochondromata, or diaphyseal aclasis has been considered a form of external dyschondroplasia projecting from the surface near the ends of the bones. However Jaffe was unable to find any relationship between exostoses and enchondromatosis.

OSTEOPETROSIS
(MARBLE BONES, ALBERS-SCHÖNBERG'S DISEASE)

This disease is characterized by a greatly increased density involving all bones of the body. It may be prenatal, occur in early childhood, or later. The cause is unknown but there has been a heredofamilial factor in about half the cases reported with consanguinity in a fifth of these. Prognosis in the early cases is poor. These children usually die but if the child survives until his bones become larger he may live a normal expectancy.

The critical defects are an overgrowth and persistence of excess perio-

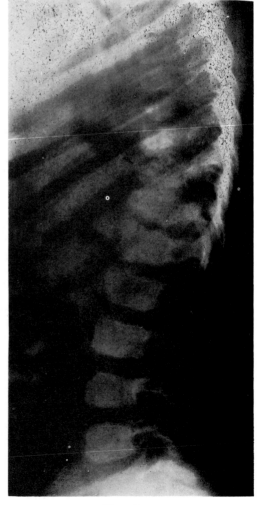

Fig. XV:15 A.

---------------→

Fig. XV:15. Enchondromatosis in a male of three years involving principally the extremities on the left side and the spine. Bone formation has been deficient because the cartilage failed to undergo provisional calcification. The masses of cartilage extend from the epiphyseal growth zone into the metaphysis. Enchondral bone growth is disturbed with a consequent shortening of the involved extremities. The epiphyses appear to be intact at this time but may become involved later after fusion occurs.

The spine is not usually involved in this process, however in this individual the cartilaginous masses have practically replaced the eleventh vertebra producing a kyphosis at that level *(arrow)*. Other vertebrae are involved to a lesser extent. (Courtesy Dr. E. B. D. Neuhauser, Boston.)

steal and enchondral bone, calcified cartilage matrix and excess osteoid. There is also a failure of the normal osteoclastic resorption process. Primary spongiosa remains and the new deposite continues as density builds up. The osteoblasts are normal or increased while the osteoclasts are diminished or absent entirely. The long bones appear dense and club shaped. The normal modeling at the metaphyses does not occur because of inadequate resorption by the osteoclasts.

The medullary cavities may be completely filled in with bone or fibrous tissue so that anaemia is a serious complication especially for the younger child. Sclerosis of the skull base and foramen encroachment may result in optic atrophy or deafness.

Macroscopically the bones are said to be heavy, hard, dense and in some cases brittle. They may or may not fracture. Some patients have shown multiple fractures, others infractions (incomplete fractures) while many patients do not sustain fractures at all.

The vertebral bodies may appear as solid bone, without trabeculae. In other

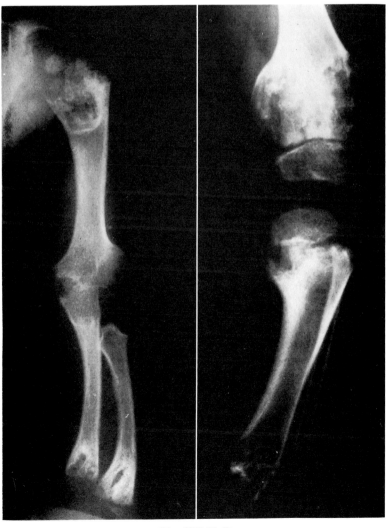

Fig. XV:15 B.

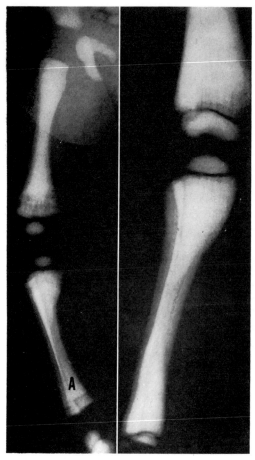

patients the vertebrae present a banded appearance. Cohen described the section of a vertebra from a child of thirty-two months as composed of two different colored hard materials. One a firm white component in the shape of an hour glass and the other a reddish, hard bony ring surrounding it (Figures XV:16 and Figure XV:17).

Transverse bands and concentric rings as seen in the ilia indicate the re-

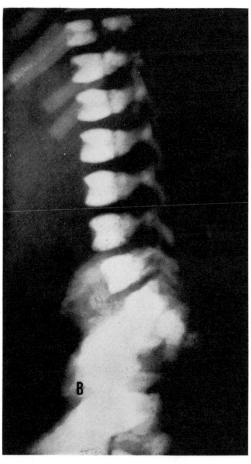

Fig. XV:16. Osteopetrosis. A, shows the lower right extremity in a female child at three months and at three and one-half years. Note the generalized increased density of all the bones and the epiphyses as indicating calcific deposit and accentuated activity of the osteoblasts. The medullary cavities are obliterated. There is some periosteal bone production along the tibial and femoral shafts on the earlier film. On the other hand, activity of the osteoclasts has been inadequate. The bones are club-shaped because modeling or tubulation has not occurred at the metaphyses. The medullary cavities are obliterated since the endosteal bone formation has not been balanced by the proper osteoclastic activity. Striations adjacent to the epiphyseal lines indicate a persistence of the primary uncalcified trabeculae.

B. A lateral projection of the spine shows the vertebral bodies to be almost solid bone. Cohen has reported that section of such a vertebra showed it to be composed of a dense white ma-

terial surrounded by a hard reddish bony ring. Sections have shown the architecture distorted, with the trabeculae greatly increased and irregular in formation. Note the enlarged ribs of ground glass appearance and the dense pelvic bones. Normal bony trabeculae are not visualized on the roentgenograms. (Courtesy of Dr. Edward Neuhauser, Boston, Mass.)

missions and exacerbations of the disease while the longitudinal striations noted in the long bones are an evidence of retained primary trabeculae.

Various authors have postulated a relationship between osteopetrosis, melorheostosis, osteopoikilosis and diaphyseal dysplasia or Englemann's disease. Certain features of these are shared in common but there is no definite proof of such a relationship. The question must await a better understanding of these different conditions. In the older patient some confusion may arise with Paget's disease. Osteosclerosis from the various poisonings by lead, phosphorous, bismuth or fluorine may require differentiation.

DIAPHYSEAL DYSPLASIA
(ENGLEMANN'S DISEASE)

This condition appearing in early childhood is characterized by fusiform enlargement and sclerotic changes involving the midshafts of the long bones. The etiology is unknown and there is no obvious heredofamilial factor.

These frail, poorly nourished, underdeveloped children with weak muscle tone complain of pains in the legs, walk with a peculiar gait and tire easily.

The condition shown by the roentgenograms is bilateral and symmetrical but without epiphyseal involvement. The cortex of the diaphysis is thickened and sclerotic. There is both subperiosteal and endosteal development of dense bone, the latter being responsible for some encroachment upon the medullary canal. Serial studies over a period of years have shown progressive extension along the shafts. Deficient osteoclastic activity is evidenced by inadequate metaphyseal modeling and narrowing of the medullary cavity.

Changes of a somewhat different character are notable in the small cuboid bones, the epiphyses and the vertebrae. In these locations the structures are traversed by coarse trabeculae corresponding in direction to the lines of force (Figure XV:18). Spinal involvement below the cervical region is not usually considered to be a feature of diaphyseal dysplasia. In fact heavy trabeculation such as visualized in this patient does not fit the appelation of that disease. However if such heavy trabeculation is encountered in roentgenograms of the spine a survey of the long bones is indicated.

Various histological studies have shown a diffuse, hard, dense, cortical hyperostosis of normally laminated bone with both osteoblastic and osteoclastic activity proceeding in a normal manner. However the latter may be deficient at certain points, as above mentioned. Cartilage cells are not present in the affected areas and some of the medullary structure is replaced by fibrous tissue.

Calcium, phosphorous and alkaline phosphatase values are essentially normal. The latter differentiates this condition from Paget's disease which it resembles somewhat altho occurring in a younger age group. Microscopically the bone of Englemann's disease is dense but does not show the mosaic pattern of Pagets (Figure X:16). Infantile cortical hyperostosis is a selflimited febrile condition resembling somewhat diaphyseal dysplasia but occurring in a less symmetrical distribution. Compare this dysplasia with the appearance noted in osteopetrosis.

ACROMEGALY

Acromegaly is usually caused by hyperpituitarism secondary to an eosinophilic adenoma involving the anterior lobe of that gland. There is increased secretion of a growth hormone which has been called somatropin. This stimulates a hyperplasia and hypertrophy of the skeletal structures and soft tissues. When occurring in childhood the disease results in giantism but in adults the victims present a coarse thickened facies with prognathism and enlargement of the hands. Headache is complained of and the roentgenogram reveals an erosion of the sella, later in the disease.

Bone growth is stimulated with resultant tuberosities and spur formations at the attachments of ligaments and muscles. There is enchondral bone growth at the condyle of the jaw which together with the periosteal bone hyperplasia causes enlargement of the mandible with malocclusion of the teeth. Active periosteal bone growth increases the transverse and AP diameters of the vertebral bodies by apposition of new bone to the anterior and lateral surfaces of those structures. Hyperplasia of the posterior spinal articulations may result in a thoracic kyphosis with compensatory low lumbar lordosis. Concavity of the posterior surfaces of the lumbar vertebrae has been reported (Figures XV:19, XV:20 and XV:21).

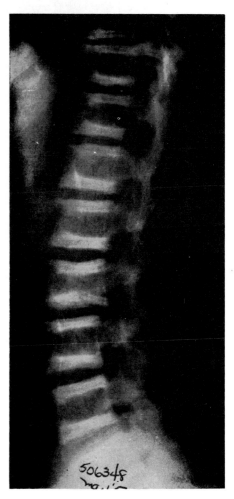

Fig. XV:17 A.

REFERENCES

Anchondroplasia

Caffey, J.: 1958, *Am. Jor. Roent., 80:*449–457.

Epstein, J. A., and Malis, L. I.: 1955, *Neurology, 5:*875–881.

Fairbank, H. A. T.: 1949, *J. Bone J. Surg., 31B:* 600.

Harris, H. A.: 1933, *Bone Growth in Health and Disease,* Oxford Medical Publications, Oxford University Press, London.

Jackson, W. P. U., *et al:* 1954, *Arch. Int. Med., 94:*871–910.

Lane, J. W.: 1960, *Am. Jor. Med. Sc., 240:*636–670, Cartilignous Dysplasia.

Slurgaard, R. K.: 1953, *Am. Jor. Dis. Child., 86:* 788–794.

Stowens, Daniel: 1959, *Pediatric Pathology,* Williams & Wilkins, Baltimore.

Osteochondrodystrophy
Morquio's Disease

Brailsford, J. F.: 1952, *J. Bone J. Surg., 34B:*53–63.

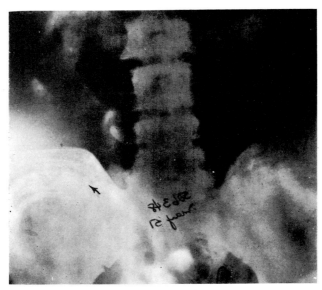

Fig. XV:17. Osteopetrosis of the banded or "sandwich" type involving the verbral bodies. The AP projection clearly visualized the alternating curved bands parallel to the iliac crests *(arrow)*. These correspond to the positions of the epiphyses at times of exacerbations or remissions of growth activity. Layering is also seen in the dense vertebral bands. (Courtesy of the Armed Forces Institute of Pathology #506348, Washington, D. C.)

Dale, T.: 1931, *Acta Radiol., 12*:337–385.

Evans, P. B.: 1952, *Jor. Ped., 41*:706–712, Cretinism.

Fairbank, H. A. T.: 1949, *J. Bone J. Surg., 31B:* 291–301.

Feldman, N., *et al:* 1951, *Arch. Dis. Chld., 26:* 279–288.

Helweg-Larsen, H. F.: 1945, *Acta Path. Microb. Scan., 22*:335–357.

Jackson, W. P. U.: 1954, *Arch. Int. Med., 94:* 871–910.

Neuhauser, E. B. D., *et al:* 1952, *Rad., 59*:637–650, Radiation effects on the spine.

Reeves, R. J., *et al:* 1941, *Rad., 36*:362–366.

Russo, P. E.: 1943, *Rad., 41*:42–47.

Toma, J. J.: 1953, *Surg. Clin. N. A., 33*:1765–1774.

Whiteside, J. D.: 1952, *Arch. Dis. Chld., 27*:487–497.

Stippled Epiphyses
Dysplasia Epiphysialis Punctata
Conradi's Disease

Allansmith, M.: 1960, *Am. Jor. Dis. Child., 100:* 109–116.

Brogdon, B. G., *et al:* 1958, *Am. Jor. Roent., 80:* 443–448.

Cohen, J., *et al:* 1956, *Am. Jor. Roent., 76*:469–475.

Fairbank, H. A. T.: 1949, *J. Bone J. Surg., 31B:* 114–122.

Ford, G. D.: 1951, *Ped., 8*:380–392.

Karlen, A. G., *et al:* 1957, *J. Bone. J. Surg., 39:* 293–301.

Mosekilde, E.: 1952, *Acta Rad., 37*:291–307.

Putschar, W. G. J.: 1951, *Bull. Hosp. Joint Dis., 12*:514–527.

Roul, L. W.: 1954, *Am. Jor. Roent., 71*:941–946.

Sheach, J. M.: 1956, *Brit. Jor. Rad., 29*:111–113.

Gargoylism, Hurler's Disease, Lipoid Osteochondrodystrophy, Dysostosis Multiplex

Caffey, J.: 1952, *Am. Jor. Roent., 67*:715–731.

Craig, W. S.: 1954, *Arch. Dis. Chld., 29*:293–303.

Dawson, I. M. P.: 1954, *Jor. Path. & Bact., 67:* 587–604.

Evans, P. R.: 1952, *Jor. Ped., 41*:706–712.

Fairbank, H. A. T.: 1949, *J. Bone J. Surg., 31B:* 302–308.

Gilbert, E. F., *et al:* 1958, *Am. Jor. Dis. Child., 95*:69–80.

Henderson, J. L., *et al:* 1952, *Arch. Dis. Child., 27*:230–253.

Lindsey, S., *et al:* 1948, *Am. J. Dis. Child., 78:* 239–309.

Neuhauser, E. B. D.: 1953, *Am. Jor. Roent., 69:* 723–737.

Reilly, W. A., *et al:* 1948, *Am. Jor. Dis. Child.,* 75:595–607.

Smith, E. B.: 1952, *Ann. Int. Med., 36:*652–657.

Strauss, Lotte: 1948, *Am. Jor. Path., 24:*855–888.

Zellweger, H., *et al:* 1952, *Am. Jor. Dis. Child., 84:*421–435.

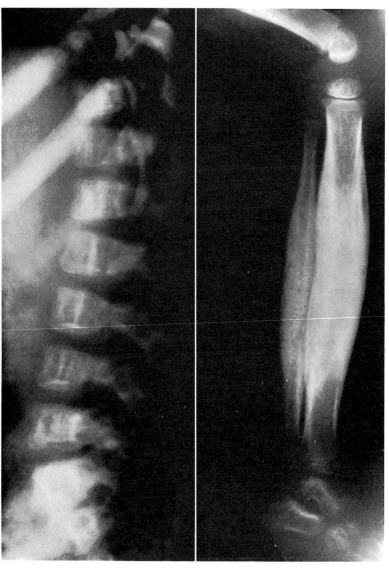

Fig. XV:18. Englemann's disease or diaphyseal dysplasia in a young female. The mid shaft of the tibia shows the characteristic fusiform hyperostosis with encroachment of the medullary cavity. Because of lessened osteoclastic–osteoblastic activity the metaphyseal modeling of both the femur and the tibia are less than normal. Of special interest are the heavy trabeculations which are present in the vertebral bodies, the epiphyses and to some extent the tarsal bones as well. It would seem that this dysplasia attempts to make unnecessarily generous provision for reinforcement at areas of possible stress. (Courtesy of Dr. Edward Neuhauser, Boston, Mass.)

Hypophosphatasia

Bethune, J. E., *et al:* 1960, *Am. Jor. Med., 28:* 615–622.

Bolton, W. D., *et al:* 1958, *J. Bone J. Surg., 40B:* 64–74.

Currarino, G., Neuhauser, E. B. D., *et al:* 1957, *Am. Jor. Roent., 78:*392–419.

Fraser, D.: 1957, *Am. Jor. Med., 22:*730–746.

Leucutia, T.: 1955, *Am. Jor. Roent., 73:*485–487, Editorial.

MacDonald, A. M.: 1957, *Arch. Dis. Chld., 32:* 304–310.

Rathbun, A. C.: 1948, *Am. Jor. Dis. Child., 75:* 822–831.

Osteogenesis Imperfecta

Bickel, W. H.: 1943, *Rad., 40:*145–154.

Brailsford, J. F.: 1943, *Brit. Jor. Rad., 16:*129–136.

Bromer, R. S.: 1933, *Am. Jor. Roent., 30:*631–640.

Caniggio, A., *et al:* 1958, *Acta. Med. Scan.,* Supp. 340, 162–172.

Chont, L. K.: 1941, *Am. Jor. Roent., 45:*850–861.

Fairbank, H. A. T.: 1948, *J. Bone J. Surg., 30B:* 164–186.

Follis, R. H.: 1952, *Jor. Ped., 41:*713–721.

Knaggs, R. L.: 1924, *Brit. J. Surg., 11:*737–759.

Lutz, J. F.: 1939, *Rad., 32:*391–402.

Schwarz, E.: 1961, *Am. Jor. Roent., 85:*645–648, Hypercallosis.

Zander, G.: 1940, *Acta Rad., 21:*53–61.

Enchondromatosis—Dyschondroplasia —Asymmetrical Chordrodystrophy Ollier's Disease

Carleton, A., *et al:* 1942, *Quart. J. Med., 11:* 203–228.

Cleveland, M., *et al:* 1959, *J. Bone J. Surg., 41A:* 1341–1344.

Cohn, I.: 1946, *Ann. Surg., 123:*673–687.

Fairbank, H. A. T.: 1948, *J. Bone J. Surg., 30B:* 689–704.

Heckman, J. A.: 1951, *Arch. Surg., 63:*861–865.

Jaffe, H. L., and Lichtenstein, L.: 1943, *Arch. Surg., 46:*480–493.

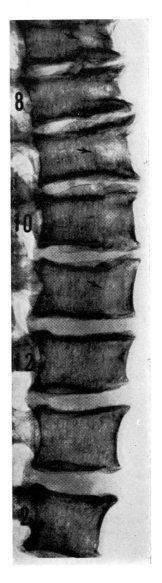

Fig. XV:19. Roentgenogram of one half of the lower thoracic and upper lumbar spine from a female of forty-eight years suffering from eosinophilic adenoma. There had been symptoms of acromegaly for the past twenty-two years. J. Erdheim in his classical description from the Vienna Pathological Institute pointed out the growth of periosteal new bone on the anterior surfaces of the vertebral bodies in this case. He mentioned the fact that the AP diameter of the thoracic vertebrae exceeded that of the lumbar and described the hyperplasia of the disc which was carried forward to the anterior margin of the new bone. The arrow points indicate the anterior margins of the vertebral bodies, originally. (Erdheim, J.: 1931, *Virchow's Arch. f. Path. Anat., 281:*197.)

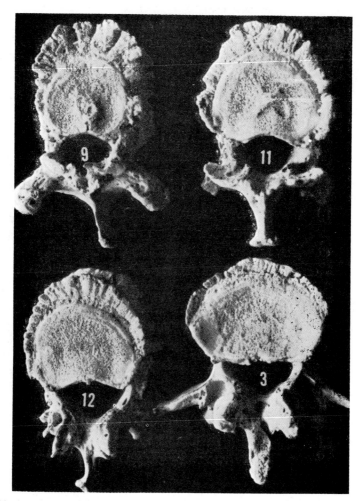

Fig. XV:20. Another case from the same report is that of a male patient thirty-nine years old with a pituitary tumor who had a history of acromegalic symptoms for eighteen years. Outlines of the original flat surfaces of the T_9, T_{11}, T_{12} and L_3 vertebral bodies are clearly shown with masses of new bone growing outward from the anterior surfaces. There is somewhat less growth of new bone laterally and the spinal canal appears to be spared. Note the lessened amount of new periosteal bone at the lower spinal levels as compared with T_9. The presence of the disease for two decades in these cases had permitted the increased amount of growth hormone to stimulate the growth of new periosteal bone. Since the disease had developed after completion of enchondral bone growth at the epiphyseal plates no additional longitudinal growth had occurred.

Murray, A. M.: 1960, *J. Bone J. Surg., 42B*:344–347.

Histology of Bone Formation

Maximow and Bloom: *Histology* (6th Edition), W. B. Saunders, Philadelphia, Pa.

Osteopetrosis—Osteosclerosis Fragilitas Marble Bones—Albers-Schönberg's Disease

Callender, G. R.: 1953, *J. Bone J. Surg., 35A:* 204–210.

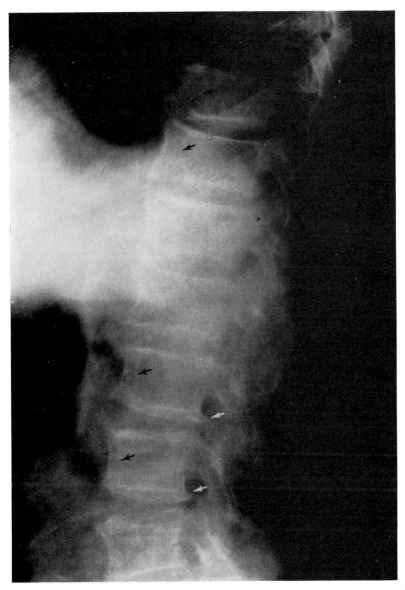

Fig. XV:21. Acromegaly, lateral roentgenogram of a patient to show the increased A. P. diameter of the lower thoracic vertebrae caused by new periosteal bone formation upon their anterior surfaces. Black arrows indicate the original surfaces of the centra. Some spur formation has occurred posteriorly *(white arrows)*. (Courtesy Dr. E. K. Lang, Indianapolis, Ind. and the *American Journal of Roentgenology.*)

Clifton, W. M., *et al:* 1938, *Am. Jor. Dis. Child.,* 56:1020–1036.

Cohen, J.: 1951, *J. Bone J. Surg., 33A*:923–938.

Fairbank, H. A. T.: 1948, *J. Bone J. Surg., 30B:* 339–356.

Hinkel, C. L., *et al:* 1955, *Am. Jor. Roent., 74:* 46–64.

Kneal, E.: 1951, *Am. Jor. Dis. Child., 81*:693–707.

Montgomery, R. D.: 1960, *J. Bone J. Surg., 42B:* 303–312.

Piatt, A. D.: 1956, *Am. Jor. Roent., 76:*1119–1131.

Zawisch, C.: 1947, *Arch. Path., 43:*55–75.

Progressive Diaphyseal Dysplasia Engleman's Disease

Bingold, A. C.: 1950, *Brit. J. Surg., 37:*266–274.

Caffey, J., and Silverman, W. A.: 1945, *Am. Jor. Roent., 54:*1–16.

Lennon, E. A., *et al:* 1961, *J. Bone J. Surg., 43B:* 273–284.

Neuhauser, E. B. D.: 1948, *Rad., 51:*11–22.

Sear, H. R.: 1948, *Brit. Jor. Rad., 21:*236–241.

Sear, H. R.: 1953, *Jor. Fac. Rad., 4:*221–234.

Smyth, F. S., *et al:* 1946, *Am. Jor. Dis. Child., 71:* 333–350.

Acromegaly

Chester, W., *et al:* 1940, *Am. Jor. Roent., 44:* 552–557.

Erdheim, J.: 1931, *Arch. Path. Anat. Phys., 281:* 197–296.

Finlay, J. M., *et al:* 1954, *Canad. M. A. Jor., 71:* 345–353.

Knaggs, R. L.: 1935, *Brit. J. Surg., 23:*69–109.

Lang, E. K., *et al:* 1961, *Am. Jor. Roent., 86:* 321–328.

Steinbach, H. L., *et al:* 1959, *Rad., 72:*535–549.

Chapter XVI

Tumors and Tumorous Conditions

IN THIS CHAPTER no attempt has been made to offer a complete presentation of all the different tumors which may affect the spine. Only a few interesting instructive cases have been selected. A more comprehensive discussion will be found in the works of various pathologists.

THE RETICULO-ENDOTHELIOSES

This is a group of related granulomatous lesions which include: eosinophilic granuloma, Schüller-Christian's disease and Letterer-Siwe's disease, the latter a fatal condition of infants.

EOSINOPHILIC GRANULOMA

This is a benign condition of unknown cause usually affecting young or middle aged people and characterized radiographically by well circumscribed areas of bone destruction. The normal tissue is replaced by granulomata made up of histiocytes primarily, together with collections of eosinophils and other elements as well as macrophages and giant cells. The punched out osteolytic lesions may involve one or more bones in any part of the body (Figure XVI:1). The cortices may be destroyed or expanded and periosteal bone formation has been reported. The vertebral bodies may be involved with resultant kyphosis. Eosinophilic granuloma has been designated as a low grade inflammatory process characterized by pain, tenderness, swelling and mild fever. The prognosis is good. The granulomata form and heal rapidly, either by spontaneous resolution or after curettage or radiotherapy. The condition is probably an early stage of Schüller-Christian's disease. In fact it may be quite difficult to differentiate these two related conditions either by the radiographs or the clinical picture. Likewise it is frequently impossible to differentiate them histologically since both may contain the so-called foam cells in the later healing stages. These are granulomatous lesions and do not metastasize.

SCHÜLLER-CHRISTIAN'S DISEASE

Described by those workers originally in 1915 and 1919 respectively as a lipoid storage disease this condition was subsequently (1940) classed as one of the reticulo-endothelioses. It is primarily a granuloma resulting from a proliferation of reticulo-endothelial cells and histiocytes. The latter secondarily take up cholestrol esthers and become the characteristic foam cells (lipophages). There is no primary disturbance of cholesterol metabolism. In this early stage however the lesions are microscopically similar to eosinophilic granuloma until the foam cells develop. These in turn are replaced by fibrosis and calcification as healing occurs.

The cause of Schüller-Christian's disease is unknown and altho it occurs principally in childhood there is no evidence of a familial or hereditary factor. The usual picture is that of a child with circumscribed areas of bone destruction in the calvarium, diabetes insipidus, exophthalmos and loss of teeth. The skull lesions are extradural, punched out and may coalesce. Involvement of the tuber cinerium is said to be responsible for the diabetes insipidus. Granulomas of the

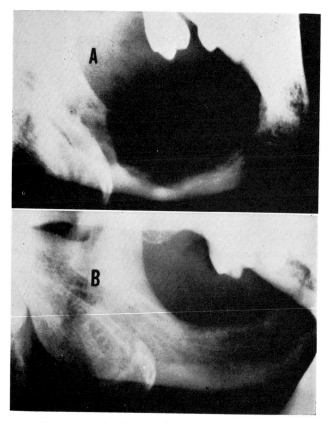

Fig. XVI:1. Female, fifty years old with reticulo-endotheliosis. The patient suddenly began losing her teeth. Radiograph of the left jaw (A) revealed a destruction of the alveolar process. The section (S) was reported as eosinophilic granuloma. The larger oval cells are histiocytes and the small dark nuclei, especially below at the right, are eosinophiles. There were no foam cells visualized. Following 1160r of radiation therapy the jaw was reexamined one and one-half years later (B) revealing a satisfactory replacement of the destroyed bone.

A lesion was discovered in the right ilium (C) one year following the initial involvement of the left mandible. A total of 2000r units was required to control this area. The reexamination (D) made 27 months later showed a filling in with bony tissue.

During the next five years the patient developed the characteristic clinical picture of Hand-Schüller-Christian's disease with diabetes insipidus mastoid involvement, and nine or ten different areas of bone destruction accompanied each time by fever and local pain.

The symptoms were promptly relieved in each case by radiation but the patient eventually succumbed to a brain tumor.

This case adds weight to the observation that eosinophilic granuloma or histiocytosis is probably an early stage of the Hand-Schüller-Christian's syndrome.

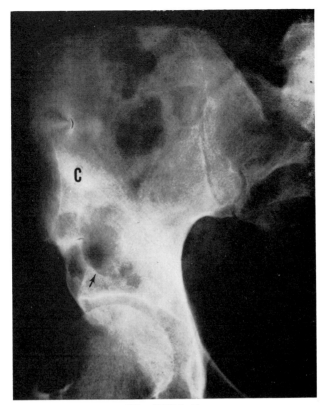

Fig. XVI:1 C.

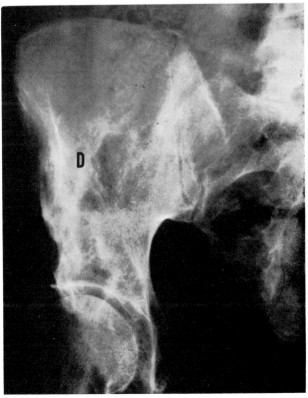

Fig. XVI:1 D.

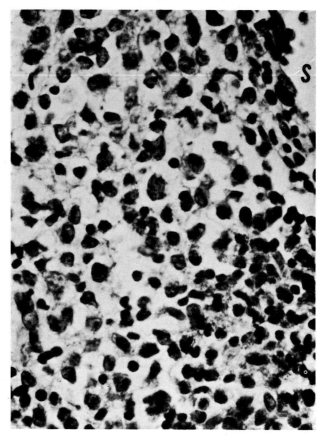

Fig. XVI:1 E.

mandible result in gingivitis causing the loss of teeth. The spine or any of the other bones of the body may be involved. These granulomas may likewise form in the organs and soft tissues of the body. Collapse of a vertebra produces the appearance of a platyspondylia as originally described by Calve (Figure XVI:2).

About one third of the cases terminate fatally from intercurrent disease or anaemia altho otherwise the course of Schüller-Christian's disease is essentially benign.

The related Letterer-Siwe's disease of infants on the other hand is an acute, fatal reticulo-endotheliosis with fever, anaemia, lymphadenopathy, rashes and haemorrhages. Otherwise with its skeletal defects and eosinophilic granuloma the pathology of this disease is similar to Schüller-Christian's altho the patients do not live long enough to develop foam cells.

OSTEOID OSTEOMA

These small, painful, bone lesions, usually encountered in young people, were first described by Jaffe in 1935 as "tumorlike" processes. The character-istic nidus is a translucent round or oval mass of osteoid tissue seldom more than 1.5 cms. in diameter. The central core of the nidus may be more or less calcified. Surrounding the nidus, either within the spongiosa or the cortex, is a reactive zone of bony sclerosis. If the lesion is cortical the overlying zone of dense periosteal bone formation may be quite extensive. Roentgenographic visualization is best accomplished by well coned, over penetrated films or by laminography. The radiolucent portion of the nidus may be narrow or wider depending upon the diameter of the dense central core (Figure XVI:3).

Clinically the lesion is characterized by severe pain and point tenderness to

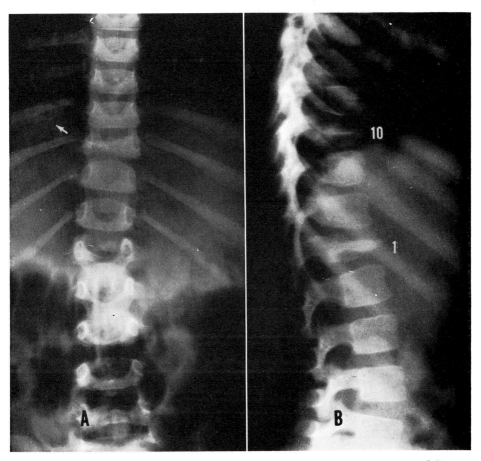

Fig. XVI:2. Schüller-Christian's disease in a young girl. Roentgenograms A and B were made at the age of four years. Deposits of the granulomatous material had occurred in various skeletal structures. The T_{10} and L_1 vertebral bodies were so weakened that partial collapse resulted especially in their anterior portions. The pedicles and neural arches were not involved. Since the epiphyseal plates were not destroyed the subsequent radiographs showed excellent growth of these involved vertebrae. Radiograph C was a preadolescent examination at eight years and D shows complete regrowth at twenty years of age (see Figure III:3). The elbow (E) at three years had healed at five years (F).

Also involved were certain other long bones, the left ninth rib *(white arrow)* and the skull. Throughout the entire calvarium were numerous punched out areas where the bone had been replaced by the granulomata. (G). After 1352r of radiation therapy, these became largely filled in with new bone (H) six months later. The child had minimal exophtalmos and diabetes insipidus. The loss of teeth was not a problem. All of the various involved areas eventually became nicely healed as the patient reached adulthood.

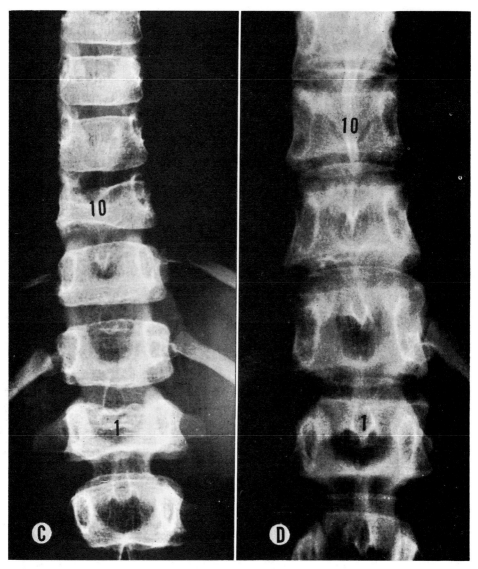

Fig. XVI:2 C, D.

deep pressure. The symptoms are entirely out of proportion to the size of the involved area. Other than pain, there is no evidence that this is an inflammatory process. The spine or any other bone may be involved but the femur and tibia account for about one half of the cases.

Microscopically the radiolucent nidus is seen to be composed of osteoid cells forming trabeculae of osteoid tissue. This occurs in a substratum of highly vascularized osteogenic connective tissue. Many of the trabeculae are partially calcified and some of them are undergoing resorption by giant cell osteoclasts as a part of the reossification process. There is no evidence of inflammatory reaction. It has been suggested that the very rich blood supply confined within the rigid wall of the osteoma may be responsible for the severity of the pain.

If unoperated an osteoid osteoma may persist for years but eventually becomes replaced by atypical new bone. Radiation is ineffective and operation is the treatment of choice. By way of diagnosis, the clinical picture and good roentgenograms should avoid mistaking the condition for a localized osteomyelitis with sequestrum formation or for an osteogenic sarcoma.

BENIGN OSTEOBLASTOMA
OR
OSTEOGENIC FIBROMA OF BONE

Histologically this unusual condition resembles osteoid osteoma but the lesions are larger, less painful and differ materially in their roentgenological appearance. They have a predilection for the vertebral column, are characterized by dull back ache and occur mostly in young people. Neurological symptoms may arise in parts distal to the lesion. The roentgenograms shows some enlargement of the bone which may gradually become expanded over a period of a few months. There is a reactive thickening and perforation may occur. With the local bone destruction and bulging of its contour the lesion may reach a diameter of 8 or 10 cms. Altho richly vascular like the osteoid osteoma, this lesion is less painful, probably because of the bone expansion and the lesser rigidity of its walls.

Histologically the similarity of the two is evidenced by the loose fibrous vascular matrix rich in osteoblasts laying down trabeculae of osteoid tissue. Many of these trabeculae are calcified at the center into primative osseous tissue with a layer of uncalcified osteoid on the surface. Some of the trabeculae are later resorbed by giant cell osteoclasts. It will be seen that microscopically the osteoid osteoma and the benign osteoblastoma are quite similar but the roentgenograms

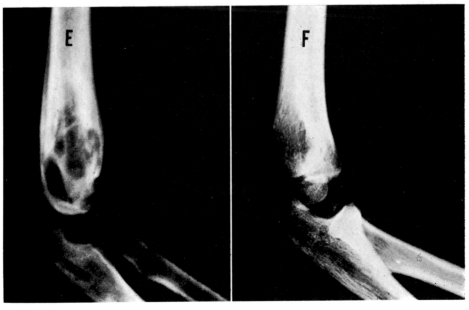

Fig. XVI:2 E & F

and the clinical pictures are strikingly dissimilar (Figure XVI:4). Like the former, the treatment of choice for benign osteoblastoma is surgical removal if possible, altho radiation therapy has proven successful where location of the lesion made it necessary.

These tumors are benign, they do not metastasize but symptoms may be produced by direct pressure.

CHONDROSARCOMA

The chondrosarcoma is a malignant slow growing bulky tumor originating from cartilage cells. It may show areas of necrosis, cyst formation or calcification. The term myxochondrosarcoma may be applied to one of these tumors showing a considerable amount of mucoid degeneration of the intercellular matrix. Sarcomatous degeneration may involve masses of cartilage cells within the bone such as enchondromatosis or the cartilaginous caps of exostoses may undergo malignant change.

The lesions are characterized roentgenographically by blotchy areas of calcification and radiopacity or bony metaplasia together with areas of spotty radiolucency. Streaky opacities may be seen radiating outward into the surrounding soft parts.

Histologically the malignant changes may not be evident at first and the lesion is diagnosed as benign. Subsequently repeated re-examinations may show increasingly malignant changes so that the tumor is finally diagnosed as malignant even years later. Such was the experience in the patient shown as Figure XVI:5 whose lesion had been diagnosed as benign seven years before his final exodus with extensive spinal destruction and cord damage.

Chondrosarcoma is less common and has a more favorable prognosis than osteogenic sarcoma. This latter tumor arises in fibrous tissue and produces cartilage as well as bone. It occurs in a younger age group while the chondrosarcoma is encountered somewhat later.

Extension, when it occurs, is by the venous channels to the lungs. These tumors proliferate in spite of heavy radiation so that the best results have been attained by early, radical surgery.

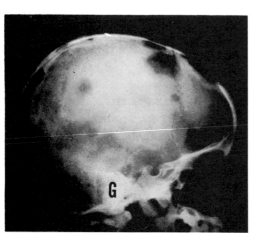

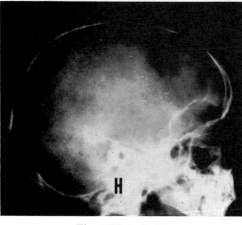

Fig. XVI:2 G, H

EXPANDING BONE DESTROYING TUMORS WITHIN THE SPINAL CANAL

These bulky newgrowths may occur at any level from occiput to coccyx. Gradual expansion destroys the inner cortex of the pedicle thus increasing the transverse diameter of the canal. Arcuate concavities develope on the posterior surfaces of the vertebral bodies and the anterior surface of the laminae may be eroded. Kyphosis, scoliosis or a combination of the two is not uncommon. It has been estimated that only a fourth of the tumors within the spinal canal exhibit bone destruction visible upon the roentgenogram. Neither is the plain film usu-ally indicative of the type of tumor. Myelography has much greater diagnostic value and the clinical picture is important. Visualization of an expanding bone destroying process within the spinal canal is good roentgenographic evidence of tumor but the absence of such evidence does not preclude a new growth. Most common is the extramedullary but intradural tumor, next is the extradural growth and finally the intramedullary gliomas such as the ependymomas, Figures XVI:8 and XVI:9.

NEUROFIBROMATOSIS

In 1882, von Recklinghausen described a disease characterized by a diffuse proliferation of the peripheral nerve elements, areas of cutaneous pigmentation and multiple soft tissue tumors or fibroma molluscum. Bone involvement occurs in a substantial percentage of cases. The condition seems to be hereditary and may appear in early childhood, often combined with various other congenital malformations and skeletal alterations. It is thought to be a deficiency of the mesodermal tissues.

The patients develop perineural fibromata involving the axis cylinders and nerve sheaths. These painless tumors are lobulated growths surrounded by a firm fibrous capsule. They produce pressure erosions in adjacent bony structures. When intradural fibromas occur the vertebral bodies may be eroded, the pedicles destroyed and the foramina enlarged. The growth may exit from the canal thru the enlarged foramen and appear alongside the spine as a so-called "dumb bell" tumor. In the thoracic region these paraspinal tumors may become quite large and even cause erosions of the ribs. Weakening of the vertebral bodies and arches result in spinal curvatures, either kyphosis, scoliosis or more likely a combination of both. These curvatures have been reported in a high percentage of cases. The partially eroded vertebrae present a scalloped appearance. Atrophy of the lamina increases the A. P. diameter of the canal while pedicle erosion increases the interpediculate diameter (Figure XVI:10). Spinal involvement may occur at any level. In the thoracic region this may result in cord pressure while in the lumbar and sacral regions, root pressure is to be expected.

Other bony changes beside erosions may be associated with neurofibromatosis. A sclerotic overgrowth of individual bones from unknown cause has been reported in certain cases of this disease. Bone atrophy may occur without osteoporosis producing slender, bowed shafts, with or without fracture. These resemble somewhat the condition noted in osteogenesis imperfecta tarda. Fibrosis of the bone marrow and radiolucent areas having a

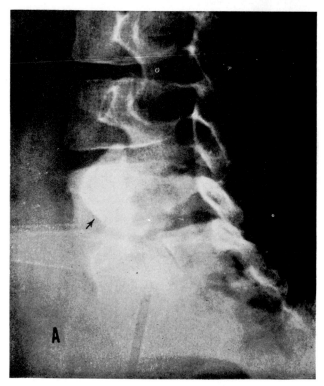

Fig. XVI:3. Osteoid osteoma of the right lamina and pedicle of L_4 This seven year old girl gave a history of lumbar pain radiating down the right leg for fifteen months before operation. She was tender to pressure over the lower lumbar spine. The oblique projection (A) visualizes the dense, smooth, sharply delineated lesion involving the 4th pedicle *(arrow)*. The laminogram (B) taken thru the center of the nidus shows the dense core surrounded by a zone of uncalcified osteoid tissue *(arrow)*. A section of the latter (S) X165 shows many trabeculae of osteoid tissue lined with osteoblasts lying within a fibrous matrix. The darker trabeculae are undergoing calcification. (Courtesy of Dr. Stephen Bastable and St. Joseph's Hospital, Syracuse, N. Y.)

somewhat cystic appearance have been encountered. These suggest the possibility of a relationship to fibrous dysplasia. Confusion with bone cyst, hyperparathyroidism, Ollier's disease and the reticuloses is to be avoided. A complete bone survey is recommended.

The tumors of neurofibromatosis are usually benign and radioresistant. Occasionally however malignant degeneration occurs and they may become sarcomatous.

CHORDOMA

Chordoma is a malignant, bulky, show growing destructive tumor originating from remnants of the notochord (see Figures I:4, I:6, I:7, and I:8). Of the reported cases about 35 per cent are said to arise at the base of the skull in the spheno-occipital synchondrosis, 55 per cent in the sacro-coccygeal region and the remaining 10 per cent at various levels of the spine. There is nothing characteristic about the roentgenogram. Serial studies reveal a slowly enlarging

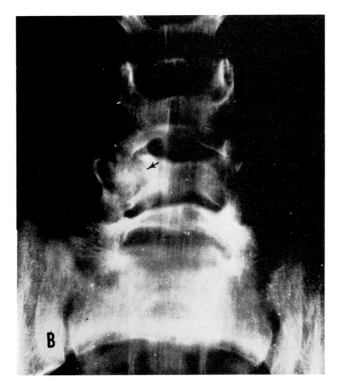

Fig. XVI:3 B.

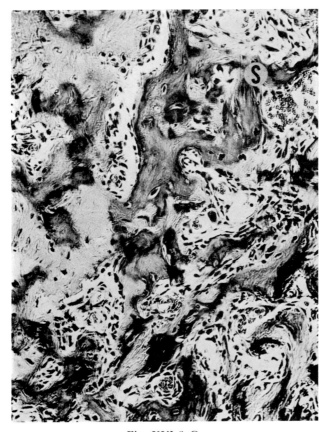

Fig. XVI:3 C.

destructive process of bone without evidence of a walling off reaction, altho at times there may be some areas of increased opacity. The lessions seldom metastasize but ulitimately destroy the patient by irresistible expansion and pressure upon adjacent vital structures. However metastases have been reported from pelvic chordomata. The initial complaint is pain from bone destruction and nerve involvement depending upon the location of the tumor. At the upper end of the spinal column the process may penerate the skull and attack the various structures at the base of the brain. Neurological complaints also result from vertebral body involvement with pressure upon the cord when the spinal canal is invaded. One or more vertebral bodies may be destroyed. The

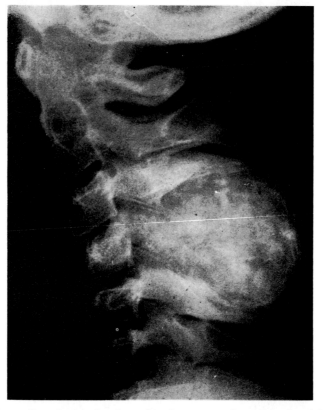

Fig. XVI:4. Expanding, destructive, bone-forming tumor, involving the right side of the 4th cervical neural arch and spinous process in a female child of six years. The 3rd and 5th spinous processes have been forced apart with angulation of the cervical spine forward and toward the left side. The right oblique projection shows the left 4th pedicle uninvolved by the disease *(white arrow)*. The section (S) X165 reveals trabeculae of osteoid tissue lined by osteoblasts *(black arrows)* lying in a richly vascular matrix of fibrous tissue. Note the occasional giant cell osteoclast lying alongside the trabeculae *(white arrows, right side of section)*. The more darkly stained trabeculae are becoming calcified. Diagnosis: Benign Osteoblastoma. Histologically there is a close similarity between benign osteoblastoma and osteoid osteoma. The latter, however, is closely confined within a dense bony shell and is painful. The osteoblastoma on the other hand expands freely and severe pain is not a troublesome problem. (Courtesy of Dr. Wm. Peacher and St. Joseph's Hospital, Syracuse, N. Y.)

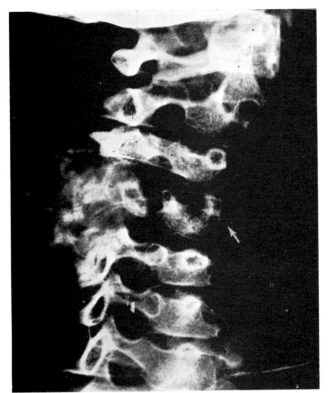

Fig. XVI:4 B.

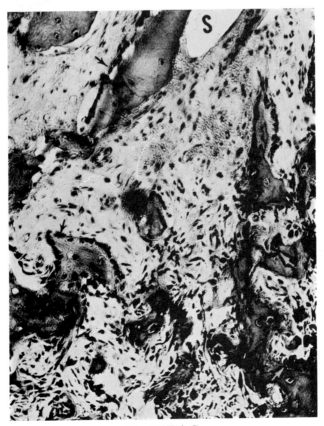

Fig. XVI:4 C.

adjacent discs may be spared or likewise invaded and destroyed.

The sacrococcygeal chordoma is a gradually enlarging mass occupying the pelvic cavity. It may eventually attain considerable size and exit laterally into the buttocks. The sacrum becomes destroyed. The tumor is soft but gradually invades and compresses with a resultant disturbance of bowel and bladder function as well as neurological symptoms.

The condition is frequently mistaken to be metastatic bone disease. A definitive diagnosis depends upon a micro-scopic examination of the tumor tissue. The characteristic histological picture is made up of the so-called physaliphorous cells. These are vacuolated cells, distended by mucin. In addition to the intracellular vacuolation there may be intercellular pools of mucinous material.

Surgical removal may at times prove to be palliative but recurrence is inevitable. Radiation therapy is of debatable value. The condition is progressive and always proves ultimately fatal irrespective of any treatment employed (Figure XVI:11).

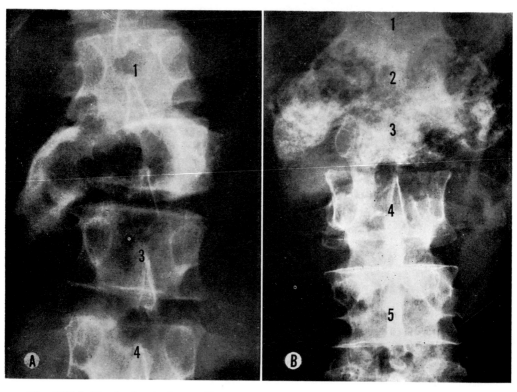

Fig. XVI:5. Slowly developing malignant tumor originating at L_2. This man had complained of increasing pain in the back over a period of thirteen years. He had been completely paralyzed for nine months before death at the age of thirty-eight. Biopsy taken at the time of roentenogram A, seven years before death, was considered benign, however during the interval it will be noted (roentgenogram B) that the destructive process had extended to include L_1 to L_4. Autopsy revealed the extension even to the disc of T_{11} and compression of the spinal cord (C). There was a complete lack of unanimity among a group of pathologists who studied the sections. In a characteristic manner the case was finally signed out as "not inconsistent with chondrosarcoma." (Courtesy of the University Hospital, Syracuse, N. Y.)

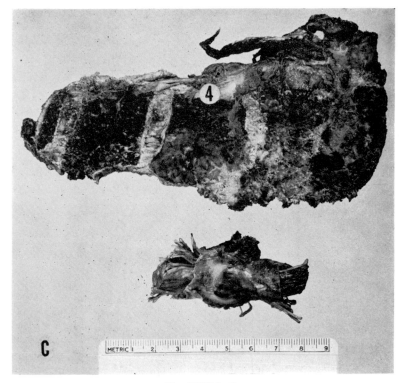

Fig. XVI:5 C.

MULTIPLE MYELOMA

This fatal disease of later life originates from plasma cells in the red bone marrow. The etiology is unknown. The principal symptom is pain of increasing severity especially in the back. This may be insidious at first with remissions and exacerbations but the suffering gradually mounts until it becomes constant and agonizing.

Multiple bones are involved in the destructive process. Greatest in order of frequency are spine, ribs and sternum to be followed by the skull, pelvis and extremities. The roentgenogram may show punched out areas, an osteoporotic appearance or a mottling of the involved bone. Pathologic fractures are common, especially multiple ones involving the ribs. Demineralization of the spine results in fracture, biconcave lumbar vertebrae or wedging in the thoracic region.

A troublesome anaemia results from the extensive replacement of hemopoietic tissue by the uncontrolled growth of plasma cells. The most important diagnostic procedure is a sternal biopsy to determine the presence of the myeloma cells.

Bence-Jones protein bodies in the urine are present in about 70 per cent of cases. However these are also found in certain other pathological conditions involving the bony and marrow structures.

Other later conditions are: chronic nephritis, n.p.n. retention, emphysema, pleurisy, intercostal neuralgia and other neurological symptoms. Cord compression with paraplegia may be terminal.

The prognosis is poor. These patients rarely live more than two or three years. Radiation therapy offers some temporary palliative relief (Figures XVI:12, XVI:13, and XII:38).

REFERENCES

Reticulo-endothelioses, Eosinophilic Granuloma, Histiocytosis, Hand-Schüller-Christian's Disease, Letterer-Siwe's Disease

Abt, A. F., *et al*: 1936, *Am. Jor. Dis. Child. 51:* 499–522.

Arcomano, J. P.: 1961, *Am. Jor. Roent., 85:*663–679.

Calhoun, J. D., *et al*: 1959, *Am. Jor. Roent., 82:* 482–489.

Compere, E. L., *et al*: 1954, *J. Bone J. Surg., 36A:*969–980.

Dundon, C. C.: 1946, *Rad., 47:*433–444.

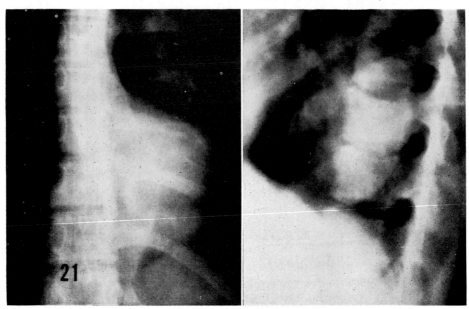

Fig. XVI:6. Female, age twenty-one. Some pain in the thoracic and left subcostal area for one year. Spine held convex toward the right side with limited movement. A. P. and lateral radiographs revealed a paravertebral shadow T_9 to T_{11} also a sharply delineated rounded mass extending outward into the left hemithorax. There were no calcifications at this time and the mass did not pulsate. There was no evidence of bone destruction involving the ribs, vertebrae or the neural arches.

At thirty-one years the mass had increased moderately in size and density. It had become somewhat lobulated and had acquired a mottled, calcified character. The patient experienced some discomfort especially after eating a heavy meal but was relatively comfortable. She had married and was living a normal useful life. However she frequently wished to have the mass removed because of the fear that "it might develop something serious." It was possible to keep her dissuaded from this course for nearly twelve and one-half years but twenty-seven months after these roentgenograms were made a firm lobulated tumor measuring 12 x 11 x 7 cm. was removed from the spine. Diagnosis: osteochondromyxoma.

The final roentgenograms at thirty-four years, fourteen months post operative, shows the recurrence of the tumor mass. This very rapid growth continued, forcing the heart forward against the anterior chest wall. The patient died in severe terminal pain twenty months postoperative.

Fisher, R. H.: 1953, *J. Bone J. Surg.*, *35A*:445–499–526.

Hodgson, J. R.: 1951, *Rad.*, *57*:642–652.

Jaffe, H. L., and Lichtenstein, L.: 1944, *Arch.*

Green, W. T., *et al:* 1942, *J. Bone J. Surg.*, *24:*

Path., *37*:99–118.

Laymon, C. W.: 1948, *Arch. Derm. & Syph.*, *57:* 873–890.

Lichtenstein, L.: 1953, *Arch. Path.*, *56*:84–102.

McGarvan, M. H.: 1960, *J. Bone J. Surg.*, *42A:* 979–992.

Ponseti, I.: 1948, *J. Bone J. Surg.*, *30A*:811–833.

Wallace, W. S.: 1949, *Am. Jor. Roent.*, *62*:189–207.

Weston, W. J.: 1959, *J. Bone J. Surg.*, *41B*:477–485.

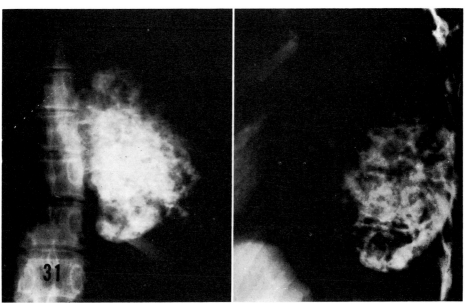

Fig. XVI:6 B.

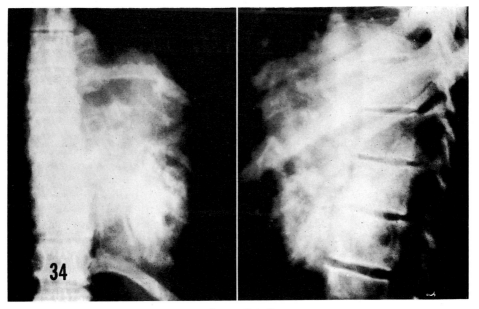

Fig. XVI:6 C.

Osteoid Osteoma

Fagenberg, S., *et al:* 1953, *Acta Rad., 40:383–386.*

Freiberger, R. H., *et al:* 1959, *Am. Jor. Roent., 82:194–205.*

Golding, J. S. R.: 1954, *J. Bone J. Surg., 36B: 218–229.*

Jaffe, H. L., and Lichtenstein, L.: 1940, *J. Bone J. Surg., 22:645–682.*

Lewis, R. W.: 1944, *Am. Jor. Roent., 52:70–79.*

Mayer, L.: 1951, *Bull. Hosp. Joint Dis., 12:174–201.*

Pugh, D. G., *et al:* 1956, *Am. Jor. Roent., 76: 1041–1051.*

Sabanas, A. O., *et al:* 1956, *Am. Jor. Surg., 91: 880–889.*

Sherman, M. S.: 1947, *J. Bone J. Surg., 29:918–930.*

Osteogenic Fibroma of Bone or Benign Osteoblastoma

Golding, J. S. R., *et al:* 1954, *J. Bone J. Surg., 36B:428–435.*

Jaffe, H. L.: 1958, *Tumors and Tumorous Conditions of the Bones and Joints,* Lea & Febinger, Philadelphia, Pa.

Jaffe, H. L.: 1956, *Bull. Hosp. Joint Dis., 17: 141–151.*

Kirkpatrick, H. J. R., *et al:* 1955, *J. Bone J. Surg., 37B:606–611.*

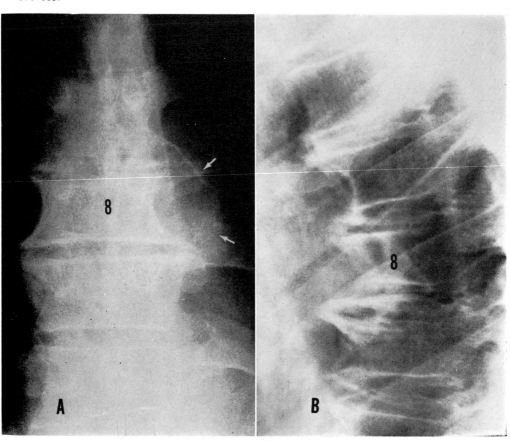

Fig. XVI:7. Luetic male of sixty years whose roentgenogram revealed a mass adjacent to the 8th thoracic vertebra. Laterally the mass was limited by a dense curvilinear shadow (*white arrows*). There was no fluoroscopic examination made. The various roentgenograms reveal bony destruction of T_7 and T_8 but the intervening disc had completely resisted the pulsation of the aneurism (*black arrow D*). The bone had developed a protective cortex adjacent to the vessel. In the photograph (C) one is able to see the posterior wall of the sac pushed forward by the disc at X. The chief complaint was pain in the shoulders.

Chondrosarcoma

Aronstam, E. M., *et al:* 1956, *Jor. Thor. Surg., 31:725–730.*

Dahlin, D. C., *et al:* 1956, *J. Bone J. Surg., 38A:1025–1038.*

Heuer, G. J., and Andruo, W. D. W.: 1940, *Am. Jor. Surg., 50:146–224.*

Lichtenstein, L., and Jaffe, H. L.: 1943, *Am. Jor. Path., 19:553–590.*

Lindblom, A.: 1961, *Acta Rad., 55:81–96.*

Phemister, D. B.: 1930, *Surg. Gyn. Obs., 50:216–233.*

Weisel, W., *et al:* 1950, *Jor. Thor. Surg., 19:643–648.*

Neurofibromatosis

Aegerter, E. E.: 1950, *J. Bone J. Surg., 32A:618–626.*

Allibone, E. C., *et al:* 1960, *Arch. Dis. Chld., 35:153–158.*

Fairbank, H. A. T.: 1950, *J. Bone J. Surg., 32B:266–270.*

Friedman, M. M.: 1944, *Am. Jor. Roent., 51:623–630.*

Heublein, J. W., *et al:* 1940, *Rad., 35:701–727.*

Holt, J. F.: 1948, *Rad., 51:647–663.*

Hunt, J. C., *et al:* 1961, *Rad., 76:1–20.*

Kessel, A. W. L.: 1951, *J. Bone J. Surg., 33B:87–93.*

Mackenzie, J.: 1950, *Brit. Jor. Rad., 23:667–671.*

McCarroll, H. R.: 1950, *J. Bone J. Surg., 32A:601–617.*

Chordoma

Baker, H. W., *et al:* 1953, *J. Bone J. Surg., 35A:403–408.*

Congdon, C. C.: 1952, *Am. Jor. Path., 28:793–824.*

Dahlen, D. C., *et al:* 1952, *Cancer, 5:1170–1178.*

Gentil, F., *et al:* 1948, *Ann. Surg., 127:432–455.*

Husain, F.: 1960, *J. Bone J. Surg., 42B:560–564.*

McCormack, M. P.: 1960, *J. Bone J. Surg., 42B:565–569.*

Morris, A. A., *et al:* 1947, *Arch. Neurol. Psych., 57:547–564.*

Poppen, J. T., *et al:* 1952, *Jor. Neurosurg., 9:139–163.*

Utne, J. R.: 1955, *Am. Jor. Roent., 74:593–608.*

Wood, E. H.: 1950, *Rad., 54:706–761.*

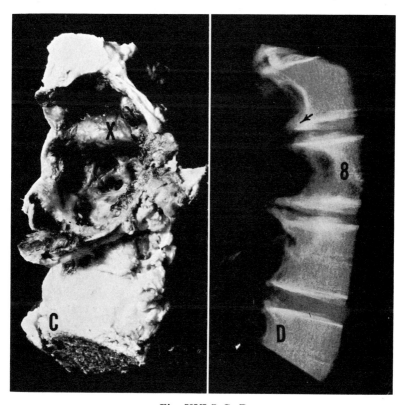

Fig. XVI:7 C, D.

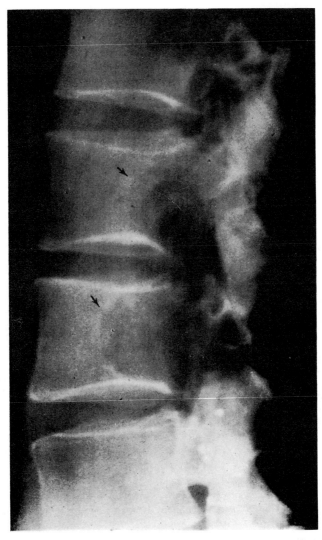

Fig. XVI:8. Recurrent ependymoma destroying the posterior surfaces of the mid lumbar vertebrae in a man of fifty-six years. The patient had been operated upon four years before. Ependymomas are one of the gliomas or supporting cell tumors. Since the ependyma is the lining of the central canal of the spinal cord, these tumors are intramedullary and therefore usually smaller than other cord tumors. In this instance however the lesion was quite bulky so that bone destruction resulted. Note as in Figure XVI:7 that the discs are more resistant to the pulsation than the vertebral bodies. The process is slowly progressive but shows some evidence of a walling off reaction in the surrounding bone *(arrows).* The necropsy report stated ". . . diffuse vertebral invasion with cord destruction." In the lumbar region these intramedullary tumors arise from the conus medularis or the filum terminale. (Courtesy of The Memorial Hospital, Syracuse, N. Y.)

Myeloma

Christopherson, W. M., *et al:* 1950, *Cancer, 3:* 240–252.

Deutschberger, O., *et al:* 1959, *Ann. Int. Med.,* 50:1309–1320.

Galgano, A.: 1955. *Am. Jor. Roent., 74:*304–314.

Geschickter, C. F., and Copeland, M. M.: 1949, *Tumors of Bone,* Lippincott, Philadelphia, Pa.

Kenny, J. J., *et al:* 1957, *Ann. Int. Med., 46:* 1079–1091.

Lichtenstein, L., and Jaffe, H. L.: 1947, *Arch. Path., 44:*207–246.

Martin, J. R., *et al:* 1957, *Canad. M. A. Jor., 76:* 605–615.

Smith, W. S., *et al:* 1958, *Arch. Surg., 76:*639–643.

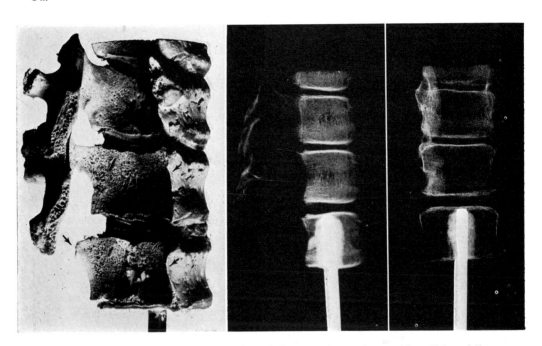

Fig. XVI:9. Specimen showing destruction of the posterior surfaces and pedicles of three lumbar vertebrae by an expanding intraspinal ependymoma in a young girl. The pedicles were completely eroded by the pulsation of the tumor as indicated by black arrows. The specimen is turned, to reveal the excavated posterior surfaces and the right lateral surfaces of the vertebrae. The supporting rod, thrust into the lowermost vertebral body, is held in place by plaster of paris.

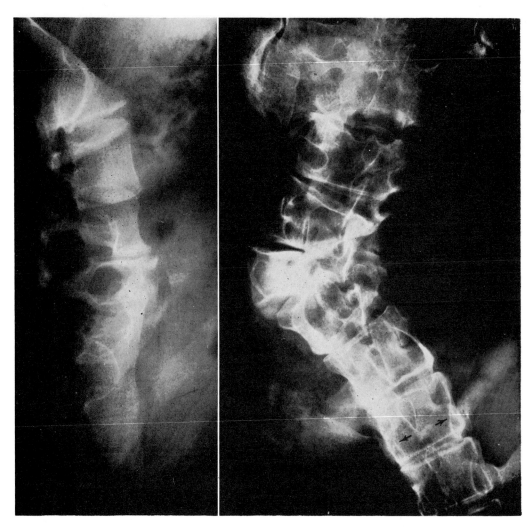

Fig. XVI:10. Neurofibromatosis (von Recklinghausen's disease) in a twenty-six-year-old female. Erosion by the pulsation of the tumorous masses within the spinal canal has destroyed the right side of the 3rd lumbar vertebral body together with that side of its arch. The resultant wedging, rotation and spinal angulation is obvious. There has also been erosion of the posterior surfaces of L_1, L_2 and L_4 as visualized by the scalloping in the lateral projection. Since growth is slow there has been some walling off reaction. Note the enlargement of the intervertebral foramina at the involved level. The spinal canal at T_{12} shows some evidence of increased interpedicular width *(arrows)*. There is some evidence that the bone erosion with a slow growing tumor may result from transmitted pulsation arising within the spinal canal. (Courtesy of The Memorial Hospital.)

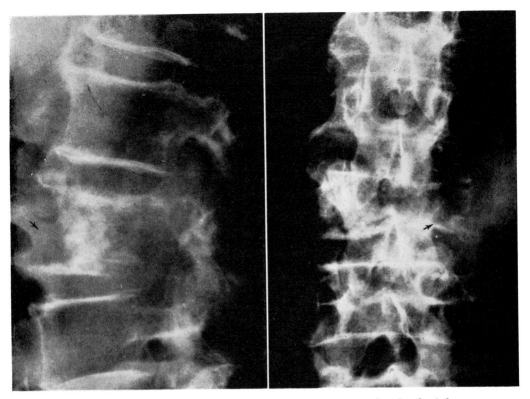

Fig. XVI:11. Chordoma in a male of sixty-four years, symptoms for the final four years with serial roentgenograms showed a slowly progressive destruction of L₃. There was a transverse myelitis for one year with paralysis and a neurogenic bladder. At necropsy the lesion was seen to have extended into the psoas muscle and into the spinal canal. The A. P. and lateral roentgenograms show the destructive process involving the 3rd lumbar vertebra *(arrows)*. There is no walling off reaction, however a vertical column of increased bone density has developed within the right side of the vertebral body. Apparently this is a compensatory supportive reaction which developes in cases of slow bone destruction, such as chordoma (see also Figure XVI:5A). The section (S) X675 shows the characteristic large vacuolated physaliphorous cells distended with mucin. Such a cell, somewhat triangular in shape, is seen just above the letter S. Many of these cells were sectioned at levels apart from their nuclei. Note the intercellular pools of mucin. Cells of similar morphology are seen in sections of the intervertebral disc in the later months of gestation (Figure I:8). (Courtesy of Dr. W. R. Redline and the Syracuse V. A. Hospital.)

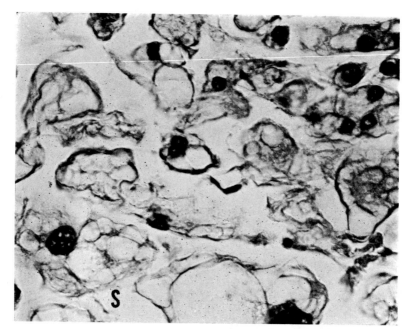

Fig. XVI:11 B.

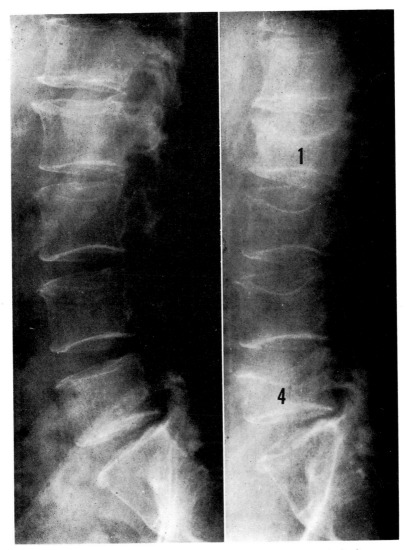

Fig. XVI:12. Multiple myeloma in a male of sixty-three years. A period of twenty months elapsed between these two roentgenograms. The trabecular structure of the vertebrae has become so weakened by the disease that the uppermost plates have bulged downward into the substance of the bodies. L_1 and L_4 have become partially collapsed. The spine has actually become shorter. (Courtesy of the Syracuse V. A. Hospital.)

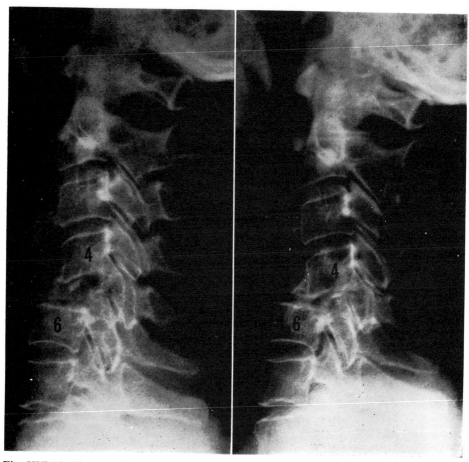

Fig. XVI:13. Plasma cell myeloma destroying the fifth cervical vertebra in a woman of fifty-two years. The neural arch is preserved but together with C_4 it became displaced backwards so that an angulation resulted. The patient had recently completed 2560r of radiation utilizing 200 k. v. p. when the first radiograph was made. The second film made thirty-two months later shows filling in with bony tissue. Collapse of C_5 had caused the neck to become shorter. The flexion-extension studies at that time revealed normal movement between the various cervical segments except at the block vertebra comprising the fourth, sixth and remaining arch of the fifth vertebra. (Courtesy of the University Hospital, Syracuse, N. Y.)

Index

539